To 'Air' is Human

Everything You Ever Wanted to Know About Intestinal Gas

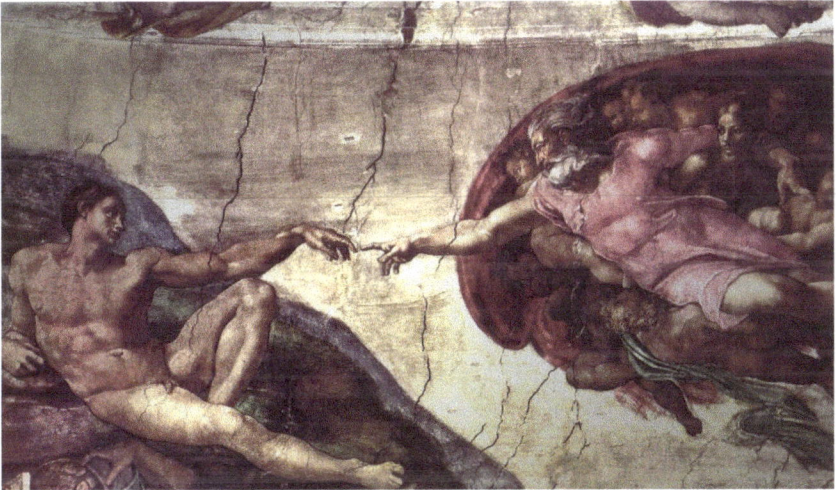

Joseph B. Weiss, MD, FACP, FACG, AGAF
Clinical Professor of Medicine,
Gastroenterology
University of California, San Diego

© 2016 Joseph B. Weiss, M.D.
        SmartAsk Books
        Rancho Santa Fe, California, USA
        www.smartaskbooks.com

ISBN-13: 978-1-943760-14-5 (Volume One)
ISBN-13: 978-1-943760-15-2 (Volume Two)
ISBN-13: 978-1-943760-02-2 (Combined Volume)

Last digit is the print number: 9 8 7 6 5 4 3

To 'Air' is Human

Dedication

This volume is dedicated to clearing the air of the misperception that intestinal gas is anything other than a normal physiologic process common to all humanity. Nature and natural processes should be universally accepted as one of the cherished principles of fundamental human rights.

I am indebted to my loved ones Nancy, Danielle, Jeremy, Courie, Lizzy, & Indy. They have offered their insights, suggestions, comments, and unwavering support throughout the long process of having this project finally come to pass. You will always be the mighty wind beneath my wings.

To 'Air' is Human

Table of Contents (Alphabetical)

Introduction

Intestinal gas has been generated and released by every human who has ever lived Very few people understand the underlying physiology of its generation or the law of physics, which play an important part in our experience of this universal condition. ***To 'Air' is Human, Everything You Ever Wanted to Know About Intest Gas*** is an informative, entertaining, and understandable volume designed to enlighten the lay public with everything they may have ever wanted to know about intestinal gas, but were too embarrassed to ask. Because of its size, over ninety tho words, and more than three hundred pages with hundreds of images, the electroni is the best value as the expense of color printing is substantial. A more economical version with a non-color interior is available.

The word fart is the correct word to use in the English language, and indeed is one it's oldest words. The alternative terms used, such as flatus and flatulence are not original English words as they have been borrowed from the Latin. There is controversy as to the derivation of the word fart. It is thought to have Indo-Europe roots in the Germanic language word farzen. One thought is that it originated as an onomatopoeia, a word that phonetically imitates the sound of the event it describe Another thought is that it was related to the term for partridge, as the bird makes a similar sound when it is disturbed in its natural habitat and takes flight.

Farts are ubiquitous, all living creatures generate gas from cellular metabolism and respiration, and humans are no exception. The bacteria of your colonic flora, part o the microbiome of living organisms that lives on and within humans, generate gas which collect in the bowel. They are joined with the air swallowed throughout the day and night, particularly at meals.

Aerophagia is universal and we swallow on average three to five cubic centimeters (one teaspoonful) of air with every swallow. Additional gasses are produced durin; the enzymatic digestive processes as well as the neutralization of gastric hydrochloric acid by pancreatic and duodenal bicarbonate. The result is a significa: volume of gasses within and transiting the bowel.

Fortunately the vast majority of the gasses produced are absorbed by the gut, then into the bloodstream through diffusion and finally exhaled when they each th alveoli of the lungs. The component gasses have very different properties of diffusion through the bowel wall and into the bloodstream. Carbon dioxide readily diffuses and enters solution and is exhaled promptly. Although it is the largest volume of gas generated, and temporarily contributes to distension and postprand (after meal) discomfort, it is the easiest to eliminate from the bowel and is only a minor contributor to flatulence.

The volume of gasses in the gastrointestinal tract is dependent on the quantity and nature of foods ingested, the body's ability to produce enzymes for the various foo types, the microbiome and gut flora, and gastrointestinal transit time. The often quoted figure of twelve farts per day is a reasonable average number of farts passe but there is a very wide range of what is considered normal.

Activated Charcoal

Commercially available products to trap and contain the dispersion of a fart have been marketed with some success. They rely on the adsorptive properties of activated carbon also known as activated charcoal, activated coal, or carbo activatus. Activated charcoal is a form of carbon processed to increase the surface area available for adsorption or chemical reactions.

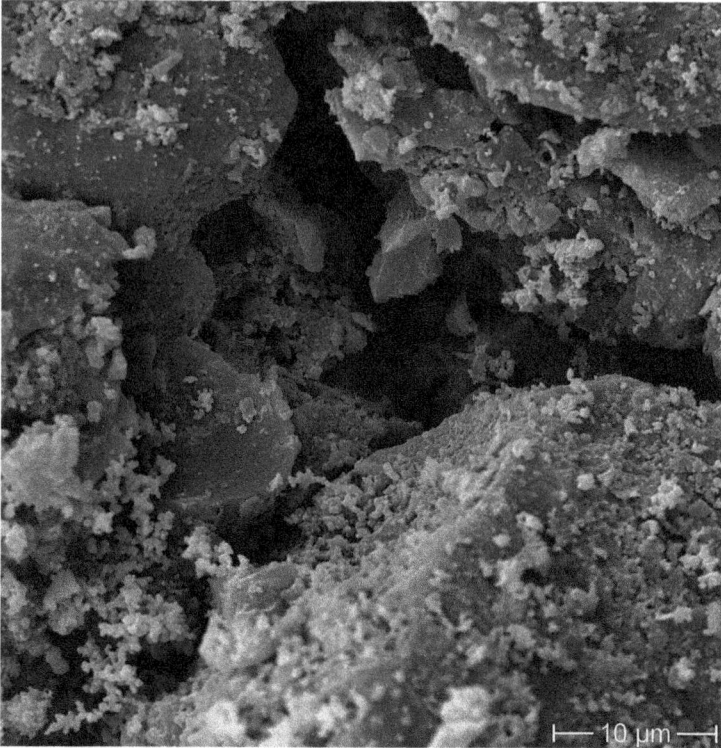

Activated charcoal, microscopic view increased surface area. Creative Commons License

The term adsorption and absorption are frequently confused. Absorption allows another material to be integrated into the volume of the absorptive matter. Adsorption is when the material being incorporated adheres to the surface of the material, and is not absorbed into its interior. An example of the difference between the two terms would be the drinking of water leads to its absorption that is it becomes internalized within your bodily tissues. Water that coats your skin in the shower or after spilling it on yourself is adsorbed, that is it is only on the outer surface of your body, and it is not absorbed.

Its very large surface area is a key concept to understanding the effectiveness of activated charcoal. A single cube of charcoal has a much smaller surface area for adsorption to take place, than an identical volume cube that has been subdivided into many smaller cubes. The following illustration helps to visualize how the surface area can be dramatically increased with the same volume of material.

To 'Air' is Human

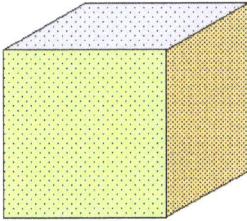

a one-meter cube has 6 square meters of suface area

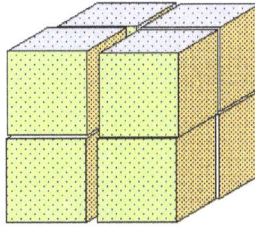

pieces half the original size have twice the surface area

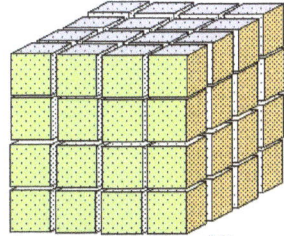

pieces one quarter of the original size have 4 times the surface area

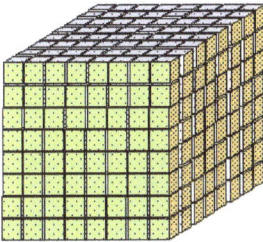

pieces one-eighth of the original size have 8 times the surface area.

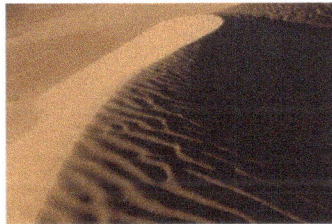

a cubic meter of fine sediment can have millions of square meters of surface area

Increase in surface area illustrated. Phil Stoffer, Ph.D. Geology Cafe geologycafe.com Creative Commons License

Activated carbon is used in the purification, decaffeination, metal extraction, water purification, and sewage treatment processes. It is also used in the air filters in masks and respirators, filters in compressed air, and to filter vodka and whiskey to remove impurities that would affect taste. In cases of the ingestion of toxins or poisons it has been used orally to bind to the toxin to prevent its absorption into the victim.

It is also effective in adsorbing offensive smelling gasses in flatus. Due to its porosity a single gram of activated carbon can have a surface area in excess of 500 meters squared, with 1500 meters squared being possible with further refining. Its adsorption ability varies amongst gasses and liquids and it is known to be a poor adsorbent of carbon monoxide, which is toxic and odorless. It is particularly effective in adsorbing most of the volatile odoriferous gasses.

The key to the success or failure of the product is the degree to which the fart can escape without having passed through the activated charcoal. The tighter the seal, the less likely for odiferous gasses to escape. The sitting pad was least effective trapping about twenty percent of gasses. Underwear pads ranged from fifty to seventy-five percent effectiveness, while the tight fitting entirely lined with activated charcoal underwear were the most effective, but also the most expensive.

odor

Flat-D activated carbon technology provides a thin barrier with sponge-like surface area for blocking the release of odor molecules.

fresh

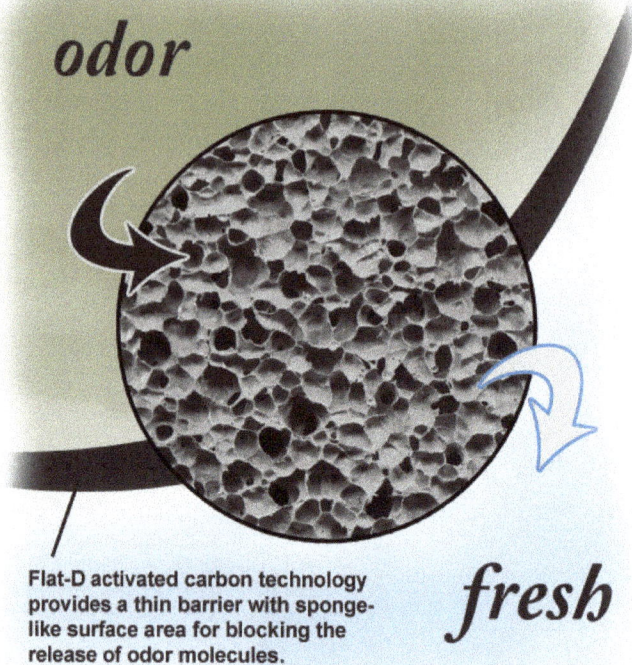

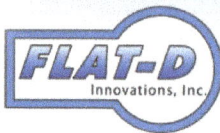

ODOR ABSORBING TECHNOLOGY

Activated charcoal pad products. Flat-D Innovations, Inc. Used with permission

Activated carbon is used to treat oral poisonings by binding to and preventing the poison from being absorbed by the gastrointestinal tract. The home remedy of eating burnt toast for food poisoning was based on the adsorptive properties of activated charcoal. Charcoal biscuits were marketed in the early 19th century as an antidote to flatulence, and are still sold today for diarrhea, indigestion, flatulence, and as a pet care product. Unfortunately orally ingested charcoal pills are not effective in appreciably reducing intestinal gas. This may be because the adsorptive capacity of the activated charcoal is fully utilized before it finally gets to the colon where its gas adsorbing properties are needed. Fortunately, bismuth products do provide a significant advantage by binding to the sulfur compounds and eliminating them without producing offensive gas.

Aerogel

Aerogel was developed by Samuel Kistler (1900-1975) at the College of the Pacific in Stockton, California in 1931. It was a silica material with a chemical structure similar to glass with gas in its pores rather than liquid. It is an open celled material that is ninety-five percent air, with pores less than one ten-thousandth of the diameter of a human hair. Further refinements allowed the air to be replaced by a vacuum, and the silica to be replaced by other materials. Kistler developed aerogels made of alumina, tungsten oxide, ferric oxide, tin oxide, nickel tartarate, cellulose, cellulose nitrate, gelatin, agar, egg albumen, and rubber. Further advancements and refinements in production have led to greater commercial applications.

The pore diameter being measured in nanometers gives it a nanoporous nature leading to the lowest thermal conductivity of any known solid. It has an extremely high surface area to mass ration with just two grams of aerogel having a surface area of a square kilometer (1,000 meters squared)

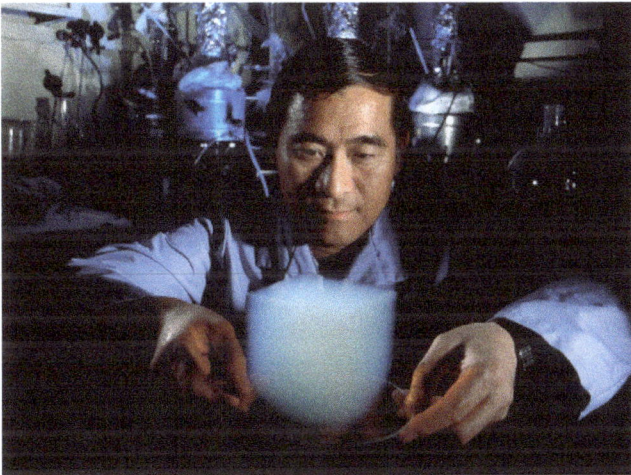

Aerogel. Stardust.jpl.nasa.gov Public Domain

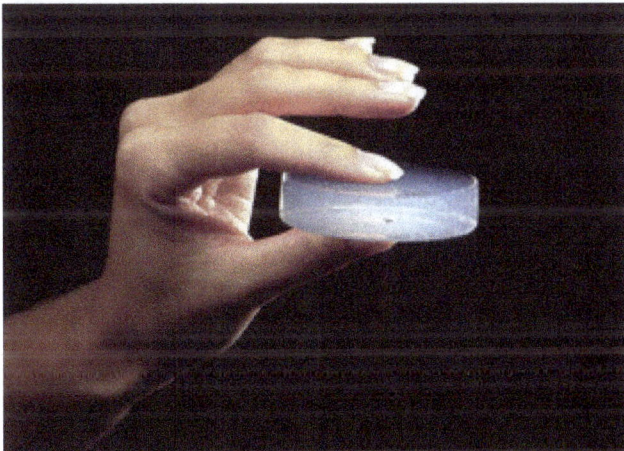

Aerogel is made from a wet gel that is dried. The substance has been described as feeling like volcanic glass pumice; a very fine, dry sponge; and extremely lightweight Styrofoam. NASA Public Domain

To 'Air' is Human

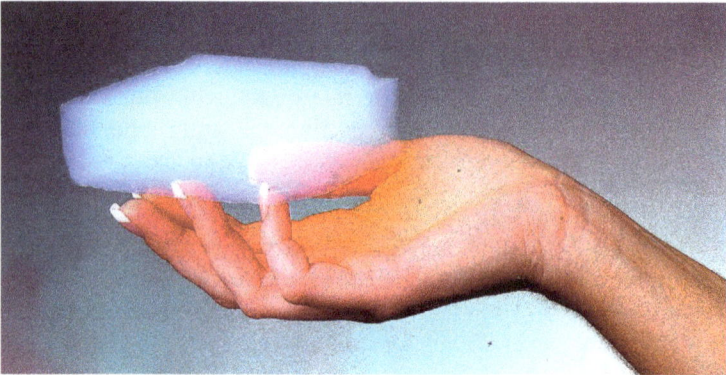

Though with a ghostly appearance like a hologram, aerogel is very solid. It feels like hard Styrofoam to the touch. Aerogel. Stardust.jpl.nasa.gov Public Domain

It is so lightweight that it has unmatched utility as an insulating material and has been utilized by NASA for the space shuttle and space exploration. The development of this product has allowed exploration of extreme environments such as outer space and deep sea exploration, where humans are exposed to the high and low extremes of atmospheric pressure that dramatically effect intestinal gas pressure and volume

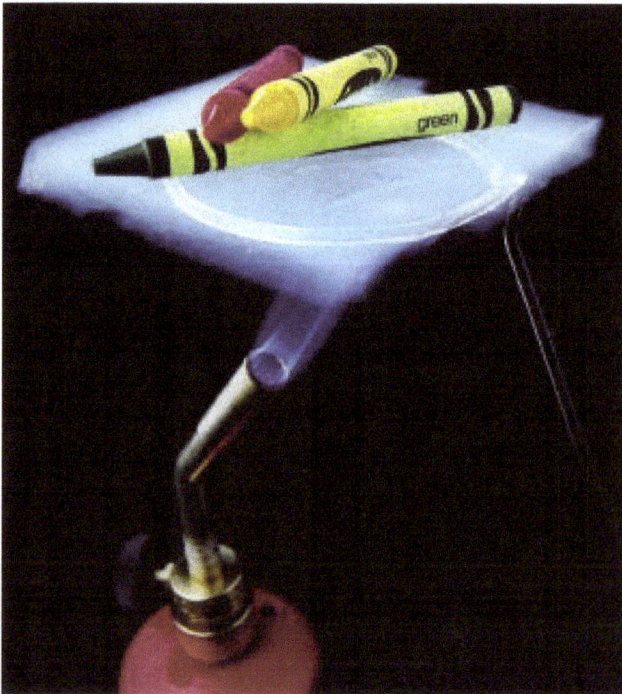

Crayons placed on top of a piece of silica aerogel will not melt from the heat of a flame. Certain types of aerogel provide thirty-nine times more insulation than fiberglass. NASA Public Domain

To 'Air' is Human

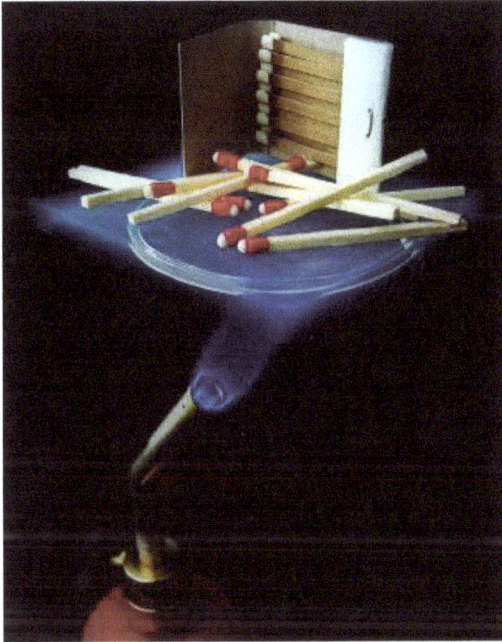

Aerogel. Stardust.jpl.nasa.gov Public Domain

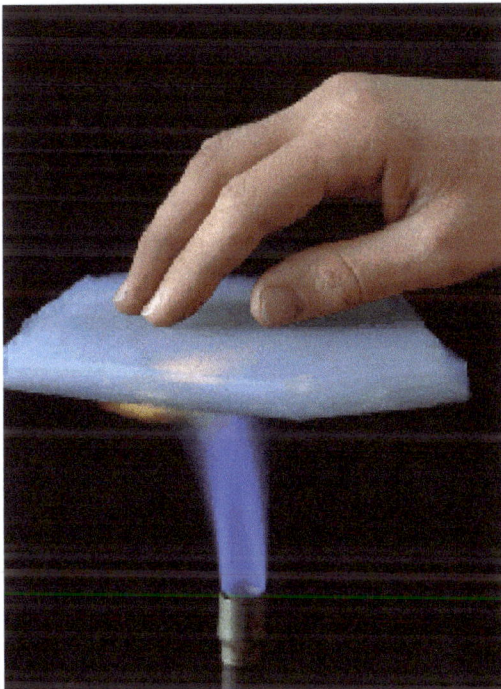

Aerogel eetd.lbl.gov Public Domain

To 'Air' is Human

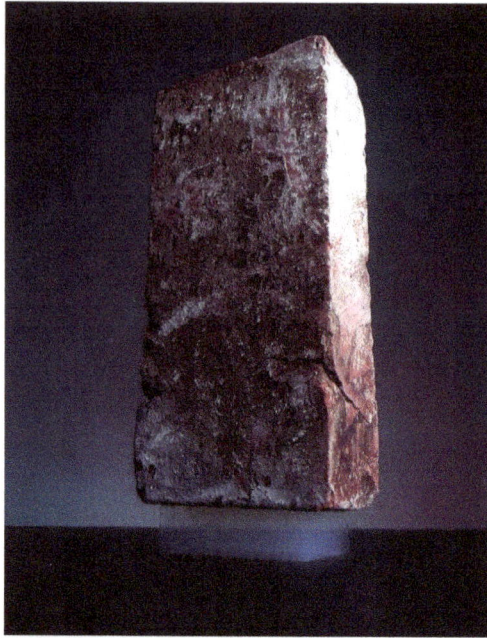

Aerogel. A five-pound (2.5 kg) brick is supported on top of a piece of aerogel weighing only 2 grams.Stardust.jpl.nasa.gov Public Domain

Aerophagia (Air Swallowing)

Air swallowing is a universal event in humans and is also known as aerophagia. We do it with every one of the on average two thousand swallows we take every day, ingesting approximately five ml (1 teaspoonful) of air with every swallow. Air is seventy-eight percent nitrogen, which is a poorly absorbed gas. If it is not released in a burp, it will contribute to bloating and distension. The volume of air swallowed is impressive, but is only a small percentage of what the digestive process can generate in terms of gas production.

Aerophagia is the swallowing of air, allowing it to enter the digestive tract, and it occurs naturally and without thinking in every individual. There is a variation of aerophagia in which the behavior becomes a purposeful, and at times obsessive-compulsive, behavior. More often, when excessive spontaneous aerophagia is occurring it is a subconscious or unconscious behavior, much like a nervous tic. The volume of air swallowed in these conditions can be impressive and a plain x-ray of the abdomen may demonstrate that the entire digestive tract is filled with air from esophagus to rectum.

Various studies have estimated the volume of each swallow as approximately twenty cc or four teaspoons. Many people swallow larger gulps of food on purpose and some even go to extremes in demonstrating their swallowing abilities. Sword swallowing is just one example where swallowing has been taken to a level of competition or entertainment.

To 'Air' is Human

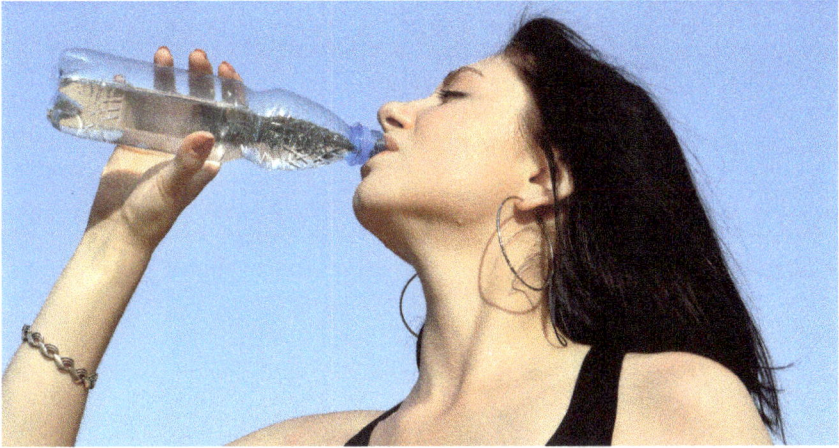

Air swallowing (aerophagia) is universal and occurs with every single swallow including swallows of food, food, saliva, etc. shutterstock/yuris

At the other extreme, some people take very small swallows and may sip foods at a teaspoon or less per swallow. They may be surprised to learn that sipping smaller volumes may actually increase the total amount of air they swallow. In general, the larger the total number of swallows, the larger the volume of air consumed.

If we took twenty ml as the volume of a normal average swallow, and the individual only took in small five ml sip of soup, each twenty ml swallow would include an additional fifteen ml of air. This is why hard candy and chewing gums, which generates small volumes of saliva and frequent swallows that mainly consist of air, lead to excessive aerophagia.

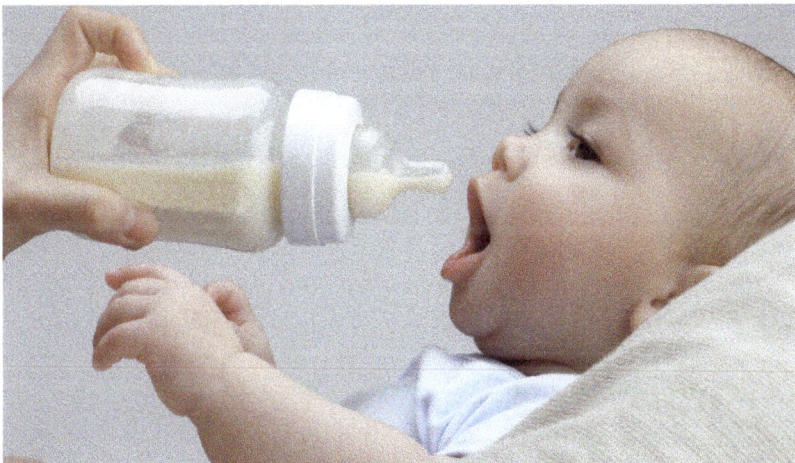

Baby bottles are a common source of aerophagia in infants. If the milk or formula does not completely cover the nipple of the bottle the baby will suck in and swallow air. shutterstock/Nicolesa

To 'Air' is Human

Since the digestive tract of the newborn is sterile, there are no microorganisms generating gas through cellular metabolism. All of the gas the newborn infant begins to pass is swallowed air. If an infant is bottle-fed rather than breast-fed they are much more likely to swallow even more air.

The first exposure to microorganisms that will be swallowed and begin to colonize the infant digestive tract are from the birth mother if the delivery is vaginal. The microorganisms that colonize the infant become its microbiome and play a major role in its ongoing health and wellness. The gut flora is one aspect of the microbiome, with skin, ears, mouth, genitourinary, and every surface of the body exposed to the external environment developing its own unique microbiome. Infants born by Caesarean section have exposure to different organisms, which establish a microbiome that is not believed to be as beneficial as via a natural vaginal delivery.

Baby bottles are a common cause of aerophagia in infants as they suck in and swallow air if the formula does not always cover the nipple. Burping the baby after a feeding is the means of allowing the swallowed air to escape otherwise it will cause distension and discomfort. Some bottles are designed to use an internal plastic sleeve to prevent air from reaching the nipple, when the formula is depleted the sleeve forms a vacuum so the infant is not sucking in air.

The air swallowed is the same as the air in the atmosphere, about seventy eight percent nitrogen, twenty one percent oxygen, one percent argon, and other gasses. Included in the other gasses that make up one percent of air is argon, comprising the vast majority at zero point nine three percent. In spite of global warming carbon dioxide makes up only a fraction of one percent of air, with the remainder including trace amounts of neon, helium, methane, krypton, and hydrogen. Seventy-eight percent of air is nitrogen and the gastrointestinal tract poorly absorbs this gas compared to oxygen and carbon dioxide.

Once the nitrogen is swallowed it has only two ways to get out of the digestive tract. Coming up as a burp or belch is its closest exit, but it has to overcome the lower esophageal sphincter, the upper esophageal sphincter and the oncoming rush with peristalsis and gravity of more food, fluid, drink, saliva, and yes even more air being swallowed. With every single swallow about five ml, or one teaspoonful, of air is swallowed whether you are eating, drinking, or just resting between meals. You swallow approximately every thirty seconds while awake, and about every five minutes while asleep.

The average person swallows about two thousand times a day, but many swallow much more than that. Foods that are extremely hot or cold tend to be swallowed in smaller quantities, resulting in more swallows being necessary to eat or drink the same volume at a moderate temperature. If you chew gum, use a lozenge or sucking candy, or use any product that is a sialagogue, i.e. generates saliva you will be doing a lot more swallowing. Don't forget that with each swallow you are taking in much more air than saliva.

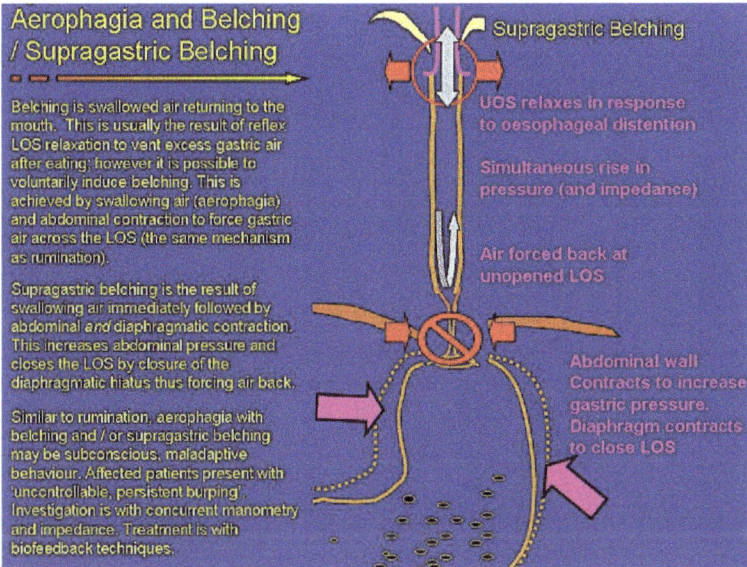

Aerophagia and Belching / Supragastric Belching

Belching is swallowed air returning to the mouth. This is usually the result of reflex LOS relaxation to vent excess gastric air after eating; however it is possible to voluntarily induce belching. This is achieved by swallowing air (aerophagia) and abdominal contraction to force gastric air across the LOS (the same mechanism as rumination).

Supragastric belching is the result of swallowing air immediately followed by abdominal *and* diaphragmatic contraction. This increases abdominal pressure and closes the LOS by closure of the diaphragmatic hiatus thus forcing air back.

Similar to rumination, aerophagia with belching and / or supragastric belching may be subconscious, maladaptive behaviour. Affected patients present with 'uncontrollable, persistent burping' Investigation is with concurrent manometry and impedance. Treatment is with biofeedback techniques.

Supragastric Belching

UOS relaxes in response to oesophageal distention

Simultaneous rise in pressure (and impedance)

Air forced back at unopened LOS

Abdominal wall Contracts to increase gastric pressure. Diaphragm contracts to close LOS

www.bmj.com

The same is true of chewing tobacco and even smoking tobacco whether as cigar, pipe, cigarette, or electronic smokeless cigarette. Do you want to hold a conversation while you are eating? Go ahead but it will cause even more air swallowing, as will drinking from a straw or tilting your head back to drink from a bottle or can. Rush through your meals, and you swallow more air than food or drink.

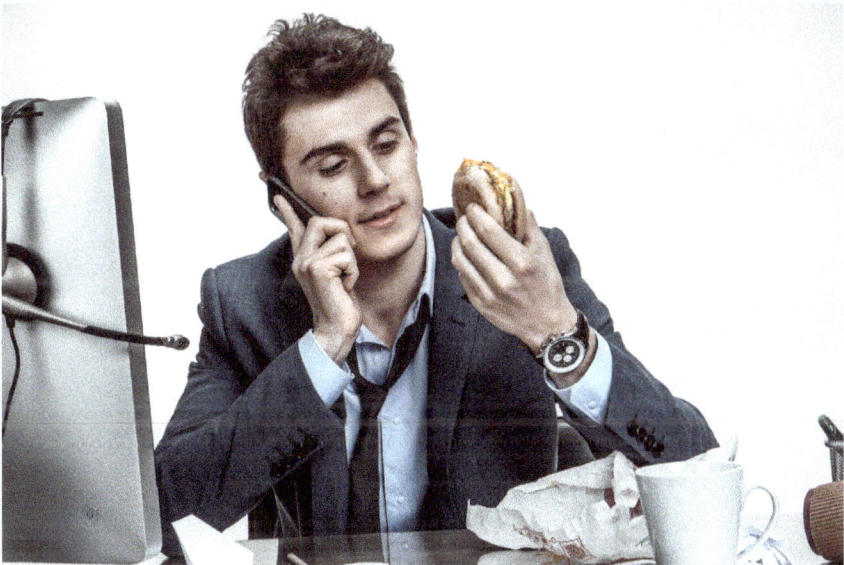

Talking while eating leads to excess air swallowing. Shutterstock/R.legosyn

To 'Air' is Human

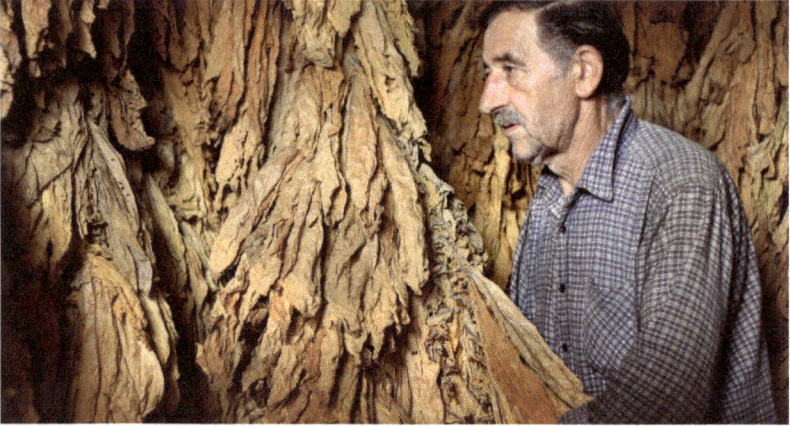

Tobacco smoked as a cigarette, pipe, or cigar, or even chewed contributes to aerophagia
shutterstock/branislavpudar

If you are a baby, just lean back and drink from your baby bottle, even those designed to keep the amount of air swallowed to a minimum. Well, the good news for babies is that most caregivers know how to get them to burp up the air swallowed after a feeding. Then again, the associated spit ups could best be avoided by changing the posture at feeding times to reduce air swallowing.

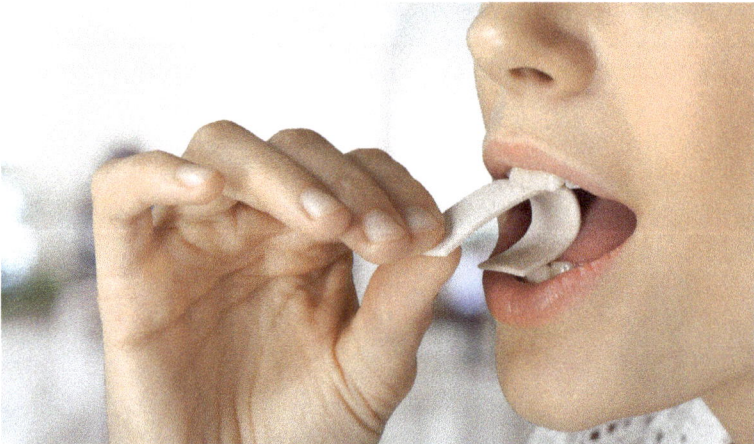

Chewing and bubble gum, as well as use of sucking candy and throat lozenges can lead to excessive air swallowing. shutterstock/billionphotos

Other conditions recognized to increase air swallowing include poor fitting dentures, not chewing food well, drinking from a straw or bottle, talking while eating, and racing through a meal. In another category is the notorious adolescent male who loves to swallow air on purpose so he can generate belches and burps worthy of a dinosaur. Although he may be proud of his newfound talent, it will take many years to achieve the maturity to recognize the sounds generated are an ineffective mating call to attract the female of the species.

To 'Air' is Human

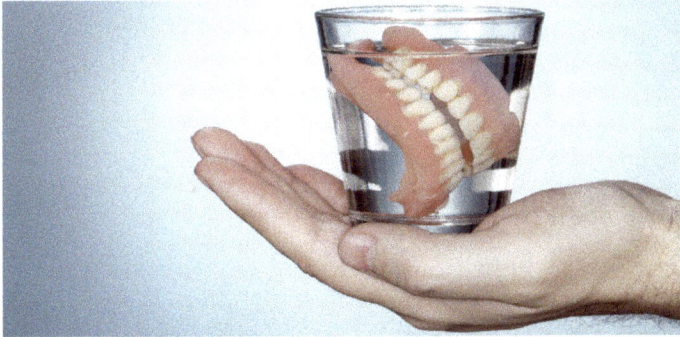

Aerophagia air swallowing is the most common source of excess intestinal gas.
Ill-fitting dentures will contribute to more air being swallowed. Shutterstock/stocksnapper

Some individuals also develop a rumination syndrome, where they subconsciously regurgitate and re-swallow food mixed in with even more air. Fortunately, it is unusual to see a different form of purposeful aerophagia since the development of the artificial larynx or voice box. Years ago, individuals who unfortunately developed cancer of the vocal cords or throat and lost their voice box, used to be taught to swallow air and generate esophageal speech. Esophageal speech was primarily air swallowing followed by controlled belching to create a modified vocalization.

Going back to the average of two thousand swallows a day we are talking about ten liters of air swallowed every single day. Even incorrectly assuming that one hundred percent of the oxygen in the swallowed air was absorbed, we are looking at about eight liters of nitrogen that has been taken in and now needs to get out. That is a lot of nitrogen, and the most direct exit, the shortest distance to travel, and the fastest way to get relief, is to burp or belch.

Sometimes the social situation or environment discourages and suppresses the natural inclination to release the swallowed air. Even if you could burp at will that is an awful lot of gas swallowed throughout the day and night. It is much more than the most frequent and dedicated burpers and belchers are able to release through eructation. The retained nitrogen will contribute to bloating and distension, before it eventually makes its way out of the other end of the intestinal tract as flatus, more commonly known as a fart.

Meals with a high fat content trigger the release of hormones that slow down gut motility. As the food spends more time in the digestive tract, continued bacterial fermentation produces increasing quantities of gas. In addition, foods that are extremely hot or cold tend to be swallowed in smaller quantities, resulting in more swallows being necessary to eat or drink the same volume at a moderate temperature. As each swallow contributes an additional quantity of air entering the esophagus and digestive tract, more swallows results in more air ingestion. Foods or snacks that require excess chewing with resultant excess swallowing of saliva, such as chewing or bubble gum, also contribute to excess air ingestion.

19

To 'Air' is Human

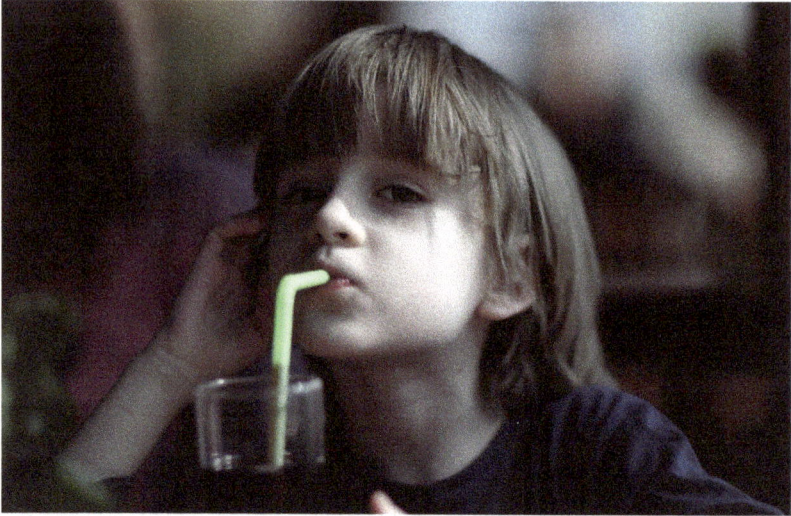

Drinking directly from a bottle or can, or using a straw, can lead to excess aerophagia.
Shutterstock/AnnaJurkovska

A hidden source of swallowed air is the air content present within many foods. Fruits contain a great deal more air than you might have imagined. If you compress an apple and add the volume of the juice and the pressed fruit together you will find that it was only sixty percent of the volume of the original fruit. In other words, of the entire fruit that you swallowed forty percent was air.

We have been in love with ice cream for thousands of years. All ice creams are not prepared in an identical manner. There is another important factor that leads to differences besides the ingredients such as cream or milk fat content, flavorings, sweeteners, stabilizers, emulsifiers, lactose, whey, casein, etcetera. It may be surprising to learn that the two largest ingredients in ice cream by volume are water (between fifty-five percent and sixty-four percent) and air (between three percent and fifty percent).

The other ingredients are measured as a percentage by weight. These include milk fat (minimum ten percent) or in premium ice creams, butter fat (up to nineteen percent). Other ingredients include sweeteners (twelve percent to sixteen percent), milk solids including proteins like casein and whey, and carbohydrates like lactose (between nine percent to twelve percent). Additional ingredients include stabilizers and emulsifiers like agar-agar or carrageenan extracted from seaweed that prevent the fat and water contents from separating (between zero point two percent to zero point five percent). Although air is a large percent by volume, it has virtually zero weight.

The finest ice creams have the lowest percentage of air, but the air is a necessary ingredient to provide a smooth, silky, creamy texture. Without the added air the ice cream would be denser, harder, and feel colder to the tongue. The size of the air bubbles is important as the smallest bubbles provide the smoothest texture. The industry term for air added to foods such as ice cream is 'overrun'. If one liter of ice cream is aerated to double the volume of the mixture to two liters, the overrun is one hundred percent. Most commercial ice creams aim for an overrun of seventy-five percent to one hundred percent, with super-premium ice creams achieving overruns of approximately twenty percent.

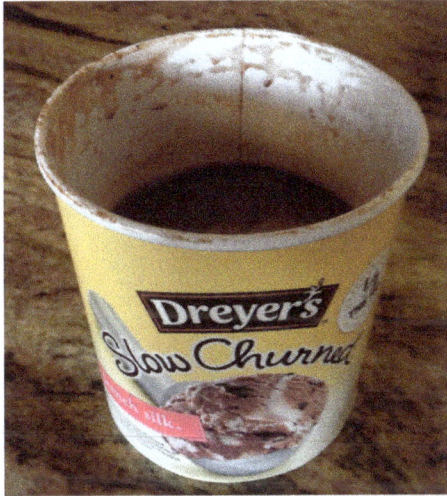

Overrun is the term used to describe air that is added into the finished food product to expand its volume as well as for texture. Air content of ice cream ranges from three percent to fifty percent and has a significant influence on texture, taste, and the value of the product purchased since ice cream is typically sold by volume, not weight. Photo by Lizabeth Weiss.

Have you ever noticed that the volume of ice cream decreases as it melts? If you have accidently left a full container of ice cream out of the freezer and it melted, you would find that it would only be about sixty percent full. You can quickly tell the difference in air content by lifting up equivalent size containers of super-premium ice creams and lower priced competitors. The super-premiums weigh much more, but also contain a lot more content, calories, and fat grams. If half of the volume of ice cream you eat is simply hidden air, you have just been spared half the calories and get the bonus of having swallowed more air to entertain your family and friends.

One of the advantages of a higher overrun, besides higher profits by selling a volume of air at the price of ice cream, is the fact that the air cells as bubbles may prevent ice crystals from forming. If you have ever had ice cream with ice crystals you know that the raspy cutting feeling on the tongue quickly ruins a pleasurable experience. The Food and Drug Administration has standardized the weight of ice cream to not fall below four and one-half pounds to the gallon. This weight standard has limited the amount of air that can be added to the ice cream to approximately fifty percent by volume.

The research team that developed the concept of aeration of ice cream included

To 'Air' is Human

Baroness Margaret Thatcher, the former Prime Minister of Great Britain and contemporary of US President Ronald Reagan. Perhaps there is a kernel of truth that it was a right-wing conservative conspiracy to allow the addition of air allowing ice cream companies to double their profit by selling half a container of air at the full price of ice cream!

Gelato and ice cream are not identical and have a different composition and nutritional value. In the U.S. ice cream is required to have at least 10 percent milkfat, with most medium- to high-end brand actually containing between 14 percent to 17 percent milkfat. Ice cream is churned at a high speed to incorporate air into the mixture to create a smooth and fluffy texture. Ice cream typically contains more than 50 percent air after the churning process both for enhanced mouth feel as well as profitability since it is sold by volume not weight. By contrast, gelato contains between 3 percent and 8 percent milkfat, and 25 percent to 30 percent air.

Gelato is denser than ice cream due to its lower air content. A scoop of gelato weighs more than the same size scoop of vanilla ice cream. Since the nutritional comparison is based on ounces of weight and not volume, a scoop of gelato that is the same size as a scoop of ice cream may have more total calories, fat and sugar than ice cream. On average, a 3.5-ounce serving of vanilla gelato contains 90 calories, 3 grams of fat and 10 grams of sugar. A typical 3.5-ounce serving of vanilla ice cream contains 125 calories, 7 grams of fat and 14 grams of sugar. The fat in content coats the taste buds of the tongue, preventing them from completely experiencing the flavors. Because gelato has a lower fat content the taste buds experience flavors more intensely, and gelato does not need as much added sugar as ice cream for sweetness

The same proposition is true for bread and most baked goods. The baking process often uses baking powder or yeast. When the dough rises you are seeing the additional volume of gasses such as carbon dioxide being produced by the yeast fermentation process. Many foods are whipped with air to increase their volume, which adds to the smoothness and creaminess of the product. It also adds to the bottom line of profitability to the manufacturer, as you are paying for a product typically sold by volume. As long as they don't push it to the detriment of flavor and texture the more air added to a product increases its volume and profitability.

Carbonated beverages are very popular worldwide. In the United States sales of carbonated beverages exceed twenty billion dollars per year, four times the sales volume of dairy products. The majority consumed today already comes carbonated with large amounts of carbon dioxide forced into solution under high pressure. As the pressure seal of the can or bottle is released the carbon dioxide forms bubbles and comes out of the solution, giving a pleasant tickling sensation on the palate, and a full at times bloated feeling in the stomach and gut.

Many soft drinks have high concentrations of simple carbohydrates such as glucose, fructose, and sucrose. Oral bacteria ferment these carbohydrates produce acidic products, which can erode the tooth enamel beginning the dental decay process. A large number of soft drinks are already acidic and have phosphoric acid added in the manufacturing process bringing their pH level to three or lower. To put this value in perspective, neutral water has a pH of seven and gastric hydrochloric acid has a pH of two. Many dentists advocate avoid the brushing of teeth shortly after an acidic beverage because of the tooth enamel is more vulnerable to abrasions after being softened by acid.

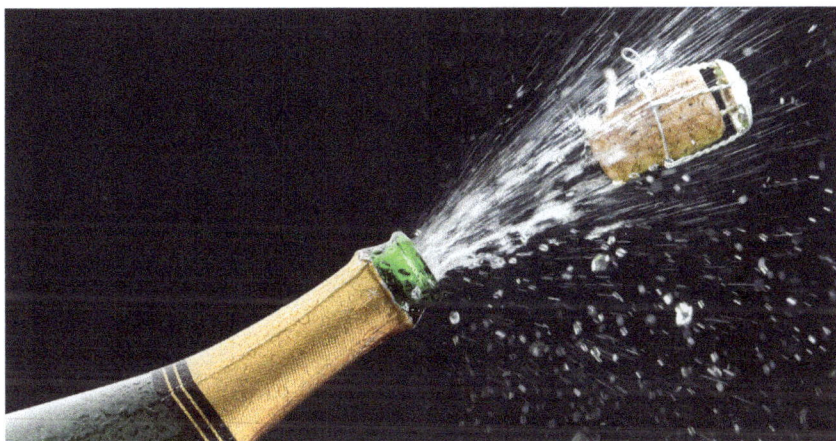

Carbonated champagne uncorking photographed with a high-speed air-gap flash.
shutterstock/lightwork

Mineral water cures were very popular in the middle ages and beyond. Going to the source of mineral springs and the drinking of its contents was referred to as 'taking the waters'. The waters had a variety of mineral content depending on source locale and included various salts and sulfur contents. The sites of such resources became well known as spas, baths, and wells and developed into destinations for the ill and infirm, as well as those who wished to preserve their good health. The term Seltzer water was originally a trademarked name for the German town of Selter that had a famous mineral spring.

The bottling of mineral waters became a profitable enterprise by offering people the opportunity to partake of the presumed beneficial waters in their own locales. An attempt to imitate the effervescent effect of the mineral waters was made by Joseph Priestley in 1767. Some fans of carbonated beverages believe this should be his claim to fame rather than his discovery of oxygen. J. J. Schweppes of Switzerland commercialized the process in 1783, moving his factory and enterprise to England in 1783.

Have you ever wondered how much carbon dioxide gas is released from a soft drink or carbonated beverage. You have already gotten a visual demonstration if the bottle or can was dropped or shaken before being opened. This agitation accelerates the release of the carbon dioxide, and it can form a jet stream of gassy bubbles to be sprayed on everyone within a dozen feet of the demonstration. This social activity is very popular amongst preadolescent boys. The quantification of how much carbon dioxide is in a one liter bottle of a carbonated soft drink is calculated using a formula known as Henry's Law.

The gas content in a one-liter bottle is a surprising two point eight liters. In other words, there is nearly three times the volume of the original container in excess gas under pressure hidden in those tiny bubbles. Do not forget another important law of the physics of gasses, Charles' Law. This law defines the activity of gasses expanding as the temperature increases. If you drink a cold carbonated beverage, and after swallowing it is warmed up to body temperature, it will exhibit another substantial increase in the volume of gasses released. The burping and belching that occurs after drinking a cold carbonated beverage may seem out of proportion to the small amount consumed. Just remember that whatever the volume of liquid carbonated beverage swallowed, there is nearly three times that volume of dissolved gas waiting to be released.

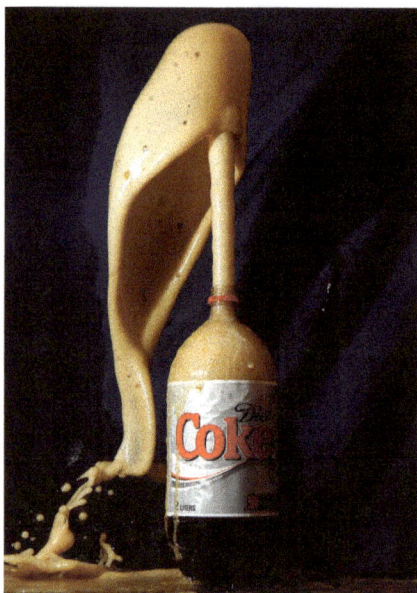

Diet Coke and Mentos Geyser by Michael Murphy Creative Commons License.

If you want further visual proof that Henry's Law is accurate take a look at the photographic evidence of another popular activity. The harmless addition of a Mentos brand mint candy tablet to a liter bottle of a carbonated beverage, such as Diet Coke, sounds like such an innocent activity. This demonstration is repeated in countless elementary school science classes. The *Guinness Book of World Records* described one thousand three hundred and sixty students in the historic university town of Leuven, Belgium creating simultaneous Mentos with Diet Coke geysers. See the entry on carbonation for more details about this process and phenomenon.

In some beverages the carbon dioxide would interfere with the taste and flavor by reacting with the ingredients, giving it an acid taste from carbonic acid. An alternative is to use nitrogen as the gas of choice as it was a neutral gas and would not interact with the beverage. The most popular example is Guinness, which uses nitrogen, or a combination of nitrogen and carbon dioxide, under pressure in kegs.

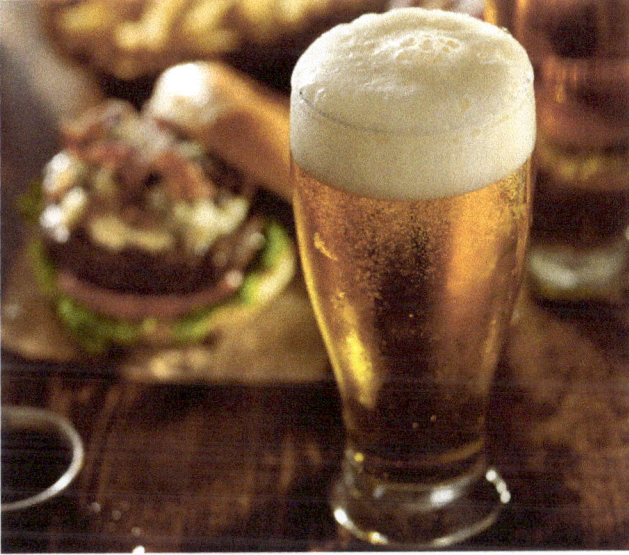

shutterstock/JoshuaResnick

The nitrogen provides smaller firmer bubbles with a smoother longer lasting head, and other companies have followed their lead. Guinness also pioneered the use of a widget, an irregularity at the base of the container to serve as the nucleation focus for gas bubbles to form at the base of cans and bottles rather than the surface.

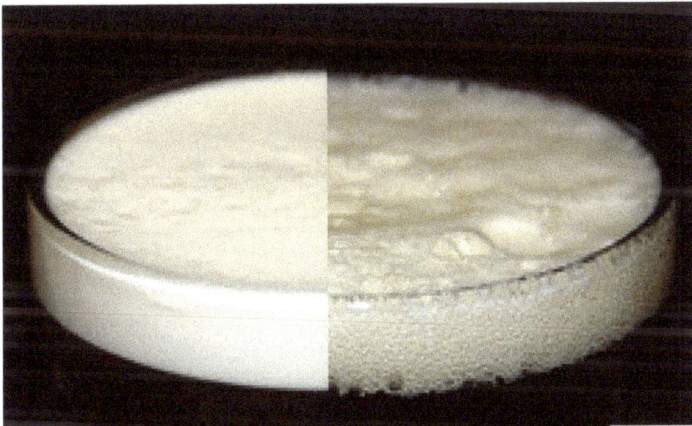

Nitrogenated   Carbonated

To 'Air' is Human

Nitrogen is poorly soluble in liquids, and the high density of bubbles contributes to a smooth creamy mouth feel. Most beers are saturated with a combination of 30% carbon dioxide and 70% nitrogen. The head serves both an aesthetic purpose, as well as accomplishing the dispersal of the beer aroma. You can get an idea of how high the nitrogen content is by looking at the size of the head created. A significant percentage of the volume of your drink is the head, and a friendly bartender will discard some of the head to give you more drink for your money, as well as to encourage a larger gratuity.

Beer drinkers are famous for the burping and belching generated. The added nitrogen gives them an edge up in competitive burping and belching contests since it is not as rapidly absorbed and eliminated via the lungs, as is carbon dioxide. Nitrogen is also used in iced coffee beverages, providing a head of bubbles very similar to that of beer.

Aerospace

Intestinal gas, like gasses everywhere, must comply with the laws of physics and the laws of nature. Boyle's law states that at a constant temperature, the product of the volume and pressure of a gas must remain constant. This requires that they maintain an inverse relationship, if one increases the other has to decrease. As such, an increase in pressure will result in the decrease of the volume of the gas, and vice versa. The atmospheric pressure on earth is defined as a standard of one atmosphere at sea level. As you go deeper down into the earth, such as happens in a mineshaft, or diving deeper into the oceans, the atmospheric pressure increases. As you go higher in elevation, whether climbing flights of stairs, ascending a mountain, or in a hot air balloon, the atmospheric pressure decreases. The atmospheric pressure is also not uniform, constantly changing along with the weather.

The changes in atmospheric pressure in aerospace are even more dramatic than in mountain climbers, both in intensity and rapidity. During World War II, flight surgeons found that at altitudes thirty thousand feet or more above sea level, aviators suffered painful abdominal distension. At that altitude, the atmospheric pressure was a fraction of that at sea level, allowing intestinal gas to balloon to nearly four times its original volume. Painful distension of the abdomen was the result of the dramatic volume expansion of trapped intestinal gas. Because the trapped gas was not near the rectum, it could not be readily released as flatus.

Popularly referred to in the military by its abbreviated acronym, High-altitude flatus expulsion (HAFE) is a common gastrointestinal syndrome seen in pilots and passengers of aircraft. It involves the uncontrollable passage of large quantities of intestinal gasses at high altitudes. As the atmospheric pressure decreases with an increase in altitude, the volume of gas in the intestine increases consistent with the principles of physics (Boyle's Law). Military pilots and astronauts have repeatedly verified the existence of HAFE, with its sensation of distension, and the need to expel the expanding intestinal gasses.

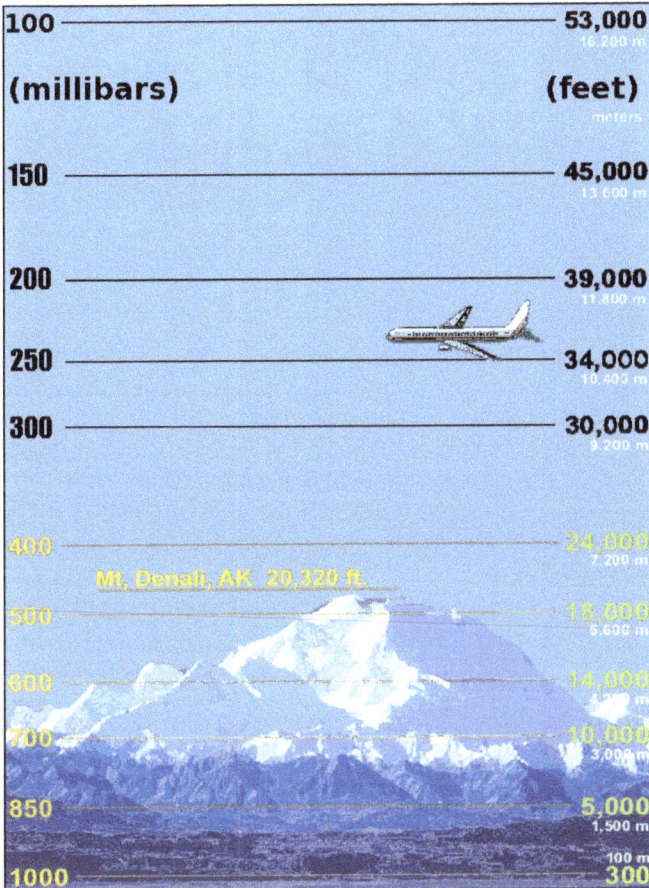

www.wpclipart.com NOAA Public Domain

With commercial aircraft commonly flying at over thirty thousand feet in elevation, the atmospheric pressure outside of the plane is a fraction of atmospheric pressure at sea level. The pressure loss at that altitude would not be tolerable to passengers, so the aircraft is pressurized to simulate what the atmospheric pressure would be at approximately eight thousand feet above sea level.

The retained pockets of air in your gut will expand quickly, and want to be released even if it comes at the expense of your embarrassment. Airlines, pilots, and flight attendants are well aware of this effect, but they rarely offer the passenger any warning or explanation. They assume that you will not comment on the natural discomfort you are experiencing, or the subsequent release of intestinal gas, either your own or of the person sitting directly in front of you. In fact, it is to be expected that there is much more air turbulence inside an aircraft than outside.

To 'Air' is Human

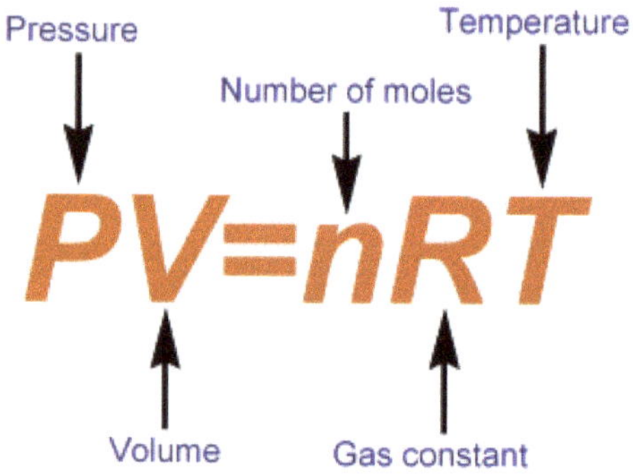

Pressure

Temperature

Number of moles

$$PV = nRT$$

Volume

Gas constant

A visual example of the differences in atmospheric pressure between beings on the ground closer to sea level, and at an atmospheric pressure equivalent to an altitude of eight thousand feet is often served to you by a flight attendant. Take a close look at what happens to carbonated beverages served at high altitude. Have you ever noticed that the release of the bubbles of carbon dioxide from a carbonated beverage is much more dramatic when flying? Flight attendants have to spend more time while pouring the carbonated beverages, pausing to let the bubbles release themselves as they fill your glass. If they did not pause to let the gasses be released, you would be handed a container of fizz and foam instead of the beverage you wanted.

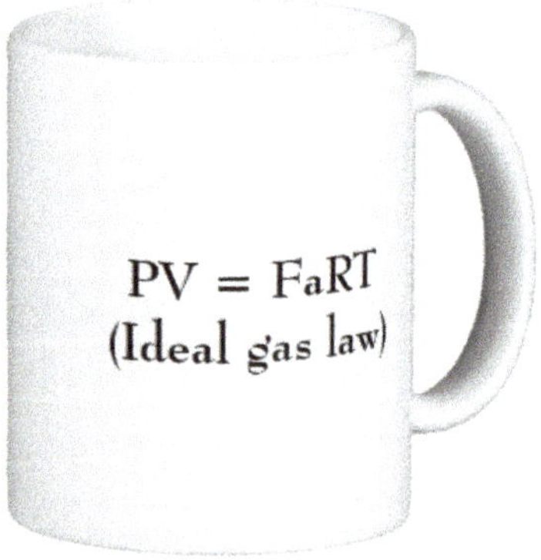

$$PV = FaRT$$
$$(\text{Ideal gas law})$$

rlv.zcache.com

Aerospace has another concern that increases the volume and frequency of farts within the tight confines of a space capsule or space station. In an environment without gravity, the weightlessness leads to muscle weakness and atrophy. As the abdominal muscles weaken, the intestinal gasses expand further distending the gut and results in an increase in fart volume and frequency. While traveling in space, even in a pressurized space capsule, there is a very significant reduction in pressure, which means that gasses must exhibit a proportional increase in volume.

For those involved in space travel, including the growing population of space tourists, the pressure changes are unparalleled. Many people are knowledgeable about the dangers of scuba and deep-sea divers, especially if surfacing from the depths too quickly. The nitrogen gas in the air that is breathed in at higher pressures dissolves in the bloodstream and body fats. When returning to the surface too quickly, the diver is subjected to a rapid drop in atmospheric pressure. The nitrogen gas comes out of solution, and forms bubbles of gas in the circulation. Decompression sickness, caisson disease, or 'the bends' is a risk for the space traveler as well.

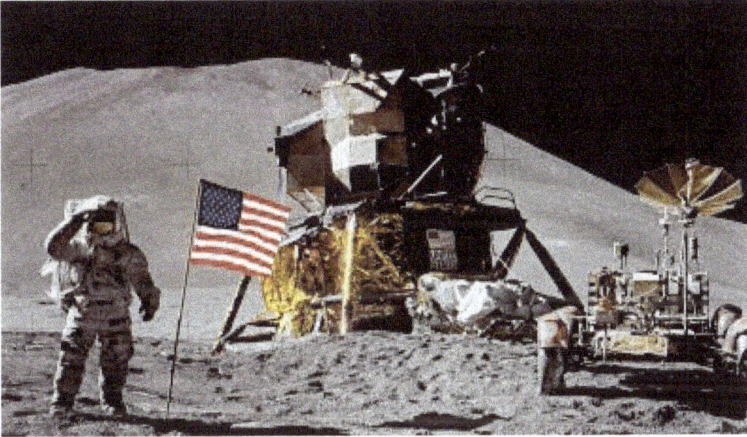

NASA Public Domain

The air and space traveler would likewise experience a rapid decrease in atmospheric pressure if not for the ability to pressurize the aircraft or spacecraft. The ambient atmospheric pressure within a spacecraft is typically maintained at fourteen point seven pounds per square inch (psi), or one hundred and one kilopascals (kPa). The most dramatic exposure to a rapid decrease in atmospheric pressure occurs when space travelers leave the pressurized spacecraft for spacewalks, more formally known as extravehicular activity.

Without the pressurized spacesuit, known more formally as extravehicular mobility units, the rapid reduction in atmospheric pressure may be life threatening. The spacesuit is typically pressurized to four point three pounds per square inch (thirty kPa). Without the spacesuit, decompression sickness also known as caisson sickness or the bends can develop in astronauts just as it does in deep-sea divers. As the atmospheric pressure is rapidly reduced the nitrogen gas that was previously in solution forms bubbles. These form in the bloodstream, nerves, joints and can cause pain, as well as circulatory collapse

Because the reductions in atmospheric pressure remain significant and put them at risk of life-threatening decompression sickness, the space travelers are given pure oxygen to breathe for several hours prior to the spacewalk. Breathing pure oxygen for several hours reduces the nitrogen dissolved in their circulation and fat stores, and further reduces the risk of nitrogen bubbles forming in their bloodstream leading to decompression sickness.

To 'Air' is Human

The early pioneers of space travel were appropriately heralded as heroes known for 'the right stuff'. They balanced the dangers and unknowns with a mixture of bravado and humor. As space travelers are at the extreme of reduced atmospheric pressure, they have a carte blanche to blame Boyle's Law for any and all gas bubbles they may wish to release. Alan Shepard, Jr. (1923 – 1998) was an American naval aviator, test pilot, and NASA astronaut. In 1961 Shepard became the first American, and second person after Soviet Cosmonaut Yuri Gargarin, to travel into space. When reporters asked Shepard what he was thinking about as he sat atop the potentially explosive Redstone rocket waiting for liftoff he replied "The fact that every part of this ship was built by the low bidder!" Ten years later, Alan Shepard was at the command of the Apollo 14 mission to the moon. Despite thick gloves and a stiff spacesuit Shepard struck two golf balls on the lunar surface driving the second golf ball "miles and miles and miles."

Benjamin Franklin was quoted as saying "Instead of cursing the darkness, light a candle." Alan Shepard created another memorable quote while waiting for the end of the interminable delays to launch. NASA engineers had delayed his first flight so many times that the Soviets were able to send the first man into orbit. On the day of his successful voyage, Shepard sat on the launch pad, waiting inside his rocket for over four hours while engineers corrected one challenging problem after another. The wait was longer than expected, and Shepard exceeded is bladder capacity. He ended up having to urinate inside his spacesuit. They had to turn off his monitoring equipment so that he did not create a short circuit. When one more problem cropped up, Shepard exclaimed, "Why don't you fix your little problem and light this candle!" The quote became the title of his biography, Light This Candle.

The U.S. space program was concerned about intestinal gas during space flight. After liftoff, while experiencing weightlessness, Shepard also experienced this other anticipated consequence of virtually zero atmospheric pressure. His internal gas bubbles expanded with the production of near continuous farting, which he graphically described over the radio communications with mission control. If you listen closely to the recording of the conversations, not all of the background noise was static!

As director of the astronaut program, Shepard received the following memorandum from astronaut John Young. "RE: Safety Issues. No less than six times have I had to listen to Borman complain about his lactose intolerance when someone stole his weird not-milk milk stuff. Additionally, when Borman drinks regular milk, he gets the farts. That's all I'm going to say about that." In the microgravity environment of space, farting results in the body being propelled when the 'digestive gas thruster is fired'. On the U.S.S.R. and Russian space station Mir, restraining devices were installed on the toilet seat, so the user would not be thrust off the seat with a fart.

Gus Grissom was scheduled to go into space two months after Shepard's inaugural flight on Friendship Seven. He insisted that the 'potty' problem had to be solved, and a naval flight surgeon was assigned to the task. He sent one of the nurses into town to buy a women's panty girdle, which was layered with absorbent pads. Grissom was the first astronaut to go into space wearing women's lingerie. Astronauts, cosmonauts, and taikonauts have to deal with bodily functions in space, and modifications have been required. The Hamilton Standard Company was the maker of the U.S. astronaut spacesuits, and male astronauts used a condom catheter under the spacesuits for spacewalks and moonwalks. Ingenuity was required to come up with a comparable solution for female astronauts.

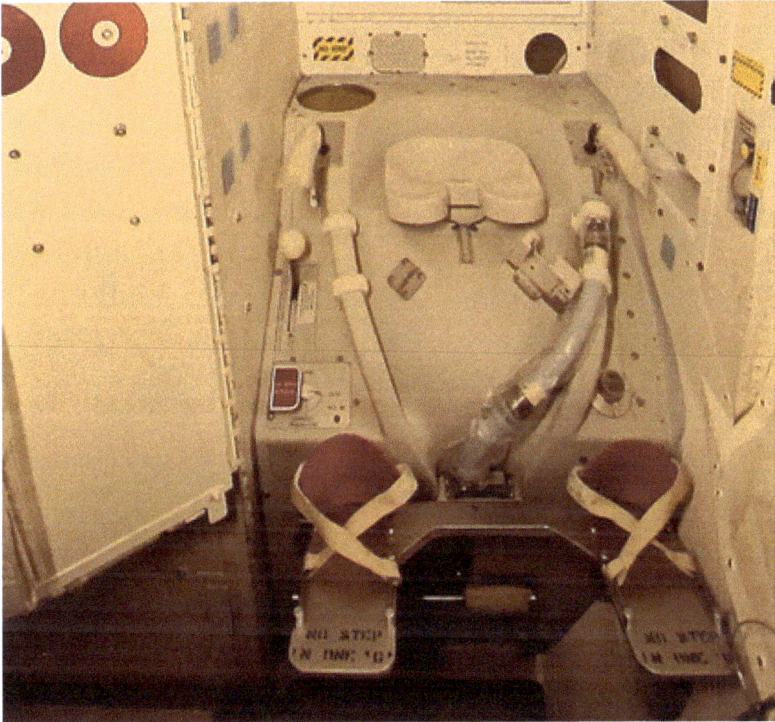

Bathroom on the space shuttle. NASA Public Domain

When the Gemini program began, the astronauts graduated to urine and fecal bags and special diapers for spacewalks. Urine waste was disposed of by an overboard dump valve. The solid waste was handled differently with a germicide placed in the storage bag, which was sealed in a locker. Since the lunar model itself was not designed with an overboard dump valve or storage cabinet, astronauts left very personal mementos of their visits behind. More than the national flag of the United States of America was deposited on the moon surface and remains there to this day. When the Space Shuttle program was being engineered, a specially designed space toilet called the "Waste Collection Facility" or WCF for short was developed. It was budgeted to cost three million dollars to develop, but with cost over-runs it ended up being the world most expensive toilet by far costing more than thirty million dollars.

To 'Air' is Human

For those living in high altitude communities such as Mexico City at over seven thousand feet above sea level, the atmospheric pressure is much lower than at sea level. Commercial aircraft are pressurized to an equivalent of eight thousand feet above sea level. With the atmospheric pressure at just over two-thirds of sea level, the gas volume expands by about forty percent. That is more than enough to cause a person to notice a significant increase in their flatulence and an increase in the flatulence of everyone else as well.

Air Enema

An air enema is often used during a barium enema study, when the air is inflated into the colon via the enema tube to provide air as a contrast to the barium. This type of barium study is called an air contrast or double-contrast barium enema. Air may also be inflated into the colon as the self-practice of the air enema that is described in the ancient yoga literature. The advanced yogi may develop anal sphincter control, and control of the abdominal muscles to create an abdominal suction effect to vacuum air into the lower intestine.

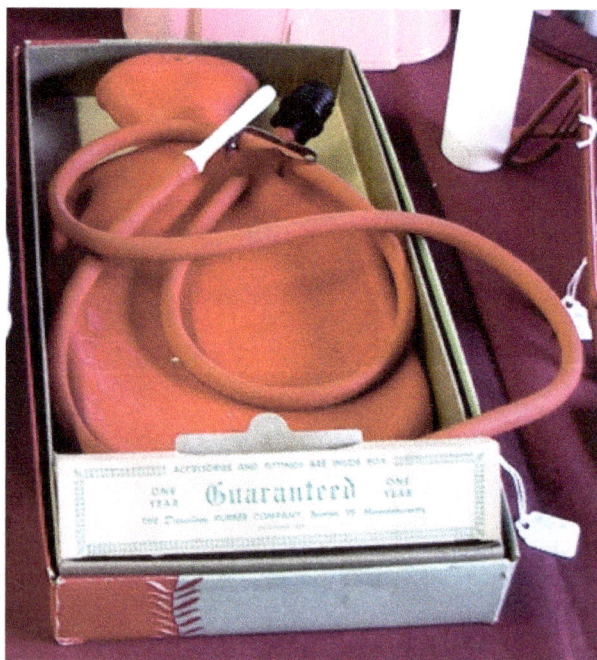

www.flickr.com Creative Commons License

Shale Baste, also called Vat Baste, Air Baste, is an air enema used as an advanced Hatha yoga technique and is best learned from an expert teacher. There are a number of different approaches and techniques, but mastery of voluntary control of the anal sphincter is a challenging practice. See the entry on yoga for more details, as well as entry on Le Pétomane a stage performer who mastered this technique to great critical acclaim and commercial success.

To 'Air' is Human

Air Fart

The ability to air fart is the common term for the ability to control the anus and muscles of abdomen and respiration, to cause air to be aspirated into the colon and then released voluntarily as a fart. It is also known colloquially as the ability to butt breathe. The air fart and butt breathe technique is known in more enlightened society as an air enema and has been practiced as a part of yoga colon hygiene for thousands of years.

Although usually considered under involuntary control these muscles can be trained, and yogis attain remarkable proficiency. At the turn of the twentieth century, the performer Joseph Pujol, under the stage name Le Pétomane, became an international sensation by demonstrating his prowess at butt breathing.

This ability is not limited to trained yogi and stage performers. According to the results of an internet-based survey on farting performed in 2001, with over one thousand three hundred participants, over fifteen percent of respondents were able to accomplish this with the benefit of being able to fart on command.

Fart survey question for men: Can you fart on command also called "Butt Breathe"?

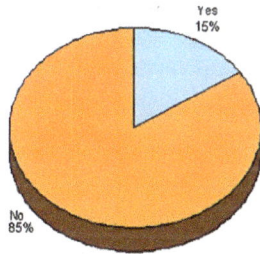

Yes
15%

No
85%

Only fifteen percent of the men surveyed can fart voluntarily by suctioning air into the colon. One-third of all men did not even know that this is possible!

Fart survey question for women: Can you fart on command also called "Butt Breathe"?

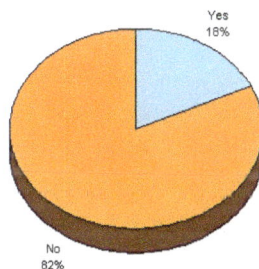

Yes
18%

No
82%

Only eighteen percent of the women surveyed can fart voluntarily by suctioning air into the colon.

To 'Air' is Human

Air, Gas Composition

If the entire abdomen is distended with air-filled loops of the intestine, a bowel obstruction may be its cause. Marked distension of the stomach can occur with gastroparesis, a neuropathy that delays stomach emptying seen most often in diabetics or when the pyloric channel or upper small bowel is obstructed. Iatrogenic is a fancy way of saying a physician was the cause. Iatrogenic air in the gastrointestinal tract is common after endoscopic procedures such as upper gastrointestinal endoscopy (esophagoscopy, gastroscopy, esophagogastro-duodenoscopy, EGD), endoscopic retrograde cholangiopancreatography (ERCP), or colonoscopy (proctoscopy, sigmoidoscopy, colonoscopy, ileoscopy, enteroscopy). The official name of the endoscopic procedure undertaken is defined by the anatomy of the organs examined.

The coming advances including capsule endoscopy will replace many of these multi-syllable, expensive, and invasive diagnostic tests. Developed initially by Given Imaging, a high-tech company based in Israel, a swallowed capsule travels through the digestive tract like a spying submarine. With remarkable visual clarity, it examines the lining of the bowel for abnormalities. Further development will allow it to obtain tissue samples and even therapeutic lasers bringing the science fiction movie *Fantastic Voyage* one step closer to reality. Other technology companies are pursuing this and other nanotechnology marvels that will travel through the body for diagnostic and therapeutic purposes.

Air is the typical gas inflated, and it may be several hours to up to a day for the excess gas to be eliminated. As described below carbon dioxide is the preferred gas for inflation since it is so readily absorbed and eliminated, but for either ease of access or costs air continues to be used by most endoscopists. The radiologist also uses air insufflation with radiographic studies such as the barium enema. When the study is enhanced by air insufflation it is called an air-contrast or double-contrast barium enema.

Barium studies are not performed as often today, but they can provide valuable diagnostic information. A number of years ago I had a patient who was scheduled to have a barium enema to examine the colon, to be followed a few days later by a barium swallow to examine the esophagus. In about twenty percent of patients undergoing barium enema, the contrast material passes through the ileocecal valve and into the small bowel. This can be useful in providing additional diagnostic information about the distal small bowel, such as the presence of inflammatory bowel disease. In this individual, the barium entered the small intestine, but before the radiologist could reduce the pressure of the barium flow it refluxed all the way into his stomach and esophagus and the patient vomited up the barium. With disgust, the patient told the radiologist to cancel the barium swallow. When asked why, the patient told him he would never be able to drink the barium because it tasted like shit!

Iatrogenic (physician caused) distension with gas is routine in the performance of laparoscopy where tube-like visual instruments are used to examine the abdomen and pelvis. The gas used to inflate the abdominal cavity, creating a pneumoperitoneum, is carbon dioxide. The carbon dioxide gas is rapidly absorbed by the body and eliminated via exhalation through the lungs. If air were used the less than one percent component of carbon dioxide would be rapidly absorbed. The twenty-one percent portion of the air comprised of oxygen would be slowly absorbed over a few days. The remaining seventy-two percent majority consisting of nitrogen is poorly absorbed. The nitrogen gas would remain within the peritoneal cavity for an extended period of time, being slowly absorbed over a period of several days to weeks.

Air, Iatrogenic

Iatrogenic is a fancy way of saying a physician was the cause. Iatrogenic air in the gastrointestinal tract is common after endoscopic procedures such as upper gastrointestinal endoscopy (esophagoscopy, gastroscopy, or esophagogastroduodenoscopy (EGD), endoscopic retrograde cholangiopancreatography (ERCP)) or colonoscopy (proctoscopy, sigmoidoscopy, colonoscopy, ileoscopy, enteroscopy). The official name of the endoscopic procedure undertaken is defined by the anatomy of the organs examined.

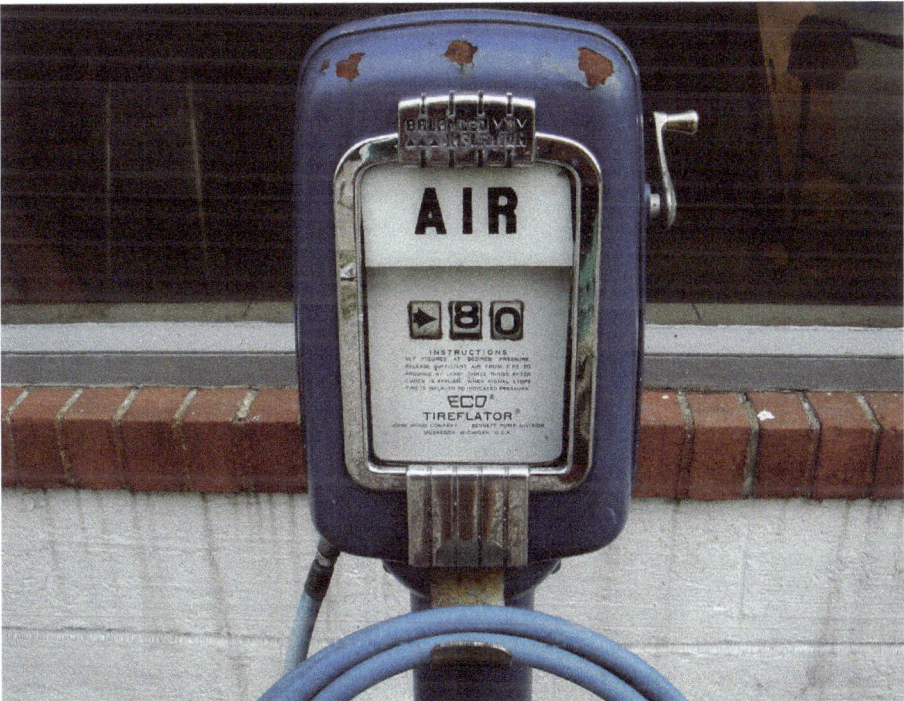

shutterstock/CedricCrucke

Air is the typical gas inflated, and it may be several hours to up to a day for the excess gas to be eliminated. As described below carbon dioxide is the preferred gas for inflation since it is so readily absorbed and eliminated, but for either ease of access or costs air continues to be used by most endoscopists. The radiologist also uses air insufflation with radiographic studies such as the barium enema. When the study is enhanced by air insufflation it is called an air-contrast or double-contrast barium enema. Iatrogenic (physician caused) distension with gas is routine in the performance of laparoscopy where tube-like visual instruments are used to examine the abdomen and pelvis. The gas used to inflate the abdominal cavity, creating a pneumoperitoneum, is carbon dioxide.

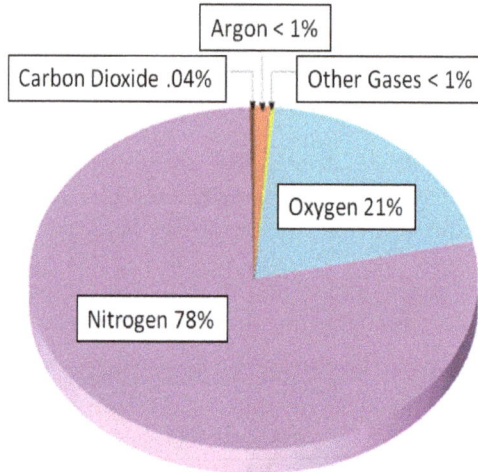

Argon < 1%

Carbon Dioxide .04%

Other Gases < 1%

Oxygen 21%

Nitrogen 78%

m7science.wikispaces.com Creative Commons License

The carbon dioxide gas is rapidly absorbed by the body and eliminated via exhalation through the lungs. If air were used the less than one percent component of carbon dioxide would be rapidly absorbed. The twenty-one percent portion of the air comprised of oxygen would be slowly absorbed over a few days. The remaining seventy-two percent majority consisting of nitrogen is poorly absorbed. The nitrogen gas would remain within the peritoneal cavity for an extended period of time, being slowly absorbed over a period of several days to weeks.

Alpha Galactosidase

Beano, Bean-Zyme, Say Yes To Beans, and competing products are an enzyme-based dietary supplement that is used to reduce the intestinal production of dietary oligosaccharides such as raffinose from legumes. Beano contains the enzymes alpha-galactosidase and invertase, which are derived from the fungus *Aspergillus Niger*. *Aspergillus Niger* and its fermentation products are 'generally recognized as safe' (GRAS) by the United States Food and Drug Administration (FDA). Because pets, such as dogs and cats, also release intestinal, the identical product was released to be marketed for pets under the brand name Curtail. Although it may be effective, it reduced the ability of guilty humans to blame a fart on the dog or cat.

To 'Air' is Human

The alpha-galactosidase is effective but must be taken with the first bite of food. Because heating inactivates it, it cannot be used in the cooking process, and must be taken when eating the food. It does not have any effect on lactose or other enzyme deficiencies. Additional doses of alpha-galactosidase will be needed if large quantities of legumes are consumed, or a substantial period has passed since the dose was taken.

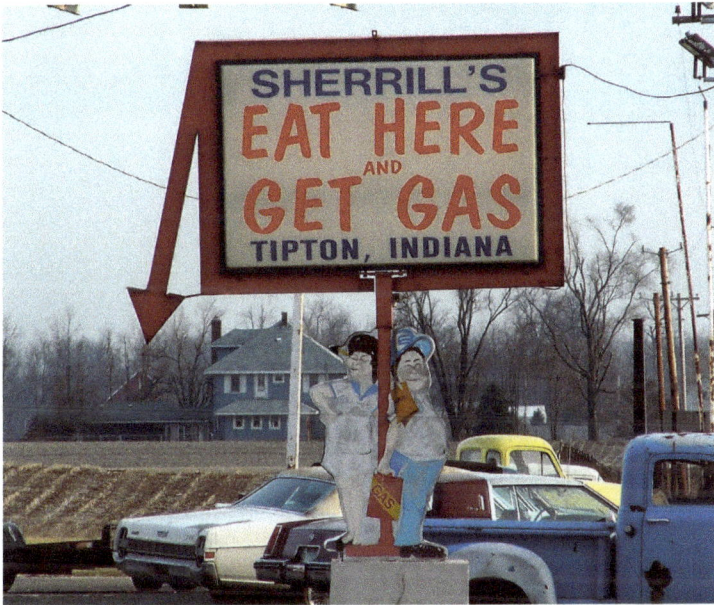

Refueling station and restaurant. Cindy Cornett Seigle www.flickr.com Creative Commons License

Another approach is to soak the beans for several hours and discard the fluid, which leaches out some of the complex sugars. Allowing the seeds to germinate allows the bean plant itself to begin to produce alpha-galactosidase. Within twenty-four hours of germination the internally generated enzyme breaks down most of the complex sugars. Using the herb asafetida can also reduce flatulence although the herb itself has an aroma that may be worse than the farts you are trying to prevent. The name of the herb itself may give you a clue as fetida has the same root as the word fetid. These words are derived from the Latin word foetidus and *foetēre* meaning 'to stink'

Certain beans are being developed that have lower concentrations of the challenging complex sugars. The enzyme hydrolyses the polysaccharides and oligosaccharides if the raffinose family including stachyose, verbascose, and galactinol found in foods such as the legumes beans and peanuts, and the cruciferous vegetables cauliflower, broccoli, cabbage, and Brussels sprouts. Beano was marketed by Alan Kligerman of AkPharma, Inc. in 1990. Originally in the dairy farm business, he was the developer of the commercially successful lactase supplement Lactaid. Beano received a US patent in 1995, which is estimated to expire in 2015. There are more than fifty competing products on the market. It should be noted that the use of these products enhances the digestibility of certain foods and increases the nutrients and calories absorbed.

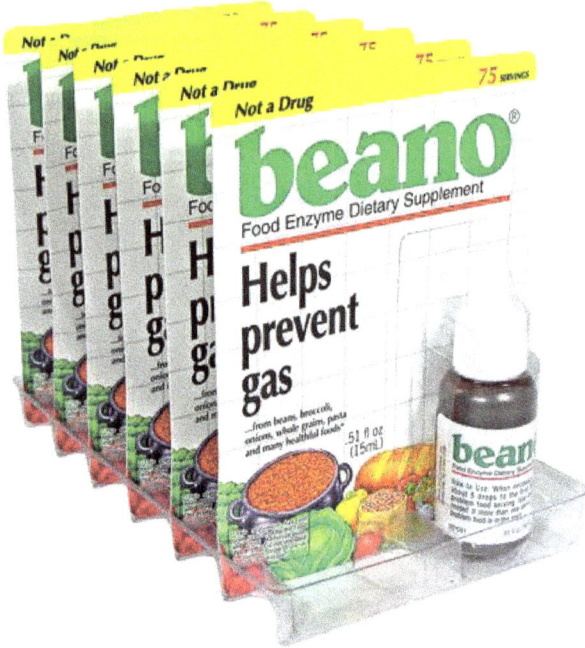

www.flickr.com Creative Commons License

The intellectual concept for a product to reduce intestinal was proposed in the 1780's by Benjamin Franklin (see separate entry). He submitted an essay "A Letter To A Royal Academy" suggesting that an award be given to the inventor of a food additive that would make the aroma of flatus attractive instead of offensive. Benjamin Franklin was known as for his sense of humor, and although some thought his proposal was serious, it was written tongue in cheek.

Simple sugars are produced in the malting process of barley to brew beer. The complex sugars not hydrolyzed or fermented and consumed by the beer drinker may contribute to its well-recognized ability to increase flatulence. Some home brewers have added Beano to the mash in an attempt to reduce this occurrence. The use of the prescription drug Acarbose or Miglitol used in the treatment of diabetes mellitus will cause a dramatic increase in flatulence because of its enzyme inhibitor activity. These drugs used to treat type 2 diabetes mellitus inhibit the glycoside hydrolases, the alpha-galactosidae family of enzymes necessary for the digestion of many starches. It specifically inhibits alpha-glucosidase enzymes in the brush border of the small intestines, pancreatic alpha-amylase, maltase, isomaltase, glucoamylase, sucrose, and invertase.

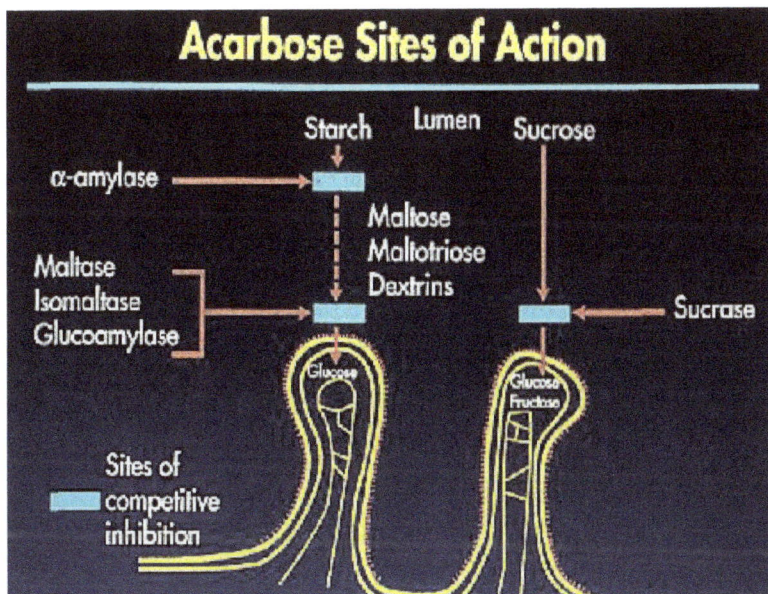

Alpha-glucosidase inhibitors are the competitive, reversible inhibitors of pancreatic ✓-amylase and membrane-bound intestinal ✓-glucosidase hydrolase enzymes. Use of these drugs leads to blocks the enzymatic degradation of complex carbohydrates in the small intestine decreasing the amount and delaying the absorption of these sugars. Acarbose, which is not absorbed by the body, has the following preferred affinity for blocking the ✓-glucosidase enzymes: glycoamylase > sucrase > maltase > dextranase and has no affinity for the ✓-glucosidase enzymes, such as lactase. Miglitol is a more potent inhibitor of sucrase and maltase than acarbose and has no effect on ✓-amylase.

Pancreatic alpha-amylase hydrolyzes complex starches to oligosaccharides in the chyme being digested in the lumen of the small intestine. The intestinal alpha-glycosidase further hydrolyzes oligosaccharides, trisaccharides, and disaccharides to glucose and other monosaccharides at the brush border of the villi in the small intestine. Inhibition of these enzyme systems reduces the rate of digestion of complex carbohydrates and decreases the amount of glucose available for absorption. It should be taken at the start of a meal, and as more complex carbohydrates pass to the colon undigested, increased bacterial fermentation will result. Increased flatulence is reported in the vast majority of patients, and approximately fifteen percent develop diarrhea. The gastrointestinal side effects may diminish with continued use over time. Adverse side effects may also include elevation of liver function tests, which usually resolves with discontinuation of the medicine.

There has been a significant increase in average size and stature of adults in a wide diversity of countries around the world over a span of only one or two generations. The obvious explanation is the improvement in access to not only additional calories but also the critical nutrition role played by vitamins, dietary minerals, and trace elements. The full role of diet, nutrition, hormones, enzymes, the gut flora and microbiome, genetics, epigenetics, and other factors is still in the process of being elucidated.

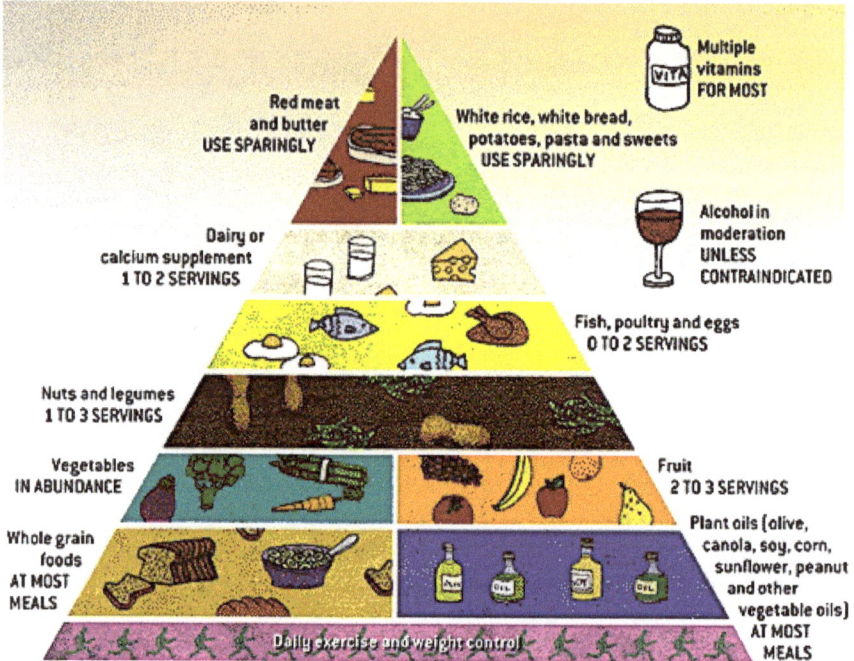

NEW FOOD PYRAMID

outlined by the authors distinguishes between healthy and unhealthy types of fat and carbohydrates. Fruits and vegetables are still recommended, but the consumption of dairy products should be limited.

Public Domain

Certain types of vegetables and fruits contain carbohydrates the sugars and starches that may be poorly digested by people but happily fermented by bacteria comprising the gut flora. The starches, including potatoes, corn, noodles, and wheat are the source of the majority of gasses generated by the gut microbial flora. Rice is the one starch exception and rarely contributes to production. Wheat has the other 'distinction' of having the protein glutamate, which contains the nitrogen base product you generate ammonia-like aromatic compounds. The most common food intolerance is for the milk sugar lactose when an individual has decreased quantities and activity of the necessary enzyme for its digestion, lactase.

Archaea (see Microbiome)

Aroma (see Fart, Aroma)

Atmospheric Pressure

Intestinal gas, like gasses everywhere, must comply with the laws of physics and the laws of nature. Boyle's law states that at a constant temperature, the product of the volume and pressure of a gas must remain constant. This requires that they maintain an inverse relationship, if one increases the other has to decrease. As such, an increase in pressure will result in the decrease of the volume of the gas, and vice versa.

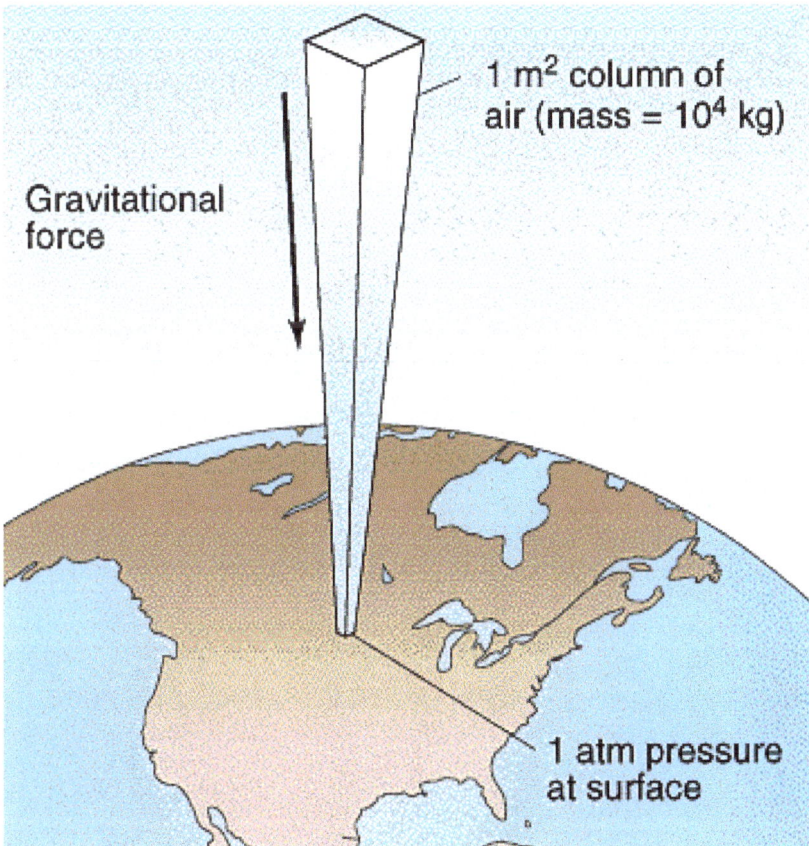

1 m^2 column of air (mass = 10^4 kg)

Gravitational force

1 atm pressure at surface

Atmospheric pressure hendrix2.uoregon.edu Creative Commons License

The atmospheric pressure on earth is defined as a standard of one atmosphere at sea level. As you go deeper down into the earth, such as happens in a mineshaft, or diving deeper into the oceans, the atmospheric pressure increases. As you go higher in elevation, whether climbing flights of stairs, ascending a mountain, or in a hot air balloon, the atmospheric pressure decreases. The atmospheric pressure is also not uniform, constantly changing along with the weather.

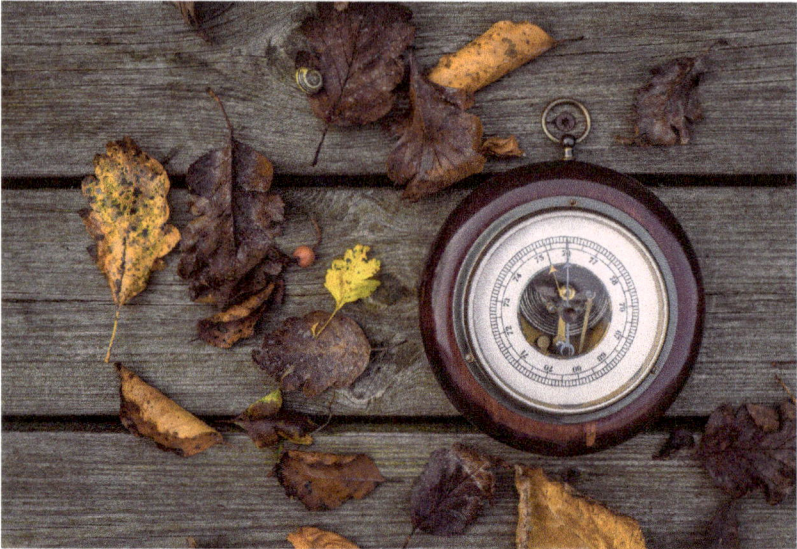

Atmospheric pressure and the weather are always changing. shutterstock/polarpx

Using Boyle's law, you can calculate how much the volume will compress as you go deeper underground or underwater and atmospheric pressure increases. You can likewise calculate how much a gas will expand, as you go higher in altitude and the atmospheric pressure decreases. If you have ever gone diving into a swimming pool or scuba diving, you can feel the increasing atmospheric pressure on your eardrums.

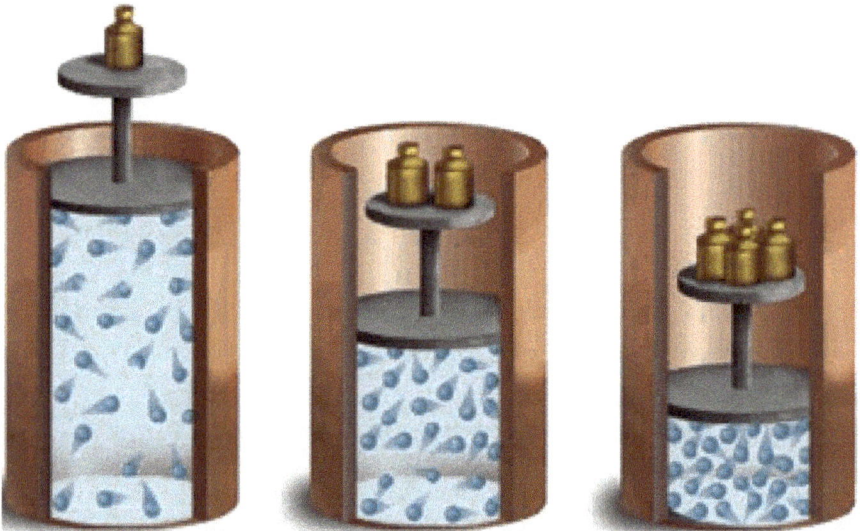

Visual depiction of the principle of Boyle's Law, as the pressure increases the volume decreases, and vice versa. Creative Commons License

To 'Air' is Human

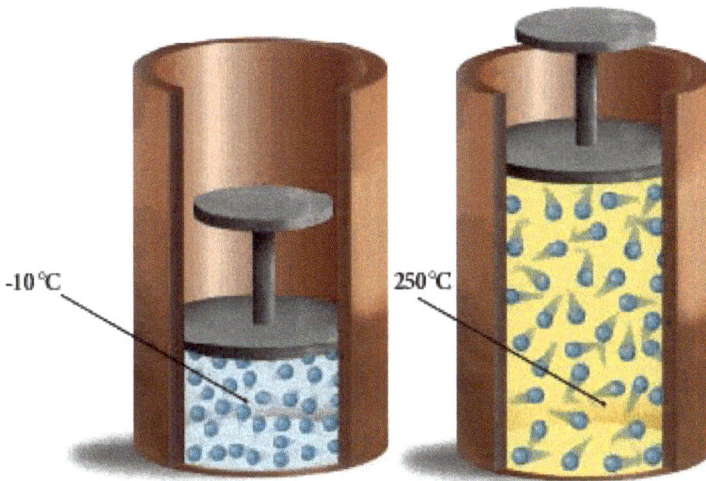

Visual depiction of the principle of Charles' Law, as the temperature increases the volume increases, and vice versa. Creative Commons License

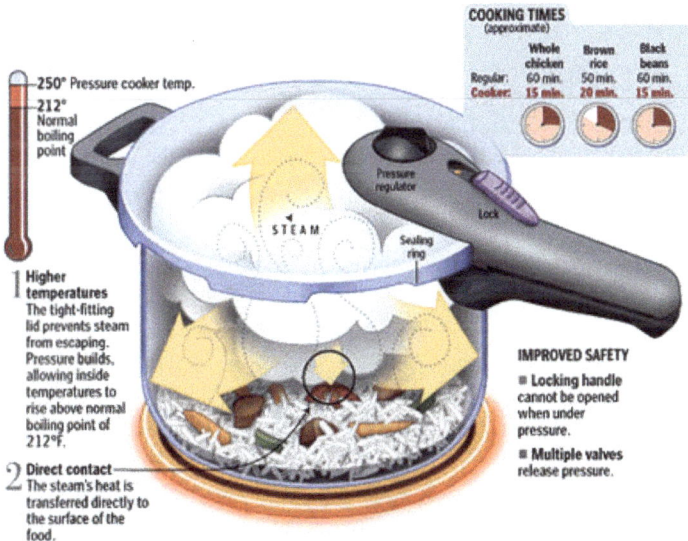

A pressure cooker is one example of the practical application of the laws of physics. As the pressure within the cooker increases the water can achieve a temperature higher than its boiling point. Creative Commons License

Aerospace

Intestinal gas, like gasses everywhere, must comply with the laws of physics and the laws of nature. Boyle's law states that at a constant temperature, the product of the volume and pressure of a gas must remain constant. This requires that they maintain an inverse relationship, if one increases the other has to decrease. As such, an increase in pressure will result in the decrease of the volume of the gas, and vice versa. See earlier entry on aerospace for more details.

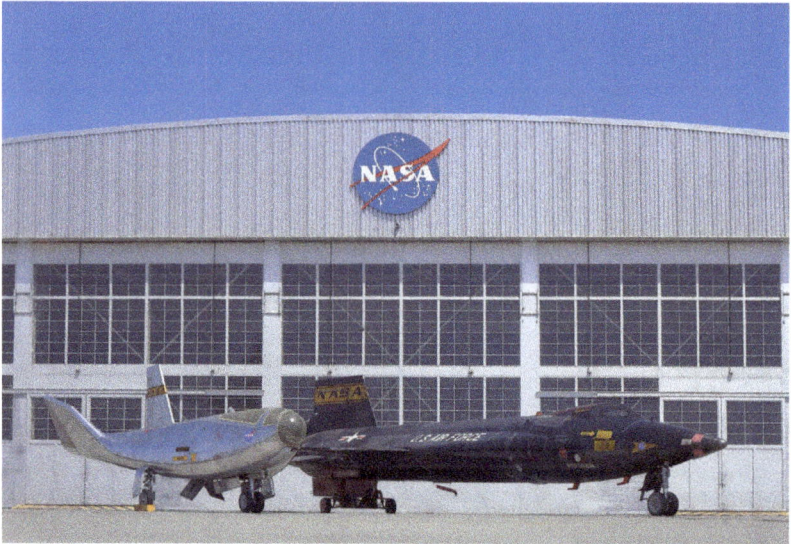

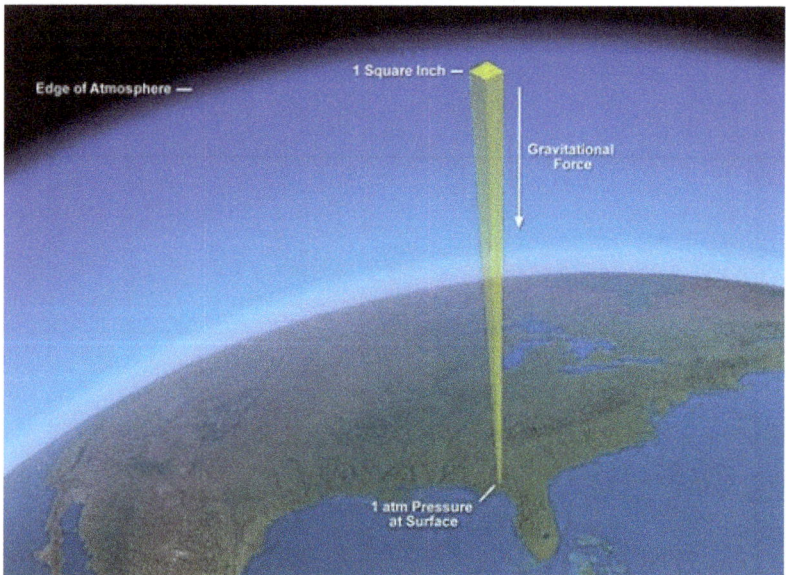

farm7.static.flickr.com Creative Commons License

Elevators

The sensation of the increasing volume of intestinal gas is most noticeable with the rapid decrease in atmospheric pressure experienced in airplane or space travel. A high-speed elevator comes close ,and you may first sense the change in air pressure by the inequality of the pressure applied to the eardrums. You may have an ear 'popping' effect from a rapid ascent in the elevator. As you rapidly ascend by the elevator in a high-rise building, driving up a mountain road, or flying in an airplane, you may feel or hear your ears 'pop' as they adjust to the decreasing atmospheric pressure. If they do not 'pop' on their own, you may feel the discomfort of the unequal pressure as the eardrum begins to bulge. Since you are not underwater you can use the more comfortable maneuver of yawning, instead of the Valsalva maneuver.

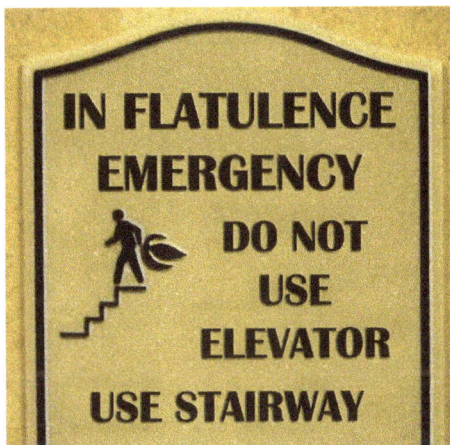

www.flickr.com Kevin Trotman Creative Commons License

Unfortunately, with the elevator's rapid ascent comes the equally rapid expansion of intestinal gasses. This may lead to an increase in the passage of intestinal gasses in the confined space of the elevator. If the elevator is crowded there are lots of people to glare at to take the suspicion off of you. Fortunately, the same risk does not occur as the elevator descends. On the descent the increasing atmospheric pressure causes the volume of intestinal gas to decrease., and the risk of being subjected to your own or someone else's fart in the confined elevator decrease.

High Altitude Communities

The majority of the world's population lives close to the seashore and have the standard atmospheric pressure of one atmosphere found at sea level. A significant percentage of the world's population lives at higher altitudes with atmospheric pressures less than one atmosphere. The higher above sea level you are, the lower is the atmospheric pressure you are subjected to. As a consequence, although the number of molecules of gas produced is identical, it will require a larger volume of space to contain it.

If you live in Denver Colorado, the mile high city with an elevation of five thousand one hundred and eighty three feet (one thousand six hundred and nine meters) feet above sea level, the volume will be larger than residing in Los Angeles or New York City. It is all relative as residing in Mexico City, which is at seven thousand three hundred and fifty feet (two thousand two hundred and forty meters), will produce a much larger volume than Denver.

To 'Air' is Human

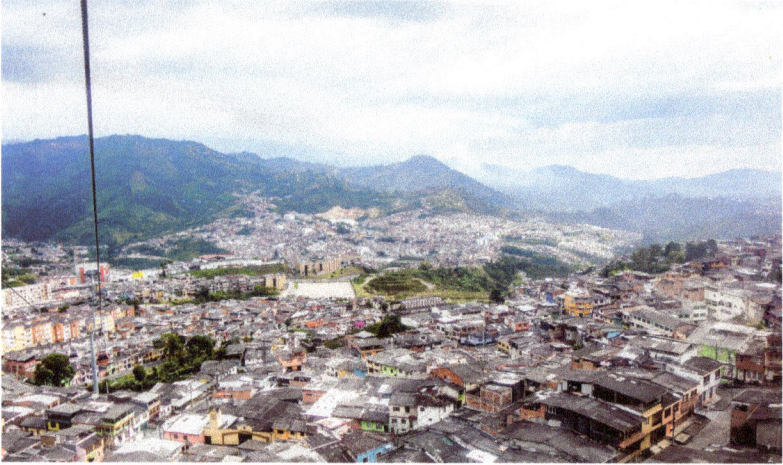

Manizales, Colombia is at an altitude of 6,690 feet (2,021 meters) above sea level.
shutterstock/fotos593

For those flying at even higher altitudes the cabin pressure in commercial aircraft limits the reduction in atmospheric pressured to the equivalent of approximately eight thousand feet above sea level high, much as if you were in Mexico City. With the atmospheric pressure at this altitude just over two-thirds of sea level, the gas volume expands by about forty percent. That is more than enough to cause a person to notice a significant increase in their flatulence and an increase in the flatulence of everyone else as well.

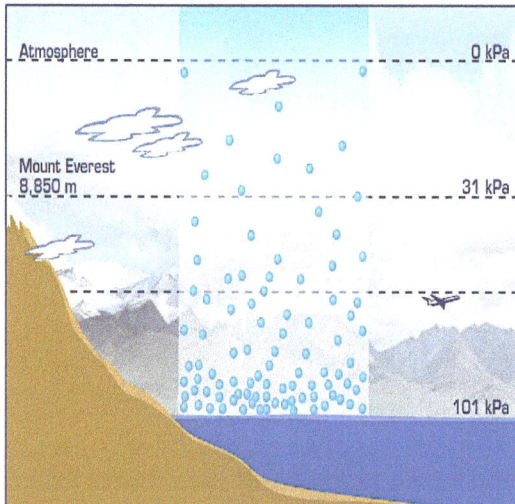

Atmospheric pressure arises from the weight of the air sitting above the observer. The mass of air in the column above the head of the observer is pulled down by the gravity of the Earth and exerts a pressure force on the observer. At the surface of the Earth at sea level the pressure is 14.7 pounds per square inch. This is also described in other measurement units as one atmosphere, 101,000 Pascals, 1kPa (kilopascal), or one bar. At higher altitudes, less air sits above an observer, so there is a lesser amount of atmospheric pressure. hendrix2.uoregon.edu Creative Commons License

To 'Air' is Human

High Rise Buildings

If you work or reside on the higher floors of an office building or residence tower, or if your place of work or residence is at a higher elevation in a mountain community the difference in atmospheric pressure may be significant. Whatever the reason for the change in altitude the resulting changes in atmospheric pressure affects intestinal gasses. They are subject to the same consequences of Boyle's Law as any other gas.

The heights of the tallest skyscrapers continue to reach new world records. Even coastal cities that are nearly at sea level will have buildings in which the changes in atmospheric pressure between those at the ground floor and those at the higher levels will be significant. This is most readily demonstrated by taking a high-speed elevator in a high-rise building. The rapid decrease in atmospheric pressure traveling from the lower to the higher floors often results in pressure changes on the eardrum (tympanic membrane). The equalization of pressure on both sides of the tympanic membrane may give rise to an ear popping sensation.

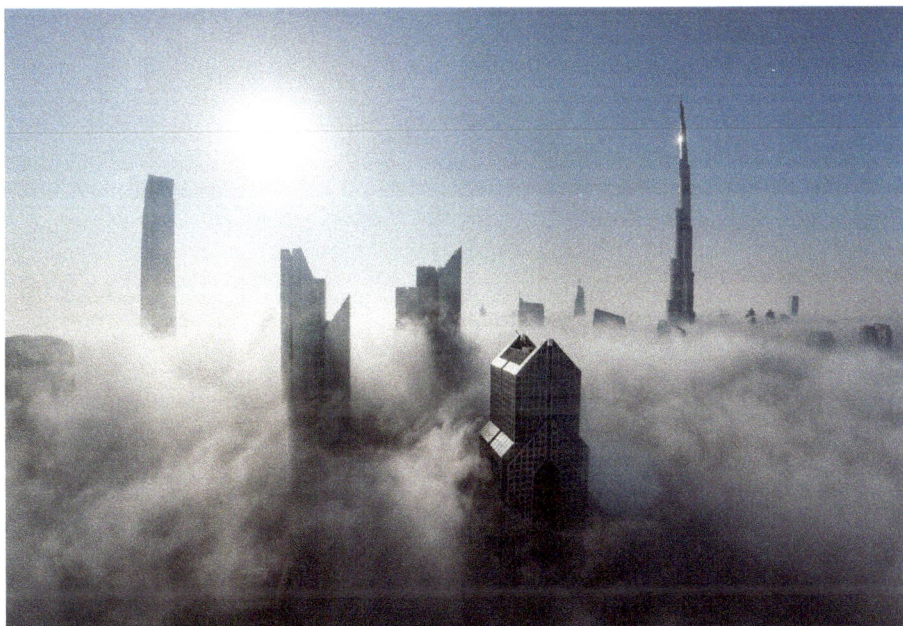

Burj Khalifa, Dubai, Tallest building in the world. Skyline is depicted above fog level.
Shutterstock/NaufalMQ

Mountain Climbing

In rock or mountain climbing, the higher the altitude, the lower the atmospheric pressure. Although the number of molecules remain unchanged gastrointestinal gasses will expand by virtue of the laws of physics. The increasing volume of gas will lead to discomfort and ultimately will find a way to exit your digestive tract. Air in the stomach may be released, as a burp or belch, but the larger quantity of gasses in the colon will come out as flatus, commonly called a fart. The higher in altitude you go, the lower the atmospheric pressure, and the more flatus you will be passing.

As you go up the elevator in a high-rise building, or drive up a mountain road, or fly in an airplane you may feel or hear your ears 'pop' as they adjust to the decreasing atmospheric pressure. To relieve the discomfort you need to equalize pressure on both sides of the eardrum. As these pressure changes occur while not underwater, a simple yawn is easier and more comfortable the Valsalva maneuver to equalize the pressure difference.

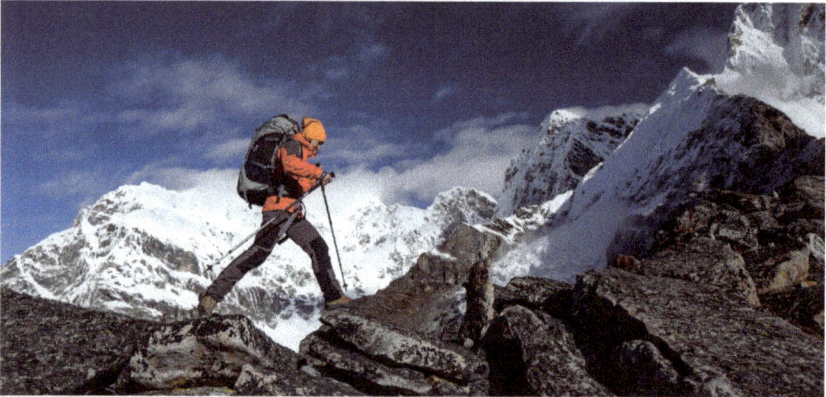
Mountain climber. shutterstock/MyGoodImages

Scuba Diving

Using Boyle's law, you can calculate how much the gas volume will compress as you go deeper underground or underwater and atmospheric pressure increases. You can likewise calculate how much a gas will expand, as you go higher in altitude and the atmospheric pressure decreases. If you have ever gone diving into a swimming pool or scuba diving, you can feel the increasing atmospheric pressure on your eardrums., also known as the tympanic membrane. If you go deep enough, the atmospheric pressure increases to such a degree that it may become painful.

To relieve the discomfort, you have to equalize the pressure on both sides of your eardrums. This equalization of air pressure is usually accomplished by performing the Valsalva maneuver. This procedure can be initiated by attempting to exhale against a closed epiglottis, much like straining during a bowel movement. The open Eustachian tube from the pharynx allows equalization of the atmospheric pressure on both sides of the eardrum.

If unrelieved, or if pressure is increased further, it may exceed the ability of the tissue to withstand it resulting in rupture or perforation. A perforated eardrum is very painful and is more likely to occur if the Eustachian tubes that must be open to equalize the pressure on both sides of the eardrum are swollen shut by infection, inflammation or other conditions. For this reason activities, which rapidly or excessively apply pressure on the eardrums, should be avoided if the individual has an upper respiratory or nasal congestion, such as sinusitis, head cold, ear infection, etcetera. The use of a nasal and sinus decongestant may be helpful but caution is still required. Scuba diving, flying, mountain climbing, and other activities require awareness of their potential effects on human health.

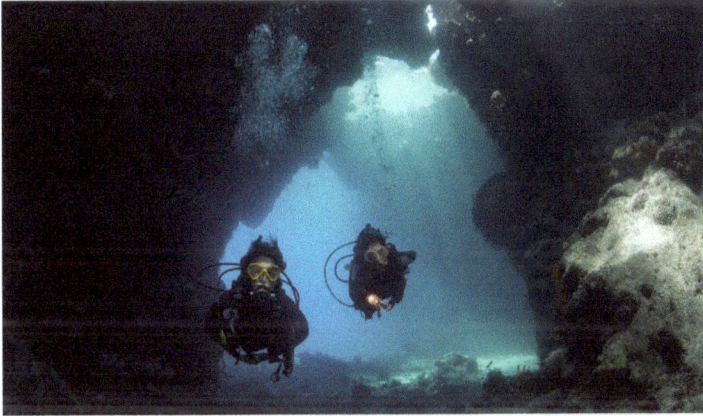

shutterstock/timsimages

Other effects of pressure changes on the gasses within human tissue are less frequent but of even greater concern. Scuba divers know better than to eat a gas producing meal, such as chili with beans and carbonated beverages, before a dive. The gas bubbles generated within the gut while at a one hundred foot dive depth are compressed into a relatively small volume by the high atmospheric pressure. Upon returning to the surface at the conclusion of the dive that small gas bubble will rapidly expand to a much larger volume as the high atmospheric pressure is reduced back to normal at the surface. As the gas bubble expands the pressure on the intestinal tract wall dramatically increases and can lead to a rupture as the result of barotrauma. Unlike a perforated eardrum, a perforation and rupture of the gut is life threatening and may lead to peritonitis and death if the perforation is not sealed or corrected surgically.

Another gas pressure related condition has to do with nitrogen dissolved in the blood under high pressure, leaving solution and forming actual physical bubbles circulating in the bloodstream. The bubbles can lead to catastrophic effects if they prevent circulation of oxygen carrying blood to vital organs as an air or gas embolism. This condition was first recognized in deep sea divers and is known as caisson disease, decompression sickness, as well as 'the bends' because it often lead to a doubling over because of joint pain within hours of returning to the surface after prolonged dives. The limitation of dive length is calculated by dive tables or computers, and is typically based on the depth of the dive and the composition of the air or inhaled gasses in the dive tanks.

Nitrox was developed to reduce the incidence of nitrogen narcosis, which can lead

To 'Air' is Human

to dangerous changes in mental awareness because of the buildup of dissolved nitrogen gas in the bloodstream. The term narcosis has the same Greek word root as the word for narcotic. The Greek word αρκωσις (narcosis) is derived from *narke*, which means a decline or loss of senses and movement. Nitrogen narcosis has also been called 'raptures of the deep', inert gas narcosis, and the 'Martini effect'.

During ascent all gases increase in volume as the atmospheric pressure decreases. As the gases in the gastrointestinal tract increases in volume they may produce symptoms cramping colicky abdominal pain, distension, belching, flatulence, and vomiting. Rare cases of rupture of the stomach and other portions of the gastrointestinal tract have occurred. Severe stomach pains have been reported during chamber dives after the divers drank carbonated beverages while under high atmospheric pressure.

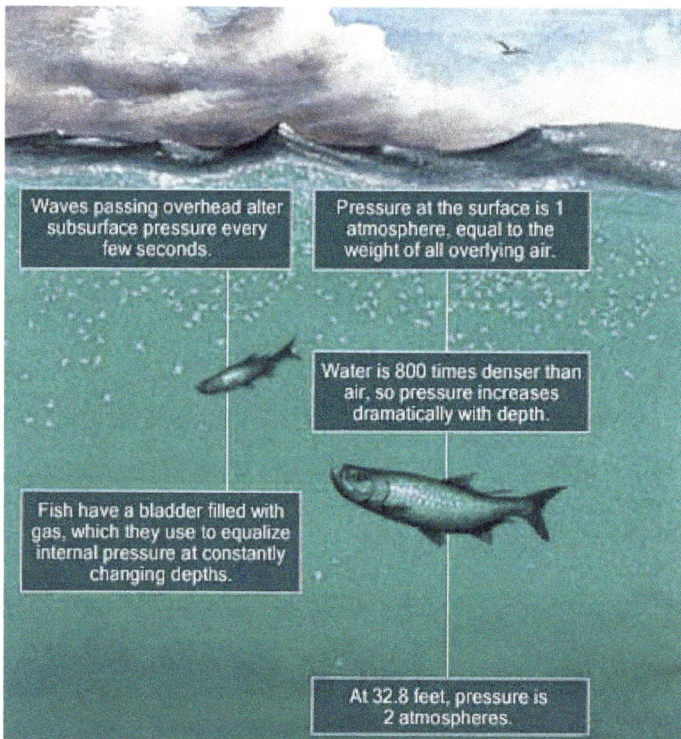

Atmospheric pressure rises quickly with greater underwater depths. Artist Jonathan Milo media.midcurrent.com.s3.amazonaws.com/wp Creative Commons License

One informative episode occurred with the grand opening of a brand new hyperbaric facility. The grand opening was toasted with champagne that was consumed while sixty feet (twenty meters) deep. The hosts and guests were disappointed that the champagne appeared to be flat without much carbonation. They decided to celebrate by drinking it even though it was flat because it tasted good. Their discomfort on ascent was exceeded only by their embarrassment.

To 'Air' is Human

During ascent the gas in the 'flat' champagne (which was present in the normal amounts) came out of solution and expanded in their stomachs leading to uncontrolled belching.

For those who enjoy scuba diving, you are already familiar with the effects of increased atmospheric pressure. The pressure on the ears can become intense unless you are able to equalize the pressure regularly in descent and ascent. To be a certified scuba diver you must be knowledgeable about the risk of potentially life threatening illness and conditions that can be associated with these pressure changes. When inhaled at pressures higher than four atmospheres nitrogen can act as an anesthetic agent causing nitrogen narcosis. This is a temporary semi-anesthetized state of mental impairment similar to that caused by nitrous oxide, commonly known as laughing gas.

Nitrogen also dissolves in the bloodstream and body fats. Rapid decompression in the case of divers ascending too quickly, can lead to life threatening decompression sickness formerly known as caisson sickness or the bends, when nitrogen bubbles form in the bloodstream, nerves, joints. Most scuba divers also know not to ingest carbonated beverages or legumes and other gas producing foods during a dive. It is not the descent that is a problem. Remember from Boyles law that as you go deeper underwater the atmospheric pressure is increasing and the gas bubbles are getting smaller and smaller in volume. The problem is on the ascent where after a half hour of diving time at 100 feet underwater, you begin your ascent. Your bowel has a modest size bubble of gas at that depth, but during the ascent this bubble expands and expands and can cause significant discomfort

Even though most experienced scuba divers know better than to fly shortly after a dive, even experienced scuba divers sometimes forget the same process can occur on land. Occasionally scuba divers will travel by land in an automobile from sea level after a dive, up a mountain road to a community or destination at a much higher elevation. Various gas mixtures have been developed for divers to reduce these risks. Trimix consists of oxygen, helium, and nitrogen, and Heliox is nitrogen free with just helium and oxygen. Hydrox is hydrogen and oxygen, an explosive combination if ignited. Nitrox is nitrogen and oxygen but is usually enriched for dives to increase the oxygen content and reduce the risk of decompression sickness.

Similar conditions can occur in miners when the mine shaft is pressurized to prevent ground water from entering, flying in unpressurized or depressurized aircraft at higher altitudes, and in space travel when the pressure in a spacesuit used for extravehicular activity is lower than the ambient pressure within the spaceship. An unusual but particularly dangerous combination is a novice scuba diver returning from a diving holiday unaware than a recent dive followed by even further reduction of atmospheric pressure by flying can lead to catastrophic consequences. Even though the dive table may suggest the risk period has ended, dive tables are calculated for a return to sea level, not the common commercial aircraft pressurization at an equivalent of an eight thousand foot elevation. See separate entry entitled Scuba Diving for more information.

Spelunking

Spelunking, the exploration of caves, has become an increasingly popular activity and can take place above or below sea level altitudes. Some of the deepest explored caves have vertical drops in excess of one thousand feet. Although changes in atmospheric pressure are noticeable, this effect is one of the least dangerous aspects of the sport activity. The exploration of underwater caves known as cave diving, combines spelunking with scuba diving, and is a particularly demanding and challenging activity. In this activity understanding the potential effects of atmospheric pressure changes becomes critically important.

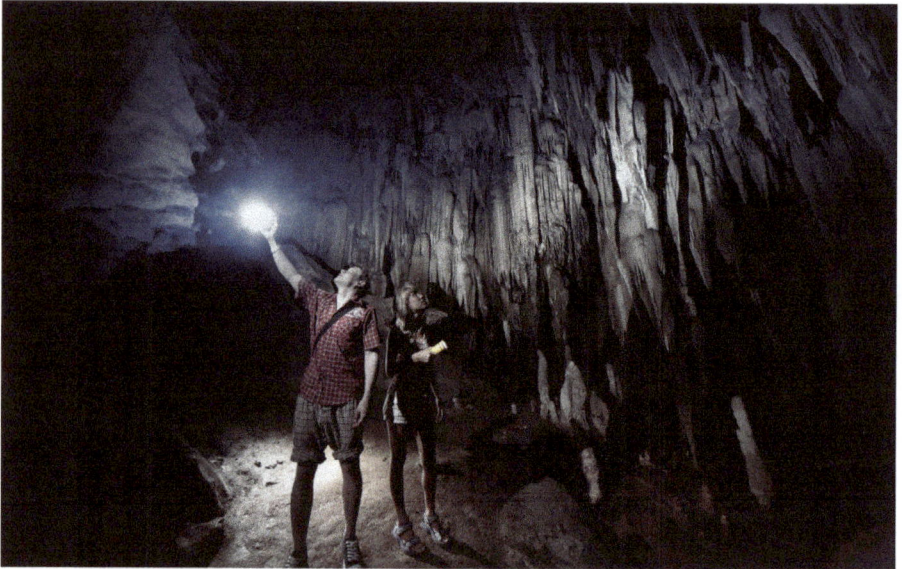

shutterstock/DudarevMikhail

Underground Miner

Mines have been present from prehistoric times but the depth of mines continues to increase. The deepest mineshaft in commercial operation to date extends two and one-half miles below the surface. As one goes deeper into the interior of the planet the atmospheric pressure increases. Just like in the diving experience, the great depth of the mine can lead to significant reduction in the volume of gasses with the increasing atmospheric pressure. In addition some mines are pressurized to prevent ground water from entering the mineshaft. The danger is on the return to the surface as the higher atmospheric pressure is reduced back to normal. With the reduction in atmospheric pressure the volume of the gasses increases, and may leave solution causing bubble formation in the blood stream.

To 'Air' is Human

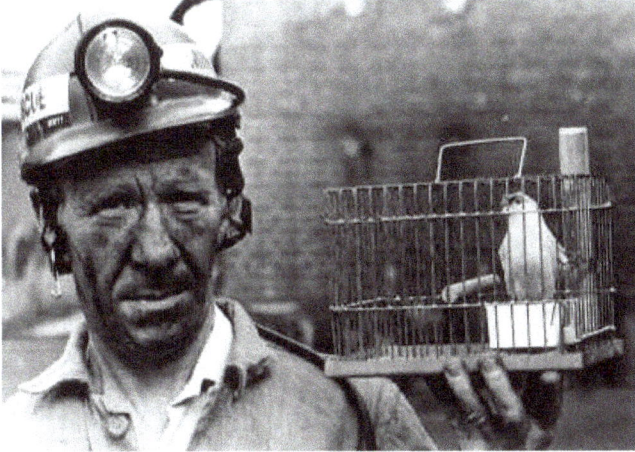
Public Domain Creative Commons License

One of the additional occupational hazards of minors is the exposure to toxic gasses, including methane. The technology has now advanced to sophisticated monitoring for such gasses, but the miner's canary still carries an image into present day folklore and humor. Canaries and similar birds were taken into the mines as an early warning sign of methane toxicity. The birds are extremely sensitive to methane and die promptly on exposure to the toxic gas. If the miner's canary suddenly toppled off its perch in an episode of sudden death the miners knew that they has to quickly evacuate the mine. Bathroom humor would have the canary as a warning of toxic methane fumes emanating from flatus. If the canary died someone farted.

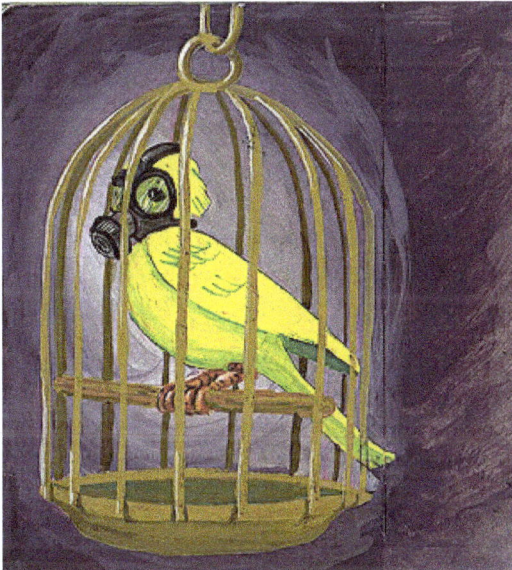
lunar.thegamez.net/coalmining/canary

To 'Air' is Human

Bacteria (see Microbiome)

Bismuth

Bismuth is a chemical element, number eighty-three on the periodic table, which has long history of being used in preparations designed to treat gastrointestinal complaints. It is a heavy metal with a low level of toxicity. Its various compound have also been used historically to treat syphilis and the severe diarrhea from cholera. Bismuthinite is a mineral consisting of bismuth sulfide (Bi_2S_3) and is an important ore of bismuth.

Bismuth subgallate, with a chemical formula $C_7H_5BiO_6$, is the active ingredient in Devrom, an over the counter product described as an internal deodorizer. The term 'sub' refers to the high oxygen content in the molecule and the presence of bismuth oxygen compounds. It is used to reduce the fecal odor arising from flatulence and fecal incontinence. Those with gastric bypass bariatric surgery, inflammatory bowel disease, irritable bowel syndrome, and ostomy appliances commonly use it. It has also been used to treat *Helicobacter pylori* infection and is in wound therapy.

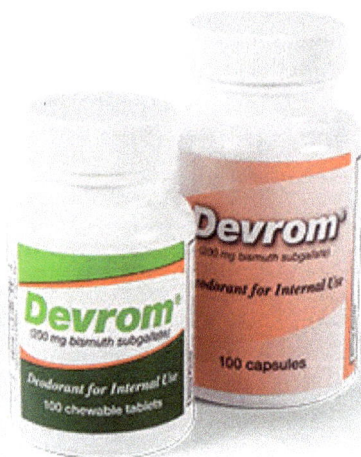

The mechanism by which bismuth works is uncertain. It may be related to its known antimicrobial activity, perhaps inhibiting the microbes that generate some of the more offensive gasses that contain sulfur as well as aromatic and volatile organic compounds. Bismuth also reacts directly with sulfur producing bismuth sulfide, a dark black insoluble compound. Bismuth sulfide may cause darkening or blackening of the tongue if sulfur is found in high concentrations in the saliva. It will also cause blackening of the stool as it binds with the sulfur that would otherwise give rise to hydrogen sulfide and other offensive sulfur gasses. The dark black color of the stool may be mistaken for melena, a sign of internal bleeding that results from the digestive process on blood cells and hemoglobin. The black coloration is not a health concern and is temporary clearing with cessation of bismuth intake.

To 'Air' is Human

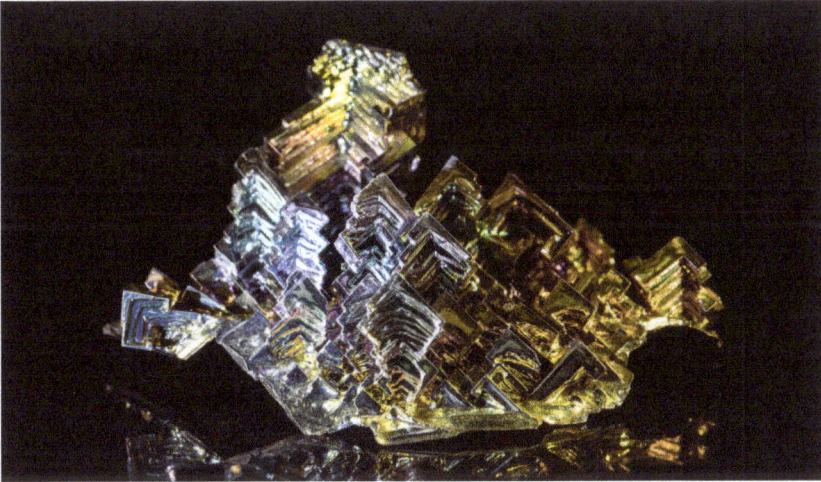
Bismuth in crystalline form. shutterstock/MiriamDoerr

Bismuth subsalicylate has a bismuth oxide core structure with salicylate ions attached to its surface. It is used as an antidiarrheal and is the active ingredient in Pepto-Bismol, as well as the U.S. version of Kaopectate since it was reformulated in 2004. It is a popular remedy for indigestion, nausea, heartburn, and as a preventative for traveler's diarrhea. It is also used to treat some other gastro-intestinal diseases and infections including the microorganism *Helicobacter pylori*, which is associated with peptic ulcer disease and stomach cancer.

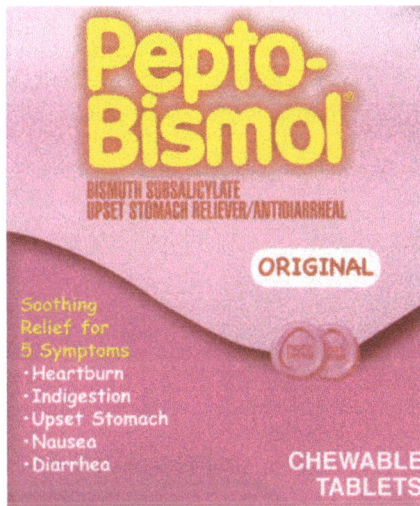

The antimicrobial property may be as a result of an oligodynamic effect, where toxic small doses of heavy metal ions are toxic to microbes. Another antimicrobial effect may arise from the release of salicylic acid as the compound is of the compound is hydrolyzed. It is believed the salicylic acid acts as an antimicrobial for toxigenic *Escherichia coli,* a principal cause of traveler's diarrhea.

As a derivative of salicylic acid, bismuth subsalicylate also displays anti-inflammatory properties as well as some adverse effects of salicylates. Because salicylate levels can accumulate and lead to toxicity any use beyond a few weeks length is discouraged. Children should not take bismuth subsalicylate while suffering from a viral infection between of the associated risk of acquiring Reye's syndrome and liver failure. Nursing mothers should not use bismuth subsalicylate as it is excreted in breast milk and may pose a risk of Reye's syndrome in nursing children.

Brain Fart

Brain fart – mental lapse, which usually results in an error while doing a repetitive activity. The actual physiological event that triggered the error was recorded on brain scans by scientists approximately thirty seconds before the event was observed.

They suspect that the brain is trying to enter a more restful state to conserve energy, and have given the brain fart the more scientific name of 'maladaptive brain activity change'. The findings were published in the *Proceedings of the National Academy of Sciences* in April 2008. Brain fart may also be used to describe a brief episode of absent-mindedness, impulsivity, or temporary inability to recall a name, word, or memory. Interestingly enough, the exact opposite of a brain fart is best described by an unusual word in the English Language, afflatus.

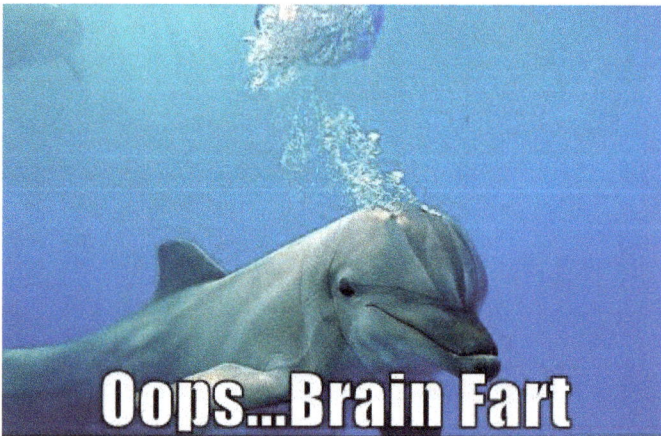

www.flickr.com/photos/ Creative Commons License

Afflatus incorporates the root word flatus, which is a commonly used as a synonym for fart. Perhaps surprisingly the definition of the word afflatus has nothing to do with a fart. Flatus is Latin for a blowing, breathing, or a wind. Afflatus is first used by Cicero in his volume *De Natura Deorum* (The Nature of the Gods). In his book, it is used as a phrase for a sudden rush of unexpected breath or fresh inspiration. The word inspiration is derived from the term inspire, to breath as well as to have a creative thought or new idea. Afflatus thus can mean a divine inspiration. The only way to associate it with a fart is to consider it to be the exact opposite of a brain fart.

Bubbles (see Surface Tension, Simethicone)

A bubble is a collection of gas, usually surrounded by a thin layer of fluid. The term gastric bubble is also used to describe the normal collection of gas within the stomach, and can be visualized on an abdominal radiograph (x-ray). Bubbles of gas within the digestive tract are called a burp or belch on eructation via the esophagus, or a fart or flatus on being passed out of the lower intestinal. The actual physical properties of a bubble are due to a concept known as surface tension. This is also visually demonstrated in watching a water glider walk across water, in water forming droplets, the tears of wine in a wineglass, the water bulging without spilling above the brim of a glass, and other physical phenomena. Please see the entry on surface tension for more details.

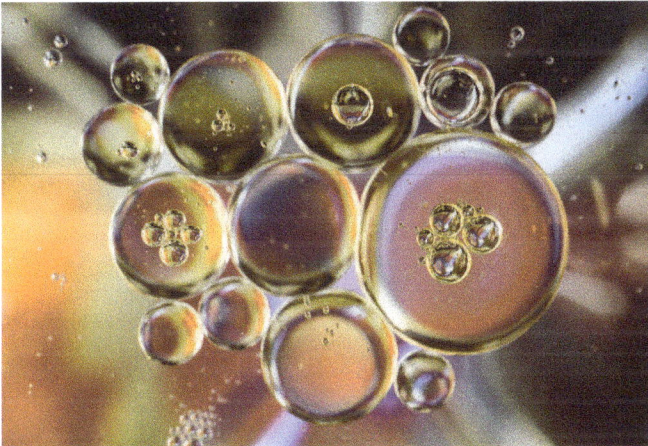

Bubbles created by surface tension. shutterstock/GiulianoDelMoretto

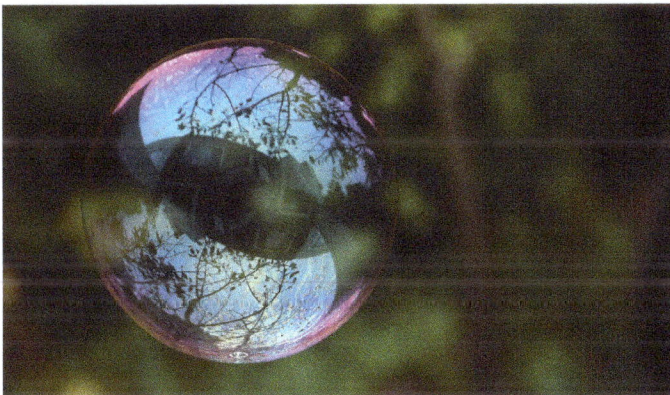

Bubble. Brocken Inaglory editing user:Alvesgaspar Creative Commons License

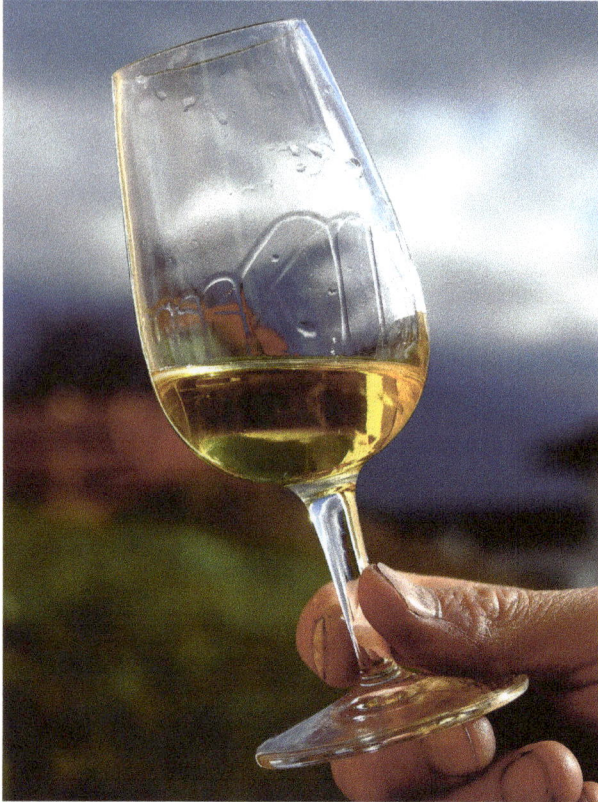

Tears of wine, also known as Marangoni effect. shutterstock/mountainpix

Belch / Burp (see Eructation, Gastroesophageal Reflux Disease)

The words burp and belch are the common terms used to describe the more scientific term eructation. Please see the entry on eructation as well as Gastroesophageal Reflux Disease (GERD) for more details. Other interesting word pairs of the common words with the less commonly known scientific terminology include chew for mastication, sneeze for sternutation, cough for tusis, pee for micturition, itch for pruritis, skin for integument, smell for olfaction, taste for gustation, and many others that fill a medical dictionary.

If a doctor wanted to know if you chewed your food well he might ask if you masticated a lot with every meal. Most people would respond incredulously "Masticate a lot with every meal? Are you crazy, do you think I want to go blind. I never masticate!". Medicine and English are much two often two separate and foreign languages. You need to insist that your doctor speak to you in a language you can understand. There is a famous quotation attributed to Sir Winston Churchill, a British statesmen, former Prime Minister, and Nobel Laureate for Literature. He said affectionately that the American and British people are divided only by a common language.

To 'Air' is Human

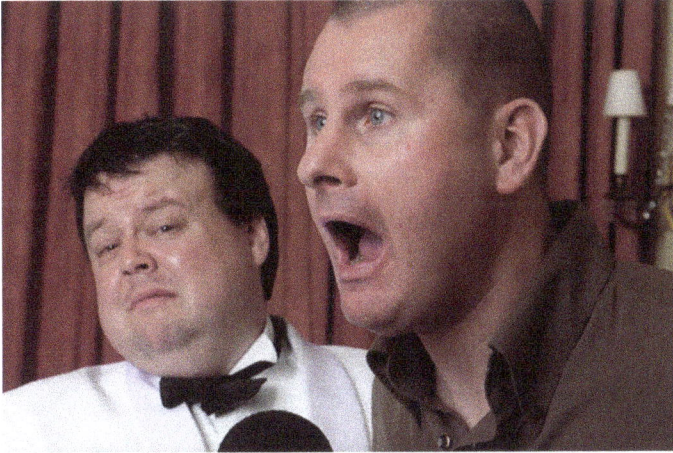

Loudest burp at 109.9 decibels youtu.be/Zt9rvaijpPY

The World Burping Federation located in Geneva Switzerland holds the annual World Burping Championship. The *Guinness Book of World Records* has a listing for the loudest burp on record. The record holder is Paul Hunn of the United Kingdom. His burp achieved a measurement of 109.9 decibels, equivalent to a car horn. The world record for the longest burp is 18.1 seconds, held by Tim Janus. To achieve this record he consumed approximately two gallons of Diet Coke and Mountain Dew. Imagine what would have happened if he swallowed a few Mentos tablets at the time of the competition.

Butt Breathe

To butt breathe is a common term used to describe the ability to air fart. An air fart is the ability to control the anus and muscles of abdomen and respiration, to cause air to be aspirated into the colon and then released voluntarily as a fart. It is also known in more enlightened society as an air enema. The air enema has been practiced for hundreds of generations as a part of yoga and as a means of achieving colonic hygiene.

Although usually considered under involuntary control, these muscles can be trained. Yogis have attained remarkable proficiency at controlling what has previously been considered involuntary muscles. At the turn of the twentieth century, the performer Joseph Pujol, under the stage name Le Pétomane, became an international sensation by demonstrating his prowess at butt breathing. This ability is not limited to trained yogi and stage performers. An internet-based survey on farting performed in 2001, had over one thousand three hundred participants. Although not a scientifically validated survey, over fifteen percent of respondents reported that they were able to fart on command.

Fart survey question for men: Can you fart on command also called "Butt Breathe"?

To 'Air' is Human

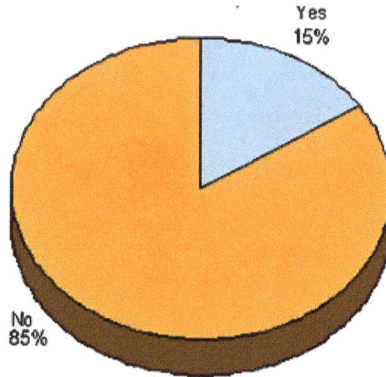

Yes
15%

No
85%

Only fifteen percent of the men surveyed can fart voluntarily by suctioning air into the colon. One-third of all men did not even know that this is possible!

Fart survey question for women: Can you fart on command also called "Butt Breathe"?

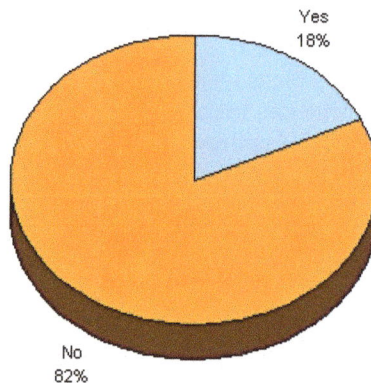

Yes
18%

No
82%

Only eighteen percent of the women surveyed can fart voluntarily by suctioning air into the colon.

Although rarely thought of as a form of butt breathe, the rare freshwater Fitzroy river turtle, *Rheodytes leukops*, found in Queensland, Australia has a unique ability. This species of turtle can breathe through its anus equivalent, the cloaca. It inspires air, or if submerged oxygenated water, into its cloaca. Through specialized highly vascular bursae it can absorb oxygen into its bloodstream. The Fitzroy turtle can obtain over two-thirds of its oxygen supply through the cloacal bursae. It pumps water in and out of the cloaca up to sixty times per minute.

Some turtles have a remarkable anaerobic capacity and can be without oxygen for up to thirty–three hours and survive. Although they are usually air breathing, they can also breathe underwater with the cloacal bursae acting like the equivalent of gills in removing oxygen from the water. This rare ability is shared with only a few other organisms, including the dragonfly nymph and the sea cucumber.

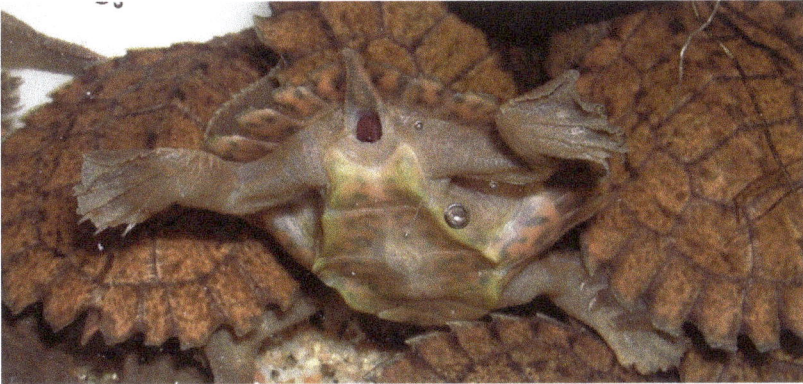

Photo by Craig Latta, freshwater turtle expert. www.tutles.net.au Used with permission.

The sea cucumber has a few other unique digestive tract features. Its anus serves as a defense mechanism and can eject sticky threads that entangle an enemy. If in danger it will expel its entire digestive and respiratory tracks that are also sticky and can ensnarl the enemy. These disgorged internal organs continue to move about independently, distracting the predator while the sea cucumber makes its escape. It then regenerates brand new respiratory and digestive tracks.

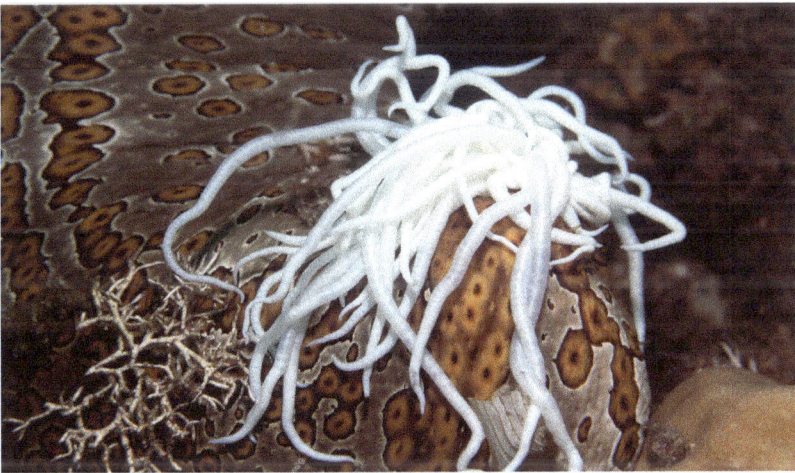

shutterstock/C.K.Ma

Carbonation

Carbonated beverages are very popular worldwide. In the United States sales of carbonated beverages exceed twenty billion dollars per year, four times the sales volume of dairy products. The majority consumed today already comes carbonated with large amounts of carbon dioxide forced into solution under high pressure. As the pressure seal of the can or bottle is released the carbon dioxide forms bubbles and comes out of the solution, giving a pleasant tickling sensation on the palate, and a full at times bloated feeling in the stomach and gut.

To 'Air' is Human

Many soft drinks have high concentrations of simple carbohydrates such as glucose, fructose, and sucrose. Oral bacteria ferment these carbohydrates produce acidic products, which can erode the tooth enamel beginning the dental decay process. A large number of soft drinks are already acidic and have phosphoric acid added in the manufacturing process bringing their pH level to three or lower. To put this value in perspective, neutral water has a pH of seven and gastric hydrochloric acid has a pH of two. Many dentists advocate avoid the brushing of teeth shortly after an acidic beverage because of the tooth enamel is more vulnerable to abrasions after being softened by acid.

Mineral water cures were very popular in the middle ages and beyond. Going to the source of mineral springs and the drinking of its contents was referred to as 'taking the waters'. The waters had a variety of mineral content depending on source locale and included various salts and sulfur contents. The sites of such resources became well known as spas, baths, and wells and developed into destinations for the ill and infirm, as well as those who wished to preserve their good health. The term Seltzer water was originally a trademarked name for the German town of Selter that had a famous mineral spring.

The bottling of mineral waters became a profitable enterprise by offering people the opportunity to partake of the presumed beneficial waters in their own locales. An attempt to imitate the effervescent effect of the mineral waters was made by Joseph Priestley in 1767. Some fans of carbonated beverages believe this should be his claim to fame rather than his discovery of oxygen. J. J. Schweppes of Switzerland commercialized the process in 1783, moving his factory and enterprise to England in 1783.

Before the commercial availability of carbonated beverages, a device for home use was popular and remains commercially available. It uses canisters of carbon dioxide under pressure that are added to beverages to create the carbonation effect. The soda siphon bottles with the carbon dioxide cartridges are making a retro look comeback in today's higher technology environment. Carbon dioxide can diffuse through the plastic container over time, which is why carbonated beverages in plastic bottles go flat and lose their carbonation over a few months' time. Glass and aluminum containers hold the carbonation for longer time periods.

Have you ever wondered how much carbon dioxide gas is released from a soft drink or carbonated beverage. You have already gotten a visual demonstration if the bottle or can was dropped or shaken before being opened. This agitation accelerates the release of the carbon dioxide, and it can form a jet stream of gassy bubbles to be sprayed on everyone within a dozen feet of the demonstration. This social activity is very popular amongst preadolescent boys. The quantification of how much carbon dioxide is in a one liter bottle of a carbonated soft drink is calculated using a formula known as Henry's Law.

William Henry was an English physician and chemist who proposed what is now

To 'Air' is Human

called Henry's law in 1803. The law states that at a constant temperature, the amount of a given gas dissolved in a liquid is directly proportional to the pressure of that gas. As the gas pressure increases, the solubility of the gas in the liquid increases. As the temperature increases, the solubility of gas in liquid decreases. The greater the pressure, the greater the quantity of a gas that can be absorbed by a liquid. The cooler the liquid, the greater the amount of gas that it can absorb. As the temperature of liquid increases, the solubility of the gas decreases forming bubbles that allow it to escape. Henry's Law explains why carbon dioxide in a pressurized container, such as in a can or bottle of a carbonated beverage remains in solution until it is opened. As soon as the container is opened the pressure is reduced causing the carbon dioxide gas to lose its solubility and escape in the form of bubbles or fizz.

The gas content in a one-liter bottle is a surprising two point eight liters. In other words, there is nearly three times the volume of the original container in excess gas under pressure hidden in those tiny bubbles. Do not forget another important law of the physics of gasses, Charles' Law. This law defines the activity of gasses expanding as the temperature increases. If you drink a cold carbonated beverage, and after swallowing it is warmed up to body temperature, it will exhibit another substantial increase in the volume of gasses released. The burping and belching that occurs after drinking a cold carbonated beverage may seem out of proportion to the small amount consumed. Just remember that whatever the volume of liquid carbonated beverage swallowed, there is nearly three times that volume of dissolved gas waiting to be released.

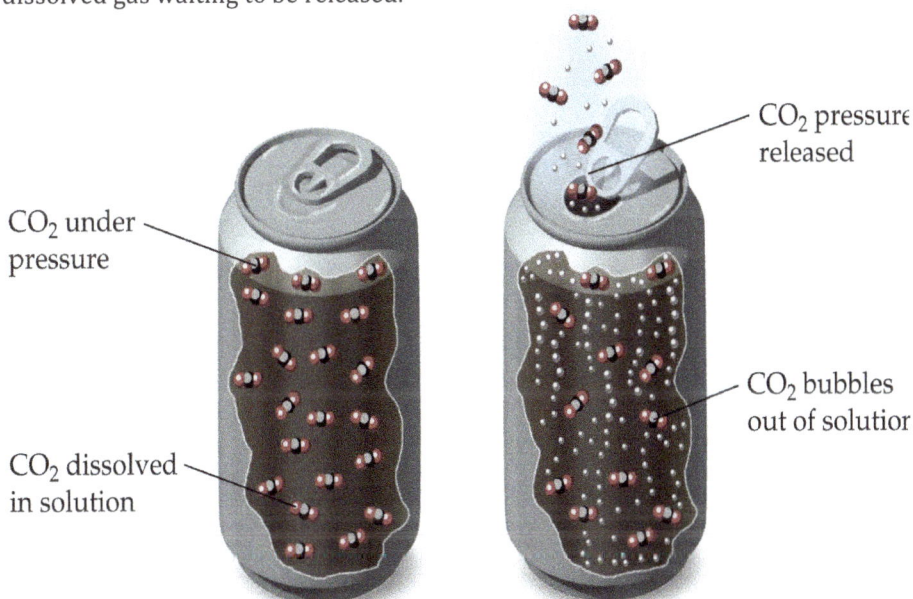

CO_2 under pressure

CO_2 dissolved in solution

CO_2 pressure released

CO_2 bubbles out of solution

Creative Commons License

If you want further visual proof that Henry's Law is accurate take a look at the photographic evidence of another popular activity. The harmless addition of a

63

To 'Air' is Human

Mentos brand mint candy tablet to a liter bottle of a carbonated beverage, such as Diet Coke, sounds like such an innocent activity. This demonstration is repeated in countless elementary school science classes. The *Guinness Book of World Records* described one thousand three hundred and sixty students in the historic university town of Leuven, Belgium creating simultaneous Mentos with Diet Coke geysers.

The instantaneous foaming effect is a dramatic virtual geyser of carbonated foam shooting many over twenty-eight feet into the air. This experiment is not without risk as the bottles will explode if not allowed to become a geyser. Scientific progress continues apace and Henry's Law was demonstrated with two thousand eight hundred and sixty-five simultaneous geysers erupted on in a mall in Manila, Philippines, breaking the previous world record.

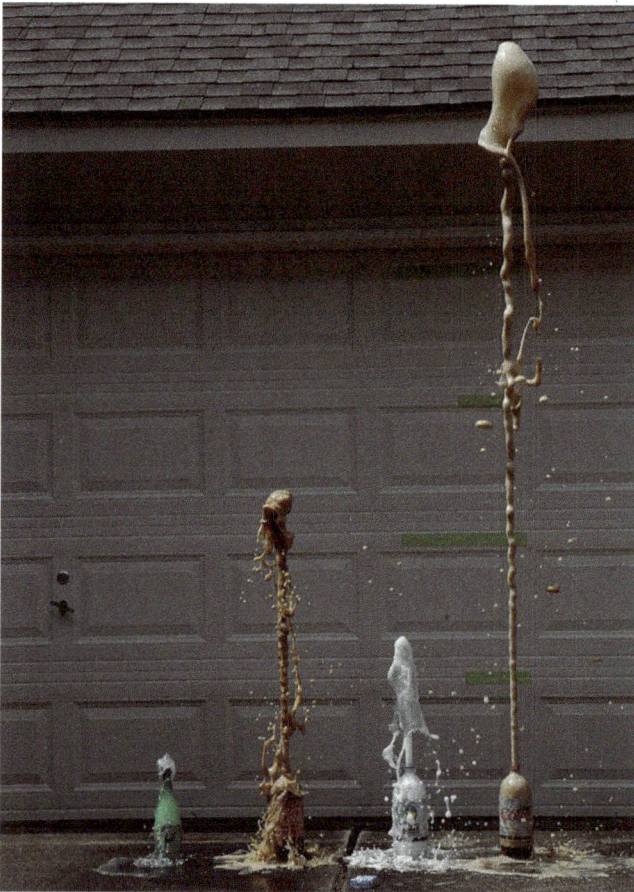

Mentos Geyser from carbonated beverages with the addition of Mentos. From left: carbonated water (Perrier), Classic Coke, Sprite and Diet Coke. The green marks in the background are at one half-meter increments. Photograph by K. Shimada Creative Commons License

Academic research physicist Tonya Coffey at Appalachian State University in

To 'Air' is Human

Boone, North Carolina analyzed why the Diet Coke created the highest geyser. She determined that the aspartame in Diet Coke lowered the surface tension of the gas bubbles allowing the interaction between potassium benzoate with the gelatin and gum Arabic ingredients of the Mentos Mint. Surface tension is a physical property exhibited when certain liquids are in contact with a gas. It is particularly pronounced when liquid water is in contact with the gasses of the air.

Each water molecule contains two hydrogen atoms and one oxygen atom, giving rise to its familiar chemical shorthand of H2O. Because of their atomic structure the negative charge of the electrons of the hydrogen atoms are attracted to the positive charge of the oxygen atom, creating was is known as a hydrogen bond. The electric charges also create an attractive force between water molecules, causing them to want to remain close together. These forces are balanced out when a water molecule is surrounded by other water molecules.

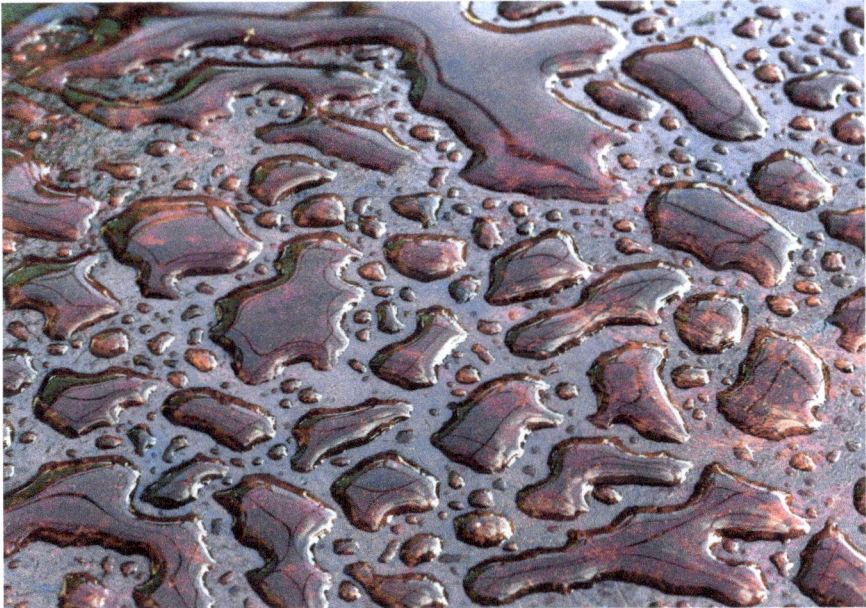

Surface tension is the physical principle, which creates islands of beaded water.
shutterstock/Kuruneko

When the water molecules on the surface are exposed to the gasses of the air above them they are no longer exposed to balanced charges. The water molecule on the surface exposed to the air is only subject to the electric charge pulling it down, keeping it in the liquid. This resistance to leaving its fellow water molecules behind gives it the property known as surface tension, a tension that prevents it from being separated from the remaining liquid. This surface tension is visible when you see water assume the shape of a droplet, or when you fill a glass to the brim and the fluid builds up above the lip of the glass before it begins to overflow.

To 'Air' is Human

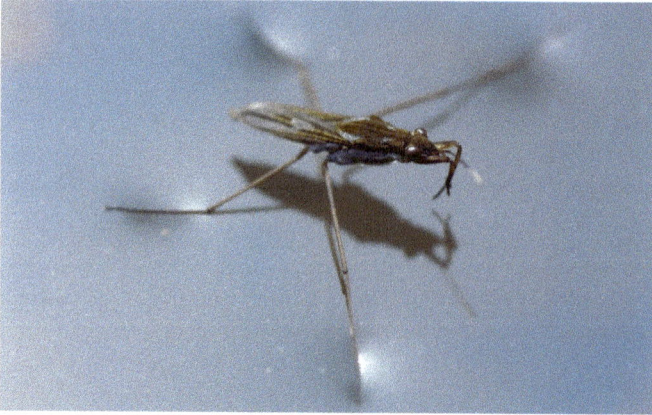

Pond skater using surface tension to walk on water Heteroptera suborder. shutterstock/optimarc

It is also the principle that allows insects heavier than water, such as the water glider, appear to walk on water because the surface tension acts as a walkable surface. Surface tension also is the force that allows the creation of bubbles. Surfactants are products that have the property of reducing surface tension and are used in detergents, as well as in anti-bubble and anti-gas products such as simethicone. Another principle of physics was also exhibited by the Mentos in Diet Coke geyser experiment. Because the mint has a microporous nature, the markedly increased surface area caused a rapid and vigorous foaming reaction. A single simple cube has a much smaller surface area for reactions to take place, than an identical volume cube that has been subdivided into many smaller cubes. The following illustration helps to visualize how the surface area can be dramatically increased with the same volume of material.

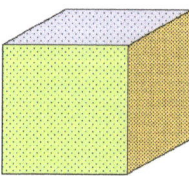

a one-meter cube has 6 square meters of suface area

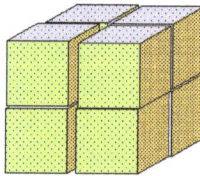

pieces half the original size have twice the surface area

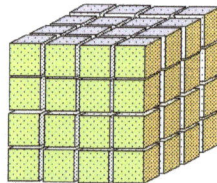

pieces one quarter of the original size have 4 times the surface area

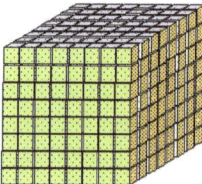

pieces one-eighth of the original size have 8 times the surface area.

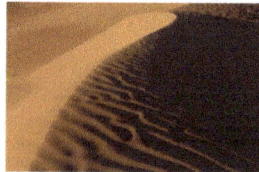

a cubic meter of fine sediment can have millions of square meters of surface area

Increase in surface area.. Phil Stoffer, Ph.D. Geology Cafe geologycafe.com Creative Commons License

To 'Air' is Human

The caffeine did not accelerate the reaction. Here is the reference for those who want to read all of the scientific details. Coffey, Tonya *"Diet Coke and Mentos: What is really behind this physical reaction?" American Journal of Physics* June 2008. 76 (6): 551–557. Competitions to see which beverage will create the highest geyser are very messy affairs that again seem to attract a disproportionate number of adolescent males in their middle years. As my spouse (who happens to be a reproductive endocrinologist, an expert on the subject) likes to remind me, there are five stages of the male life cycle: infancy, childhood, adolescence, adolescence, and adolescence.

In some beverages the carbon dioxide would interfere with the taste and flavor by reacting with the ingredients, giving it an acid taste from carbonic acid. An alternative is to use nitrogen as the gas of choice as it was a neutral gas and would not interact with the beverage. The most popular example is Guinness, which uses nitrogen, or a combination of nitrogen and carbon dioxide, under pressure in kegs.

Carbonation: The Key to the Fizz Biz

Carbon Dioxide (CO_2) consists of one carbon atom and two oxygen atoms. CO_2 is a nonpolar molecule, meaning other molecules won't stick to it easily.

Water (H_2O) consists of one oxygen atom and two hydrogen atoms. It is a polar molecule. Uneven distribution of electrons results in sticky spots — areas where molecules form weak bonds. The loose clinging results in a liquid.

Under normal conditions, it's common for CO_2 to dissolve into water. The activity of gas molecules overcomes the bonds in the H_2O chain. CO_2 escapes.

Temperature is dropped. The activity of the molecules slows. The hydrogen bonds become stronger. CO_2 can't break the H_2O chain and is retained in the water. Molecules do not, however become locked. If they did, they would become a solid — ice.

Pressure is increased. More CO_2 is crammed into the water until the mixture is supersaturated, meaning more CO_2 is dissolved in the liquid than would be possible under normal conditions. H_2O molecules squeeze in an form cages around the CO_2 molecules. CO_2 is trapped.

The water is carbonated. Syrups and flavorings are added, and the mixture then is put in a bottle. The bottle is capped, which maintains an equalized pressure inside and keeps the CO_2 in its cages until the bottle is opened.

By George Frederick for Life's Little Mysteries

i.livescience.com Creative Commons License

To 'Air' is Human

Carbon Dioxide

Carbon dioxide (CO_2) is a naturally occurring compound composed of two oxygen atoms bonded to a single carbon atom. It is a gas at standard temperature and pressure and exists in Earth's atmosphere as a trace gas at a concentration of 0.039 percent by volume. It is heavier than air, and when used as a fire extinguisher the dense ground-hugging layer of carbon dioxide prevents the flames from accessing oxygen.

As part of the carbon cycle, plants, algae, and cyanobacteria use light energy to photosynthesize carbohydrate from carbon dioxide and water, with oxygen produced as a waste product. However, photosynthesis cannot occur in darkness and at night some carbon dioxide is produced by plants during respiration. Carbon dioxide is exhaled in the breath of humans and land animals. It is also released from the fermentation of organic matter, volcanoes, hot springs, geysers and the combustion of hydrocarbons used as fuels. It contributes as a greenhouse gas to global warming. It is also a source of ocean acidification since it reacts with water to form carbonic acid.

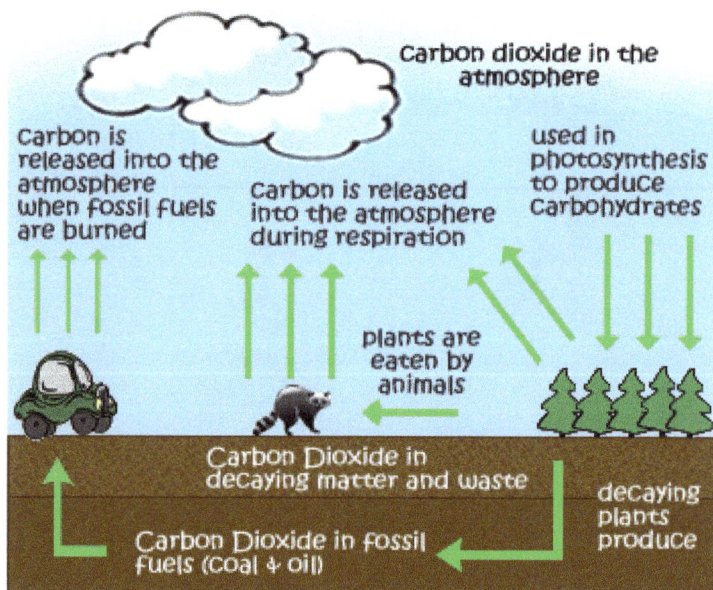

Carbon dioxide in the atmosphere

Carbon is released into the atmosphere when fossil fuels are burned

Carbon is released into the atmosphere during respiration

used in photosynthesis to produce carbohydrates

plants are eaten by animals

Carbon Dioxide in decaying matter and waste

decaying plants produce

Carbon Dioxide in fossil fuels (coal & oil)

www.realtrees4kids.org Creative Commons License

A gas subsequently identified as carbon dioxide was identified by the Flemish chemist Jan Baptist van Helmont in the seventeenth century. In the 1750's Scottish physician, Joseph Black studied the gas more thoroughly. In 1772, English chemist Joseph Priestley published a paper entitled *Impregnating Water with Fixed Air*. The paper described how he forced carbon dioxide to dissolve in a bowl of agitating water, inventing what eventually became known as soda water. Soda water was the original product from which the major industry of carbonated beverages evolved.

To 'Air' is Human

Carbon dioxide is produced in large quantities in the digestive tract. The human stomach generates about 1.5 liters of very potent hydrochloric acid. With a pH of 1.5 it can make quick work of dissolving metal coins. The stomach lining is designed to handle the intense acidity, as well as the potent digestive enzymes released as zymogens and then activated as enzymes. The lining of the stomach is under constant attack and constant repair.

In fact, the turnover is so high that your stomach lining has been regenerated over the course of any three-day period. The gastric contents of food, acid, and enzymes transits through the pyloric channel and enters the duodenum. As it enters the duodenum it is in a brand new environment, and the digestive material is now known as chime. The material leaving the stomach requires prompt action from the duodenum to neutralize its high acid content. The duodenum neutralizes the acid by releasing sodium bicarbonate from its mucosal lining. It also receives a solution of pancreatic juices with a high concentration of alkaline sodium bicarbonate. The one and one-half liters of stomach acid is neutralized by one and one-half liters of sodium bicarbonate.

Do you remember from basic chemistry lessons what happens when you add an acid to an alkaline base? Did you ever perform or watch the school experiment of mixing baking soda (sodium bicarbonate) and vinegar (weak acetic acid) to create a fire extinguisher? In the demonstration a lit candle is placed on the bottom of a glass container. In a different glass pitcher the mixture of baking soda and vinegar were reacting with an impressive display of foaming and bubbling. They were reacting as expected from the mixing of an acid and a base, generating carbon dioxide as a free gas and neutral water.

Carbon dioxide is heavier than air so although it was invisible the rising level of carbon dioxide in the glass container was pushing the lighter air out and over the top. After just minutes of bubbling, the pitcher now full of heavier carbon dioxide was tilted over the glass containing the lit candle. Although it appeared that the tilted pitcher was not adding anything to the glass with the candle, the heavier but invisible carbon dioxide was displacing the air with carbon dioxide. As soon as the invisible carbon dioxide reached the level of the flame the supply of oxygen was cut off, and the candle flame went out like magic.

By the way there is another interesting fact about carbon dioxide and human respiration. It is the level of carbon dioxide in your blood, not the level of oxygen that derives the respiratory center that controls breathing. The sensation of air hunger that arises when one is short of breath or suffocating is from carbon dioxide buildup, not from a lack of oxygen. That is why the trick of making your voice squeaky by breathing helium is actually dangerous. If you breathe in and out pure helium your body is happy to get rid of its carbon dioxide and it thinks everything is just fine, even though it is not obtaining any oxygen.

To 'Air' is Human

Main symptoms of
Carbon dioxide toxicity

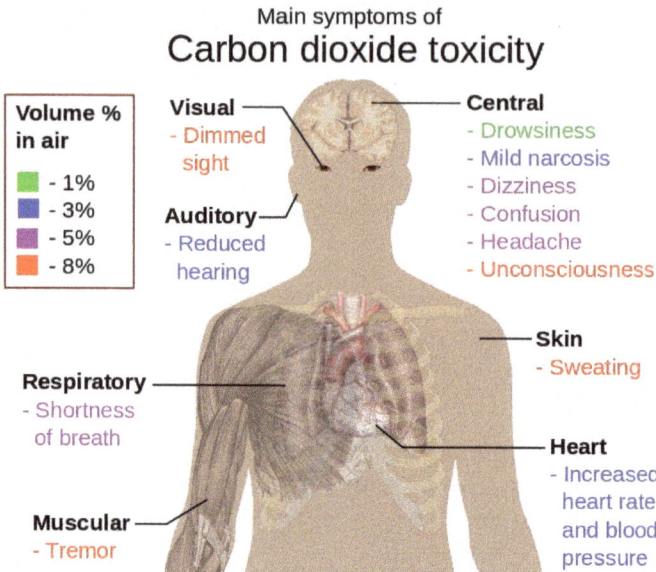

**Volume %
in air**

- ■ - 1%
- ■ - 3%
- ■ - 5%
- ■ - 8%

Visual
- Dimmed
  sight

Auditory
- Reduced
  hearing

Central
- Drowsiness
- Mild narcosis
- Dizziness
- Confusion
- Headache
- Unconsciousness

Skin
- Sweating

Respiratory
- Shortness
  of breath

Heart
- Increased
  heart rate
  and blood
  pressure

Muscular
- Tremor

Main symptoms of carbon dioxide toxicity. Wikipedia. Mikael Häggström Creative Commons License

The person breathing pure helium does not experience air hunger or suffocation because that sensation is only triggered by carbon dioxide which continues to be exhaled. Death occurs quickly, and because there is no sensation of air hunger is supposedly very peaceful. Advocates of capital punishment and euthanasia argue this would be a very humane, inexpensive, and simple way to end a life.

The one and one-half liters of potent hydrochloric acid and one and one-half liters of strongly alkaline sodium bicarbonate generate dozens of liters of carbon dioxide gas. The gas volume increases rapidly and dramatically and will lead to a bloated distended feeling within the small intestine. One may need to loosen a belt or tight clothing after a meal but fortunately the distended sensation is fairly short lived. The reason for this is that carbon dioxide gas in the in intestines is rapidly absorbed and dissolved into the bloodstream. It travels to the lungs where the carbon dioxide is released via the alveoli into the airway and exhaled. The carbon dioxide present in intestinal gas is generated by colonic bacteria and other gut flora. It averages about ten percent of passed intestinal gas by volume. This figure can change significantly dependent on diet and the gastrointestinal microbiome.

Carminative

A carminative, also known as carminativum, is a herb or preparation that promotes the prevention or elimination of gas from the gastrointestinal tract. Many carminatives have been shown to work by releasing the air swallowed (aerophagia) by reducing the pressure of the lower esophageal sphincter to promote eructation (burp). This relaxation of the sphincter can also promote reflux, regurgitation and heartburn and can aggravate Gastroesophageal Reflux

Disease (GERD), which may have atypical symptoms that are unrelated to heartburn. Many folk medicines and remedies have a long tradition of being used as carminatives. They are often mixtures herbs, spices, and essential oils. Many foods, social, and recreational products also relax the lower esophageal sphincter and encourage eructation, although one would not ingest them specifically for this carminative effect. This category includes onion, garlic, fried foods, fatty foods, chocolate, tobacco, alcohol, and marijuana.

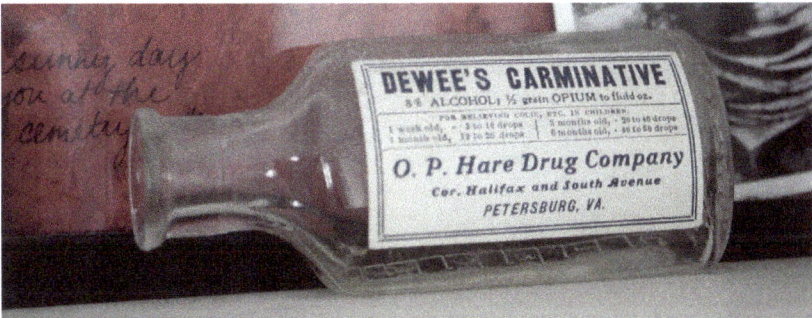

www.flickr.com Tess Shebaylo Dewee's Carminative Creative Commons License

In Western culture, the most common product that people see and use for its carminative property is mint, which relaxes the lower esophageal sphincter to encourage eructation. Chocolate can have a similar effect, so it is common to see the two combined as a traditional after dinner chocolate mint. Indian and Asian restaurants may offer other traditional carminative herbs and seeds usually found on the counter by the exit.

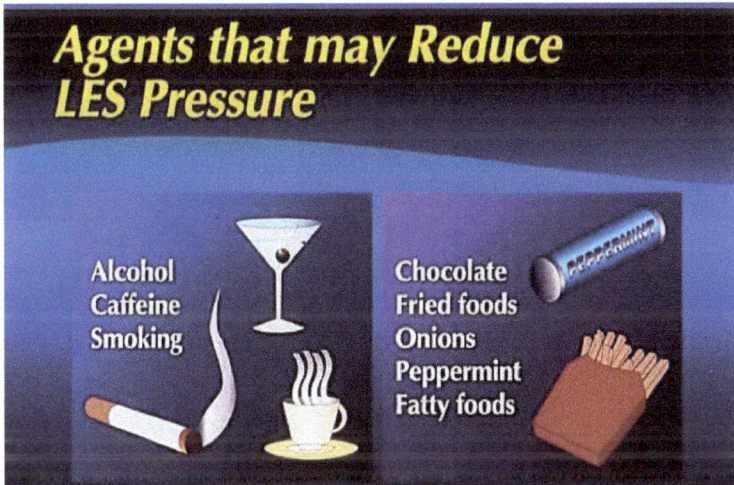

Carminatives and other agents reduce the lower esophageal sphincter (LES) pressure, allowing the easier release of gasses and air from the stomach but at the same time make regurgitation and heartburn more likely. Restaurateurs want their customers to have enjoyed their meals, and they recognize that distension from the universal aerophagia of eating can cause discomfort. Most people have no idea that the air they swallowed, and not necessarily the meal, might be the cause of their distress. The carminative mint is offered to give prompt relief, but notice how it is offered on leaving the restaurant. They do not want eructation to occur where others are dining in their refined accommodations. They prefer that the eructation occurs later to impress your 'significant other' or in the presence of your family and friends.

The following have all been described as having value as carminatives: Alcohol, Angelica, Anise, Asafetida, Basil, Black Pepper, Caffeine, Calamus, Capsaicin, Caraway, Cardamom, Chili (Cayenne) Pepper, Chocolate, Cinnamon (potency decreases with cooking), Cloves, Coriander, Cumin, Curcumin, Dill, Epazote, Eucalyptus, fatty foods, Fennel, Garlic (potency increases with cooking), Ginger, Goldenrod, Hops, Lemon balm, licorice, Lovage, Marjoram, Mint, Motherwort, Muña, Mustard, Nigella, Nutmeg, Onion, Oregano, Parsley, Pepper, Pennyroyal, Peppermint, Rosemary, Saffron, Sage, Savory, Spearmint, Theobromine, Thyme, Tobacco, Turmeric, Valerian, Wintergreen, Winter Savory, Wormwood, and others.

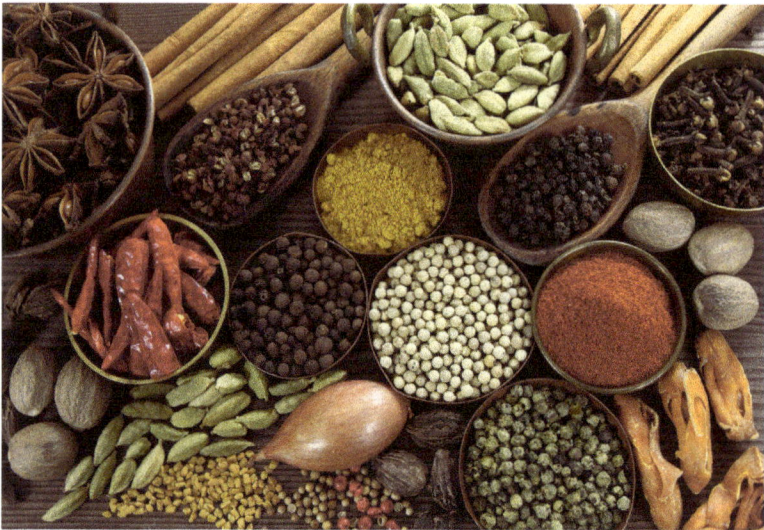

Herbs & Spices shutterstock/KrzysztofSlusarczyk

As this exhaustive list confirms, a large number of herbs and spices have been described as having carminative benefits. The problem with anecdotes and folk traditions is that it is hard to separate true beneficial properties from those that did so as a result of a placebo effect. The business of selling spices and supplements is very lucrative, so there is a strong financial interest to keep the status quo and not investigate these herbs scientifically. Although many prescription drugs can affect the tone of the lower esophageal Sphincter and promote eructation the carminative property is a side effect, and not an indication that the product should be used for that purpose. To encourage eructation avoid lying down after a meal. Sitting upright lets the air swallowed rise above the food in the stomach and when the lower esophageal sphincter relaxes air, rather than food, and escape the stomach.

Carminatives relax the lower esophageal sphincter and can be used to allow burping or belching of swallowed air to give relief of gastric distension and bloat. Mints and chocolate are often combined into an after dinner mint and offered as you exit a restaurant to induce a burp to release swallowed air to impress your significant other on the way home. Fried foods, greasy, fatty foods, alcohol, onion, and tobacco can also act as carminatives as can a number of herbal preparations. A number of pharmacologic agents used in the treatment of a wide variety of medical disorders can also act as carminatives by relaxing the lower esophageal sphincter. Female hormones such as progesterone and estrogen are in this category. During natural periods of higher hormone levels, such as during a pregnancy, reflux is more common. One reason is that the hormones have an effect on the lowered esophageal sphincter, causing relaxation that may lead to reflux. A second reason is the increasing intra-abdominal pressure from a growing child and uterus.

Chili Con Carne

Chili con carne is the Spanish name for a meal made as a stew that usually contains beans, chili peppers, tomato, and meat. Often other seasonings are added such as onions, garlic, and cumin. A wide variation of the ingredients and recipes often leads to competitions typically known as chili cook-off. It is often referred to by its abbreviated name chili in American English. It is the official culinary dish of the US State of Texas.

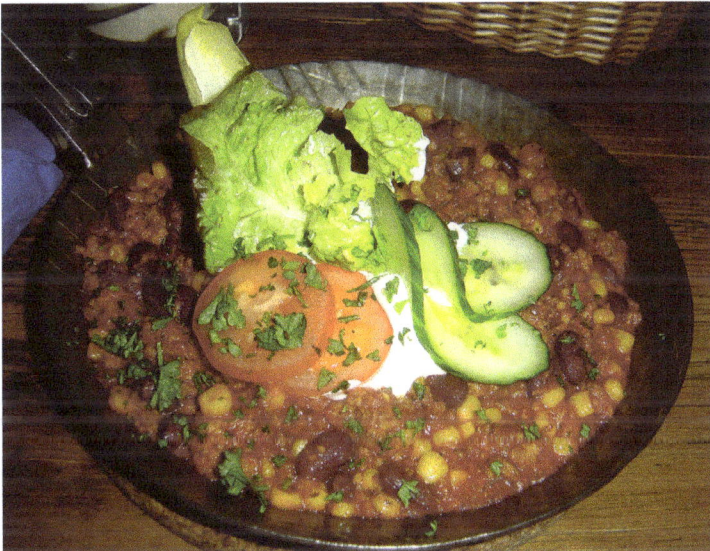

www.flickr.com Creative Commons License

To 'Air' is Human

The high legume content has led to its recognition as a potent source of intestinal gas. The variety of spices, seasonings, and animal fat leads to an equally intense variety of subsequent farts, often of startling pungency. The use of chili as a staple of the diet of cowboys on the range has led to several comedic scenes. .A famous example includes the infamous campfire scene in Mel Brook's movie Blazing Saddles.

Crepitation Contest

Attributed to the staff of the Canadian Broadcast Corporation in the 1940's, a record called *The Crepitation Contest* was produced. Canadian Broadcast Corporation sportscaster Sidney S. Brown narrated it, with sound effects credited to his producer, Jules Lipton. The recording is a parody of a radio broadcast of a live sporting event with pre-game interviews of the contestants.

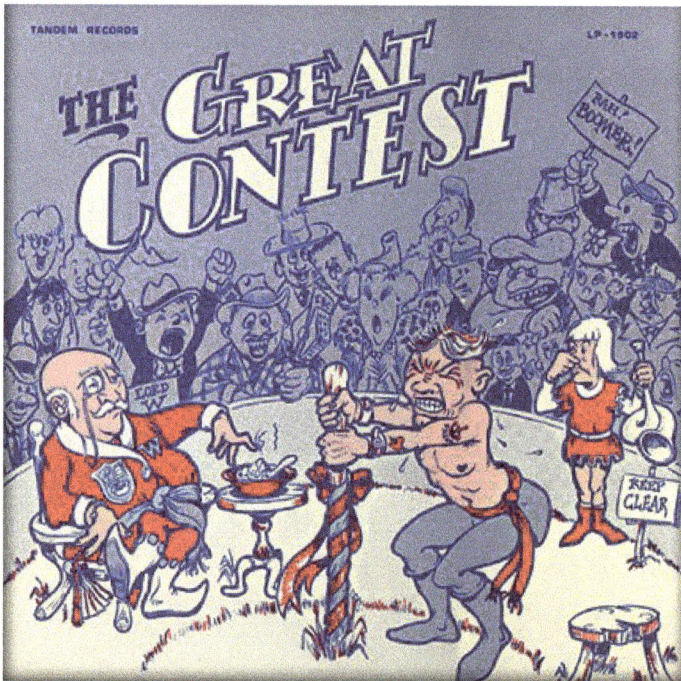

www.wfmu.org

The reigning champion is Lord Windesmear, and the challenger is Paul Boomer. The broadcast parody includes detailed descriptions of the competition including the rules, traditions, play-by-play reporting if the event and audience sounds and reactions. Reportedly the original recording was played at a New Year's Eve party in 1943 that was attended by an admiral of the United States Navy. He believed it would be a great morale booster for American serviceman. The original master recording at RCA Victor Studio in Toronto was obtained, and lacquer, and vinyl 78-rpm discs were pressed.

Diet

Diet obviously plays a major role in intestinal gas production. Certain types of vegetables and fruits contain carbohydrates the sugars and starches that may be poorly digested by people but happily fermented by bacteria comprising the gut flora. The starches, including potatoes, corn, noodles, and wheat are the source of the majority of gas generated by the gut microbial flora.

Rice is the one starch exception and rarely contributes to gas production. Wheat has the other 'distinction' of having the protein glutamate, which contains the nitrogen base product you generate ammonia-like aromatic compounds.

Common Foods that Cause Bloating and Gas

- Cabbage
- Cauliflower
- Beans
- Oats
- Apples
- Milk
- Fluffy wheat
- Broccoli
- Onions
- Corn
- Potatoes
- Pears
- Soft cheese
- Peaches

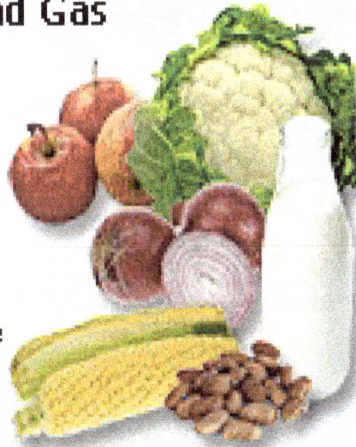

www.34-menopause-symptoms.com Creative Commons License

There are many specific enzymes required in the process of digestion, and deficiency in the quantity or activity of an enzyme can lead to food intolerance. The most common food intolerance is for the milk sugar lactose when an individual has decreased amounts and activity of the necessary enzyme for its digestion, lactase. The age of discovery is still in its infancy. Dozens of hormones, over one thousand and six hundred enzymes, over ten thousand species of gut microbes, and over one million genomes are just the beginning. Of the thousands of variables, we still have a clear understanding of only a few dozen. By the way, with so much remaining unknown and awaiting discovery, opportunity abounds if you have an interest in pursuing or supporting research activities.

If you are looking for a novel, practical, legitimate, and socially responsible way to avoid jury duty this may be your answer. A sincere desire to avoid inflicting your fart issues on fellow jurors may provide you with an excellent reason to be excused from jury duty. If you honestly believe you have excessive gas from an inherited enzyme deficiency you can bring the matter up with the clerk of the court and the presiding judge. If the court wants further clarification describe the scene of your intestinal gas leading the other jurors to flee the jury box complaining that it was a cruel and unusual exposure to a gas chamber. The judge just might have to declare a mistrial, stating that although justice is blind, she has not lost her sense of smell or hearing. A letter explaining the nature of your condition can go a long way to securing a permanent excuse from jury duty, and probably an invitation to use an absentee ballot to stay out of the voting booth on Election Day!

<u>Chili con carne</u>

Chili con carne is the Spanish name for a meal made as a stew that usually contains beans, chili peppers, tomato, and meat. Often other seasonings are added such as onions, garlic, and cumin. A wide variation of the ingredients and recipes often leads to competitions typically known as chili cook-off. It is often referred to by its abbreviated name chili in American English. It is the official culinary dish of the US State of Texas.

The high legume content has led to its recognition as a potent source of intestinal gas. The variety of spices, seasonings, and animal fat leads to an equally intense variety of subsequent farts, often of startling pungency. The use of chili as a staple of the diet of cowboys on the range has led to several comedic scenes. A famous example includes the infamous campfire scene in Mel Brook's movie Blazing Saddles.

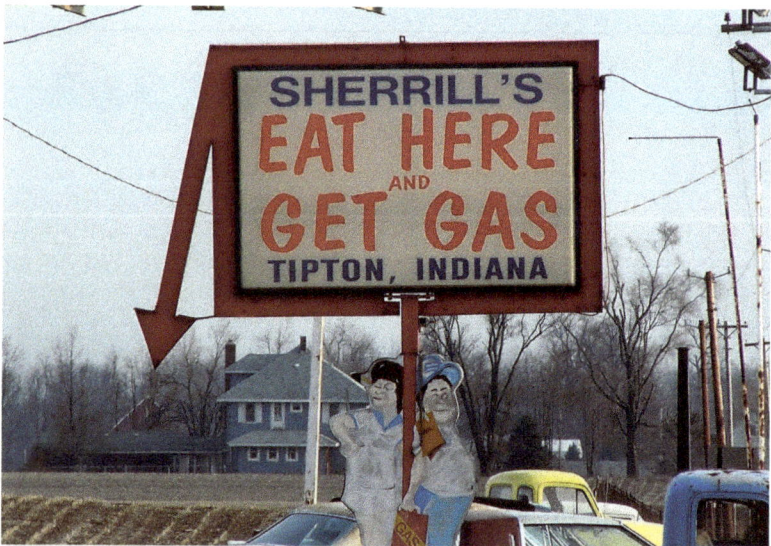

Refueling station and restaurant. Cindy Cornett Seigle www.flickr.com Creative Commons License

<u>Legumes</u>

"Beans, Beans, The Musical Fruit" is a schoolyard saying and children's song about the capacity for beans to contribute to flatulence.

To 'Air' is Human

Beans, beans, the musical fruit
The more you eat, the more you toot
The more you toot, the better you feel
So we have beans at every meal!
There are also several alternative versions, such as the one below:

Beans, beans, they're good for your heart
The more you eat, the more you fart
The more you fart, the happier/better you feel
So let's eat beans with every meal

Beans have a well-deserved reputation for contributing to intestinal gas production. Recent medical literature suggests that the degree of subjective complaints that legumes cause gas may be somewhat exaggerated. The bean is rich in the raffinose sugars, verbascose and stachyose. As humans do not produce the enzyme required for its degradation, alpha-galactosidase, these sugars undergo fermentation by the gut flora. The US Department of Agriculture is working on the development of a bean with lower levels of these sugars, and so far the Anasazi bean has been the leading candidate but no breakthrough yet. With genetically modified organisms (GMO) and foods being introduced in the marketplace, it is only a matter of time before products labeled as low-gas are promoted.

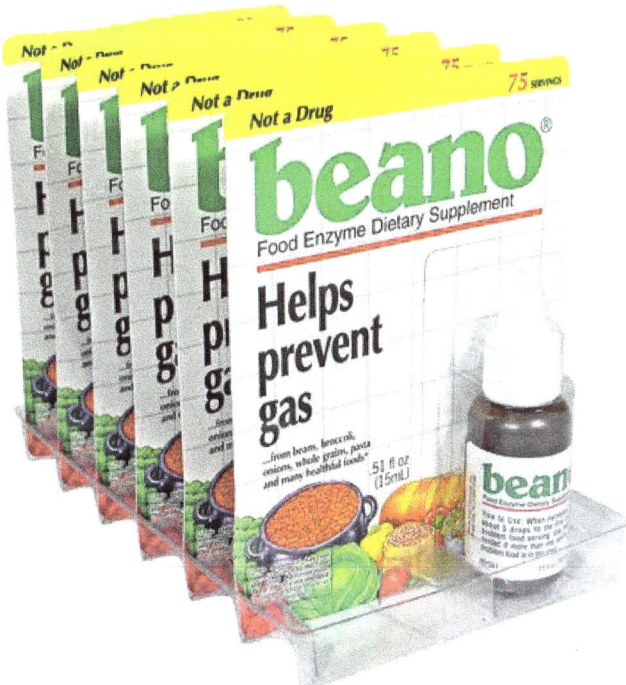

www.flickr.com Creative Commons License

To 'Air' is Human

Thankfully there are alpha-galactosidase enzyme supplements that can provide relief. The enzyme is not heat stable, so that it will be inactivated by the heat of cooking. The enzyme should be added to the first bite of the beans consumed and if a large portion is ingested additional enzyme intake during the course of the bean meal is recommended. An alternative approach is to soak the beans for several hours, leeching out some of the sugars into the water, which is discarded. The best approach is to soak the beans until they begin to germinate. With germination the seed itself begins to release alpha-galactosidase to break down its complex sugar content for the nutritional use of the newly germinated bean plant. With germination approximately 80% of the complex sugars are digested.

A legume is a plant in the family Fabaceae (or Leguminosae), grown agriculturally for their food grain seed, livestock forage and silage, and soil enhancement. Most legumes harbor the symbiotic bacteria Rhizobia in their root nodules, which convert nitrogen in the atmosphere into ammonia and ammonium. This source of nitrogen contributes to the plant's production of amino acids and high protein content. Legumes include alfalfa, clover, peas, beans, lentils, lupins, soybeans, and peanuts and a number of trees and shrubs. In farming crop rotation the growing of legumes near non-legumes is common. Legumes are sometimes referred to as 'green manure' because their symbiotic bacteria enrich the soil with nitrogenous products. A legume fruit is typically a pod that opens along a seam. They are an excellent source of protein but contain lower quantities of the essential amino acid methionine.

Like many legumes, the seemingly innocent lima bean should not be eaten raw, doing so can be lethal. Also known as butter beans, the legumes can contain a high level of cyanide, which is part of the plant's defense mechanism. In the United States there are restrictions about cyanide levels in commercially grown lima bean varieties, but not so in less developed countries, and many people can get sick from eating them. Even so, lima beans should be cooked thoroughly and uncovered to allow the poison to escape as gas. Also, drain and discard the cooking water to be on the safe side.

Many a granny came armed with a spoonful of castor oil to heal all ills, and studies show that it does indeed have health benefits to offer. Just be sure not to eat the beans from which the oil came. If castor beans are chewed and swallowed, they can release ricin, one of the most toxic poisons known to man. Eating just one or two castor beans can easily cause the demise of the eater. Ricin has been investigated as a warfare agent and has even been employed by secret agents and assassins.

Pumpernickel (Devil's Farts)

Pumpernickel (German Devil's Fart) is a heavy dark brown bread traditionally made with coarsely ground rye flour and whole rye berries and has been long associated with the Westphalia region of Germany for over 500 years. Like most rye breads, it is traditionally made with an acidic sourdough starter, which inhibits the rye amylase enzymes. The name is associated with the coarse bread-giving rise to flatulence.

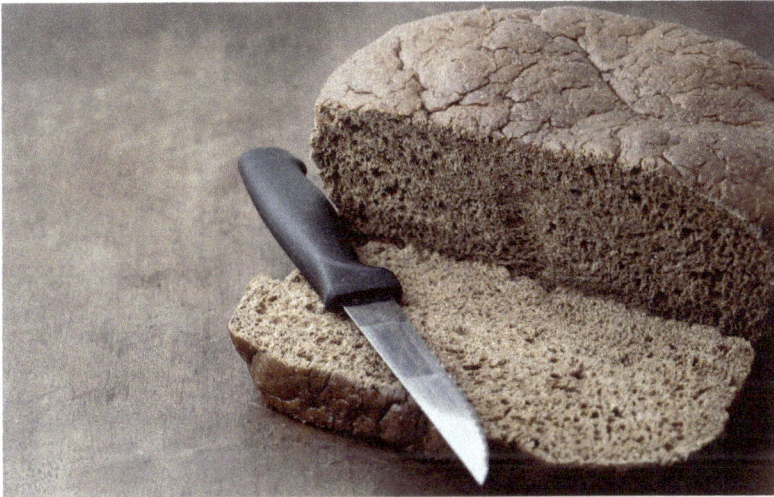

shutterstock/eclipticblue

Pets de Nonne (Nun's Farts)

Pets de Nonne, also called Pets de Sœur, is translated as a nun's farts. They are a dessert puff pastry dating from medieval times and made from butter, milk, flour, sugar, eggs and sometimes honey is added. They are traditionally pan-fried in lard and then baked. Their lightness inspired their name in French, pets de nonne and Pets de Sœurs.

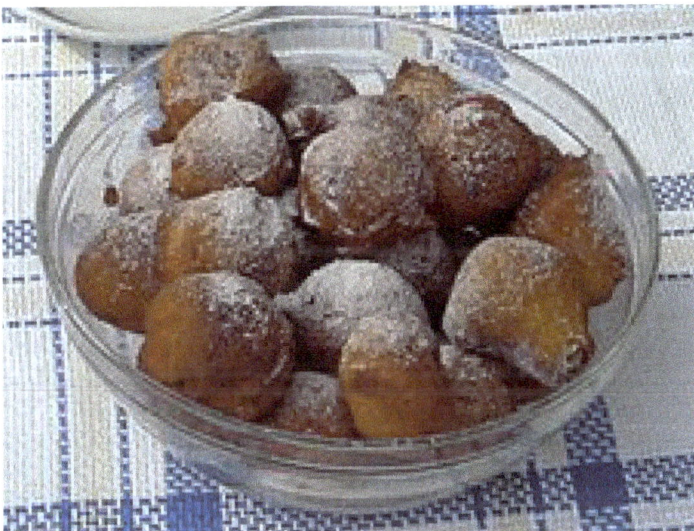

Pets de Nonne, also called Pets de Sœurs (Nun's Farts) French and Canadian Dessert Food photo by Ziga Creative Commons License

To 'Air' is Human

Digestion

The purpose of the digestive tract is to support life by providing the nutrition and energy we need for all of our body functions. Intestinal gas is simply a natural waste product and is rarely of consequence. Perhaps the analogy is not the best not the best one, but think of the digestive tract as the reverse of the assembly line, a disassembly line. A factory has a goal to be efficient and profitable, and may not win too many awards for architectural beauty. So too with the digestive tract, the process has been refined over eons of evolution, yet still have its primitive origins and end products.

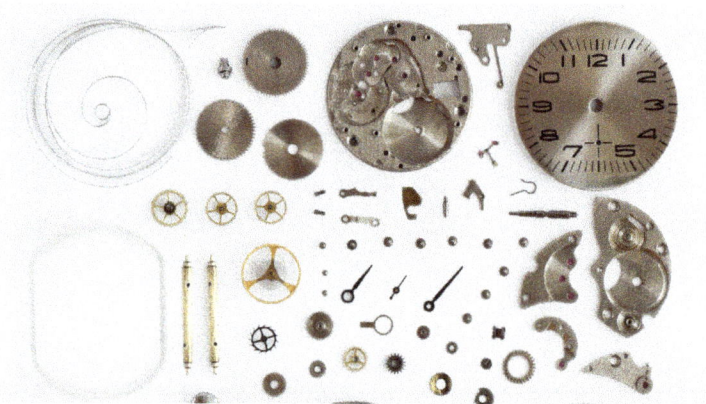

Digestion as disassembly shutterstock/yomka

We begin our factory tour with a view much like you would get sitting in your car going through a car wash. Before you even go to the car wash, your brain has to make the conscious decision that this activity is what it wants to do. In the same manner, the mind begins the digestive process with the decision to satisfy its hunger call, or because an appetizing opportunity presents itself. When thinking about food and eating, the brain may activate the secretion of saliva and prime the digestive processes of the stomach and internal organs.

Much like the water hoses and spray that greet your vehicle as you enter the beginning of the car wash tunnel, the entrance of food to the mouth receives a similar welcome. Jets of saliva are secreted from the ducts of the salivary glands located strategically around the oral cavity of the mouth. Saliva that is in the resting mouth is viscous and coats and protects the teeth and the inner surface of the mouth. The secreted saliva with eating or drinking is of a thinner more watery consistency. It has digestive enzymes including amylase to digest carbohydrates and lipase to digest fats.

If your carwash is as sophisticated as your digestive tract, it will have a crew to make sure your side mirrors are tucked in. It will also provide a prewash scrub of your tires to remove residue that would otherwise be difficult for the machinery to reach. The teeth, jaws, and tongue work together in a remarkable and powerful dance with very few of the missteps which would be the dance equivalent of stepping on toes, the biting of the tongue.

The food has to be processed into smaller more manageable portions than that what is found on your plate. Your dining utensils of fork, knife, and spoon are just the preliminary, as the teeth do the real work in preparing food for the process of digestion. The teeth are subdivided into distinct categories that have unique functions. The incisors cut the food as you bite into an apple and the canines tear the food apart as you dig into your pastrami sandwich. The molars crush and grind the salad and crunchy vegetables that you have as a side dish. The grinding and crushing break the plant cell walls apart that would otherwise protect its internal nutritious content from our digestive enzymes. They also increase the surface area of the food increasing their exposure to digestive acid and enzymes.

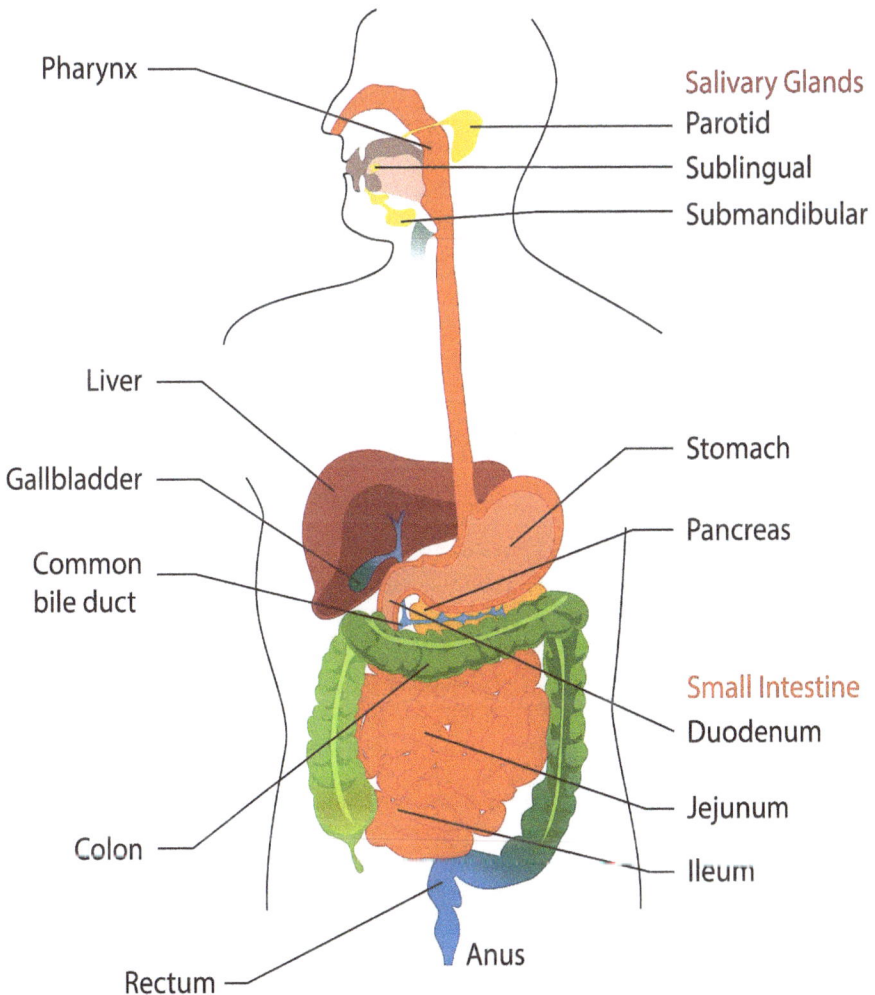

shutterstock/yaruna

To 'Air' is Human

The chewing process assures that the saliva and its active enzymes are well mixed with the increased surface area of the food. They begin the process of breaking down the carbohydrates and lipids into their essential components to ready them for further digestion and absorption. The saliva also moistens the food and lubricates it for the coordinated swallowing motion of the tongue, teeth, palate, and pharynx. These muscles and organs work together to roll it into an easy to swallow food bolus. The muscles of the swallowing process include those that protect the larynx and airway. The epiglottis closes off the passageway to the trachea, bronchi, and lungs, to prevent aspiration into the airways as the food and saliva swallow takes place.

The coordinated action is developed with age, which is why small children should avoid foods, such as nuts, grapes, larger oval or rounded candies. These foods, if inappropriately swallowed into the airway, can lead to fatal choking episodes. Tragically a number of children die because the oval or rounded shape can completely block the airway. An irregular shaped object, which can be life threatening, rarely completely obstructs the airway and usually allows some air to pass. The complicated swallowing neuromuscular coordination can also be affected by neurological disorders, stroke, surgery or other conditions, which may lead to the risk of aspiration. Once swallowed, the food bolus is propelled down the esophagus by coordinated snakelike muscular action, known as peristalsis. It is not recommended, but the swallowing mechanism is so efficient that you can swallow against gravity while standing on your head.

The muscular valve at the junction of the esophagus and stomach is called the lower esophageal sphincter. The lower esophageal sphincter is designed to allow food and fluid to enter the stomach, with the door closed behind them once they leave the esophagus. If the valve opens at the wrong time, gastric acid, digestive enzymes, and food can flow back into the esophagus. The reflux of stomach contents into the esophagus can lead to symptoms of heartburn or mucosal damage. If the refluxed material goes all the way into the airway hoarseness, sore throat, aspiration, choking, or pneumonia can develop. If it occurs frequently gastroesophageal reflux disease (GERD) can predispose to a change in the tissue lining the esophagus. The growth of intestinal type tissue is called a Barrett esophagus, and is at a higher risk of cancer development than the usual squamous lining tissue. Individuals with Barrett esophagus are treated for GERD and monitored carefully for pre-malignant changes.

The stomach is a churning caldron of muscular mixing contractions, concentrated acid secretion, and potent digestive enzymes. The vagus nerve and gut hormones play a crucial role in the intricate balance of enzymes, acid, nutrients, and motility. When the conditions are right, the pyloric sphincter of the stomach opens to allow the acid, enzyme, and food mixture to exit. This digestive material is now called chyme as it enters the first portion of the small intestine, known as the duodenum. In Greek, this means the width equivalent to twelve fingers, which is what its small size would measure using your digits. For its small size, the duodenum plays an amazing and complex part.

The highly acid chyme would quickly damage the lining of the duodenum if it did not respond quickly with the pouring on, much like a fire extinguisher, of sodium bicarbonate. The sodium bicarbonate is produced in the duodenum as well as by the pancreas. The sodium bicarbonate produced in the pancreas is released through the pancreatic duct, which empties into the duodenum through the Ampulla of Vater.

The fire extinguisher analogy shares another aspect of the story. Perhaps you made a fire extinguisher in a science class, or home experiment, by adding baking soda that contains sodium bicarbonate and vinegar that contains acetic acid. This neutralization of acid is the same type of reaction that takes place in the duodenum, when the hydrochloric acid of the stomach meets the sodium bicarbonate released to neutralize it. When the two react they produce water, sodium chloride (salt), and large quantities of carbon dioxide. The carbon dioxide is released as large volumes of gas that appears as bubbles arising from the reaction. The carbon dioxide is used as a fire extinguisher in the science experiment since it is heavier than air and cuts off the oxygen supply that the flame requires.

In the human duodenum, the carbon dioxide generated as a side product of acid neutralization only serves to bloat and distend the gut with gas. The body is pretty remarkable in getting rid of the bloat relatively quickly, in that it absorbs the carbon dioxide into the bloodstream where it travels to the lungs and is exhaled. The bile ducts from the liver join the duct from the pancreas bringing digestive enzymes and bicarbonate that enter the duodenum through the Ampulla of Vater. Within the ampulla lies the muscular sphincter of Oddi. The name sounds like a character from the story of the Wizard of Oz, and that would be an appropriate analogy. The coordinated release of hormones, enzymes, motility and vagal input is nothing short of wizardry.

Subconsciously, your body can sense what nutrients you have ingested. The body responds by releasing the correct recipe of enzymes, potent acid in the stomach, and bicarbonate in the duodenum, adjusting the pH as necessary. It adds just the right amount of bile to the mix, controls the timing and volume of stomach emptying, and controls the speed of transit and intensity of mixing contractions through the length of the intestinal tract. The majority of the sensing and control feedback takes place in a small confined space the width of twelve fingers, the duodenum

The breakdown products of the digestive process are absorbed by a sea of finger-like projections called the villi. It looks like a field of waving wheat stalks; each upstanding villus is ready to use its enzymes and absorptive capacity to absorb nutrients. If you looked under the microscope, you would find that each villus has thousands of even smaller villi on its surface, given the appropriate name of microvilli.

To 'Air' is Human

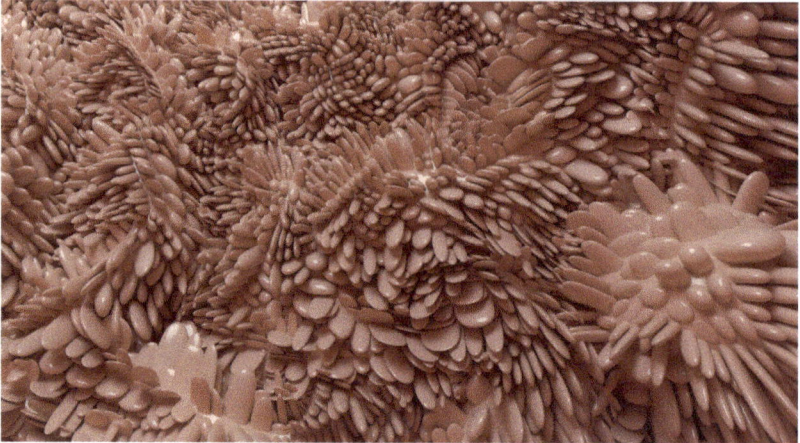

Villi shutterstock/modella

All of these folds of absorptive tissue, if flattened out, would provide the equivalent absorptive capacity of a championship tennis court. A quote from Mark Twain also illustrates the concept of surface area: "If Switzerland were ironed flat it would be a very large country". The long intestinal tunnel of eagerly awaiting absorptive villi is about twenty feet long, and it is an amazingly efficient system of digestion and absorption. If injured, the ability of the small bowel to digest and absorb nutrients is compromised. A condition that temporarily damages the small intestine, such as a viral or bacterial gastroenteritis often called stomach flu, can cause a blunting or shortening of the villi. The villous blunting will also lead to the loss of digestive enzymes that reside on the villi.

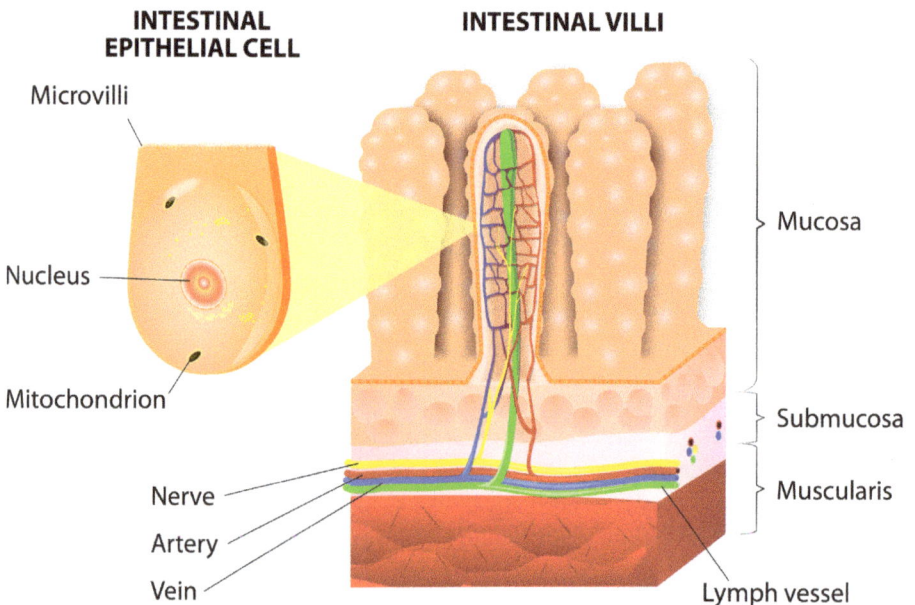

INTESTINAL EPITHELIAL CELL

INTESTINAL VILLI

Microvilli

Nucleus

Mitochondrion

Nerve

Artery

Vein

Mucosa

Submucosa

Muscularis

Lymph vessel

shutterstock/designua

To 'Air' is Human

Without the ability to digest and absorb nutrients, the unabsorbed material can cause what is known as an osmotic diarrhea. People are often advised to avoid dairy products for a week or so after stomach flu to allow the villi and enzymes to recover. If you eat or drink lactose without waiting until the recovery is complete, you may end up with symptoms of temporary lactose intolerance such as gas and diarrhea. When the liquid chyme leaves the jejunum and ileum of the small intestine, it goes through the ileocecal valve to enter the colon. In the cecum of the colon lies the infamous appendix, which for thousands of years mystified science as to its purpose. It looks like its function has finally, and only very recently, been identified. It stores a reservoir of intestinal bacteria, representing the healthy gut microbiome, from which the gut flora can be replenished after a bout of intestinal dysentery.

The gut microbiome is much more important than most people know. The microbes of the body far outnumber the number of human cells. In fact, if you just go by the number of cells and not their mass, they outnumber human cells by ten to one. In other words, you as a living system are only ten percent human and ninety percent microbes! The vast majority of the microbes living within and on us are commensals. The term commensal is used to describe a symbiotic relationship from which both parties benefit. They are able to process foods that would otherwise be indigestible, and convert them to absorbable nutrients and metabolites. It is not an understatement to say that they are a requirement for our health and wellbeing. The gut microbiome also plays a critical role in the gut-brain-microbiome-axis, which provides for the communication of information between the three. Many experts now include food as the fourth component of this important communication axis.

The colon, unlike the small intestine, is less involved in the digestion of foods and nutrients. It is primarily involved in the absorption of water and sodium, as well as some fat-soluble vitamins such as vitamin K. The colon removes the excess moisture from the watery chime solidifying the stool as it transits the gut. The ability to conserve water is necessary, and without this ability the risk of dehydration would be substantially increased. The fecal material of the stool is stored in the rectum, and sigmoid colon, awaiting the right opportunity to be eliminated through defecation. A process or illness that impairs the colon's absorption of water will lead to more fluid in the stool and diarrhea. The loss of water and electrolytes as a consequence of diarrhea, unfortunately, remains a life-threatening condition in many parts of the world, especially for infants and children.

If the elimination of the feces is delayed, the moisture continues to be absorbed, and the stools can become harder resulting in constipation. Constipation itself can be self-perpetuating as it aggravates the situation because the stools become harder and more difficult to pass the longer they remain in the colon. The more common treatments for constipation attempt to increase the moisture content of the stool. The feces excreted can provide information about bowel health. For most people going about their daily activities, the passage of the feces itself is the end of the story of digestion. The human digestive system, like that of other animals, does not remove all of the contained nutrients from food. For other organisms, including the common housefly, the feces are thus an available source of nutrition. For them, the elimination of feces is just the beginning of their story of digestion and can play an important role in the transmission of disease back to humans.

Farts are ubiquitous, all living creatures generate gas from the cellular respiration of metabolism, and humans are no exception. The bacteria in your colonic flora produce microscopic nanofarts and microfarts, which collect into larger bubbles of gas in the bowel. They are intermixed with the atmospheric air swallowed throughout the day and particularly at meals.

Distension

Distension and its synonymous term bloat are the familiar sensation that the abdomen is distended or overly full. There are many causes of bloating ranging from simple overeating and the regular production of intestinal gasses to abdominal ascites fluid buildup from an underlying tumor. Common causes of abdominal bloating include overeating, gastric distension, lactose intolerance, fructose intolerance and other food intolerances. Other causes include food allergy, aerophagia (air swallowing), irritable bowel syndrome, partial or complete bowel obstruction, and gastric dumping syndrome or rapid gastric emptying. The list continues with gas-producing foods, constipation, visceral fat, and obesity.

Less common causes include splenic flexure syndrome, menstruation, dysmenorrhea, premenstrual syndrome, polycystic ovary syndrome and ovarian cysts, and Alvarez' syndrome. The possibilities are an extensive list of ailments, infections, and disorders including intestinal parasites (e.g., *Ascaris lumbricoides*), diverticulosis, celiac disease, prescription medications such as phentermine, intra-abdominal tumors such as cancer of the ovary, liver, uterus, stomach, and colon.

Temporary bloating is common after gastrointestinal endoscopic procedures. Rarely a megacolon, which is an abnormal dilation of the colon, can be caused by ulcerative colitis or Chagas disease caused by the parasite *Trypanosoma cruzi*. After surgical repair of a hiatal hernia or treatment for gastroesophageal reflux with a procedure known as a Nissen fundoplication, the ability to burp and belch is restricted resulting in uncomfortable bloating and distension.

A number of lifestyle and dietary factors can also affect the frequency and intensity of the sensation of bloating. Exercise stimulates the releases of hormones that encourage peristaltic activity in the bowels. In a similar fashion, Caffeine containing beverages and food such as coffee, tea, cola, and chocolate also stimulate peristalsis and improve the transit time of food through the digestive tract. A rapid gastrointestinal transit gives the gut flora less time to ferment the material in the lumen of the bowel, with a resultant decrease in the total volume of gas produced by bacterial fermentation. Even a walk after a meal may help to move the contents along helping to ease the volume of gas produced. If nothing else, it at least allows you to release it outdoors!

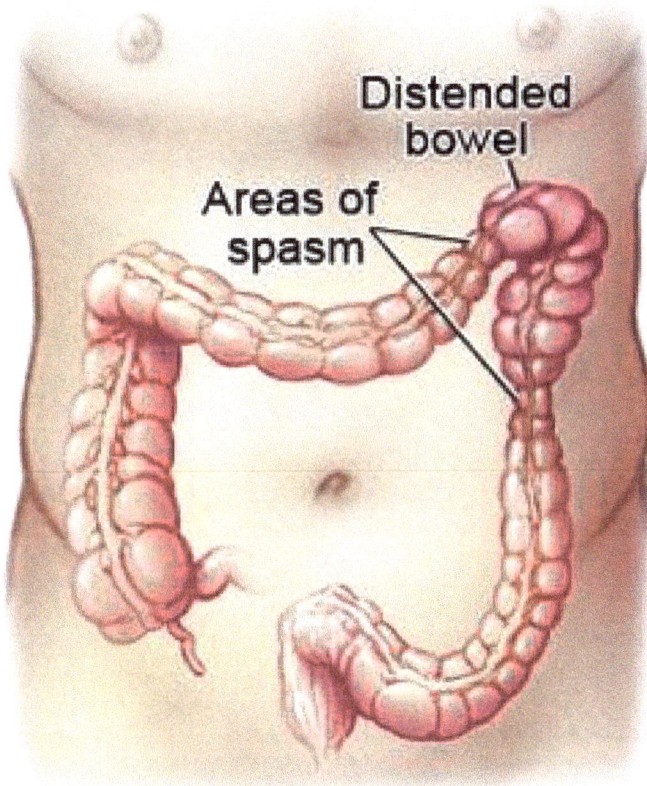

Meals that are high in fat create the exact opposite effect as fat causes the release of hormones and slows down gut motility. As the food spends more time in the digestive tract continued bacterial fermentation produces increasing quantities of gas.' In addition, foods that are extremely hot or cold tend to be swallowed in smaller quantities resulting in more swallows being necessary to eat or drink the same volume at a moderate temperature. As each swallow contributes an additional quantity of air entering the esophagus and digestive tract, more swallows results in more air ingestion. Foods or snacks that require excess chewing with resultant excess swallowing of saliva, such as chewing or bubble gum, also contribute to excess air intake. Certain types of vegetables and fruits contain sugars and starches, which may be poorly digested by people but happily fermented by bacteria comprising the gut flora. The most common food intolerance is lactose intolerance.

The treatment is always directed at the underlying cause. Empiric trials of carminatives, probiotics, dietary restrictions, enzyme replacement therapy, simethicone, etcetera can be attempted. Alternative health approaches to treating bloating include acupuncture, homeopathy, and hypnosis. Sometimes the underlying bloat is not bloating from the air but from the increased body fat of obesity. Now that is a real challenge, but the benefits of eliminating that bloat can be profoundly beneficial to health and longevity.

Another contributor to gastrointestinal bloat is reduced gut motility. With the reduction in peristaltic activity, the intestinal gasses accumulate and distend the bowel. Diabetes mellitus, neuropathy, various drugs including opiates, and other causes may lead to a reduction in peristaltic activity. Bowel obstruction leads to distension of proximal portions of the gastrointestinal tract because of accumulating gas, fluids, and undigested food residue.

Bloating and distension continue even after death. As there is no longer any gastrointestinal peristalsis or motility, the gasses rapidly accumulate. In the cases of victims of drowning the body, which initially descended deeper into the water, begins rise as the gasses accumulate. After a day or so enough gas has collected so that the body floats to the surface and remains there for a week or so. In cold water or colder climates the microbial metabolism is slowed so it takes longer for sufficient gas to be produced to float a body from submerged depths. In the San Francisco Bay area the Golden Gate Bridge is a frequent location for tragic suicide leaps into the frigid waters below. The water is so cold it often takes a week for gasses to accumulate to allow retrieval of the body. The cold temperature also involves Charles Law, which dictates that the lower the temperature the smaller the volume the gas will occupy.

At some point the pressure of the gasses that are accumulating through the microbial metabolism and the decomposition process result in rupture of the body. This event can be explosive in nature and injury and death have occurred from proximity to decomposing bodies and animal remains. In most societies, early burial prevents exposure to the decomposition process. In Western and other cultures a body may be displayed prior to burial. As the intestinal gas production does not cease with death, and indeed accelerates, gas may continue to escape as an audible fart. Part of the mortician practice is to perform a procedure that seals and secures the anus of the deceased so that the audible release of gas does not occur. Most people are not aware that the dead can fart, and when an uninformed person is exposed to a deceased person farting they are frightened, often believing that they are partly alive. Perhaps this has given rise to a belief in a zombie like state between life and death.

Elevator (see Atmospheric Pressure, Fart Aroma, Fart, Diffusion)

Elevators are a source of frustration and humor when it comes to intestinal gas in confined small places. There is an underlying science as to why farts are more likely to occur when going up as opposed to coming down. Additional insights can be gathered by reading the entries on atmospheric pressure, altitude, ideal gas laws, fart aroma, and diffusion.

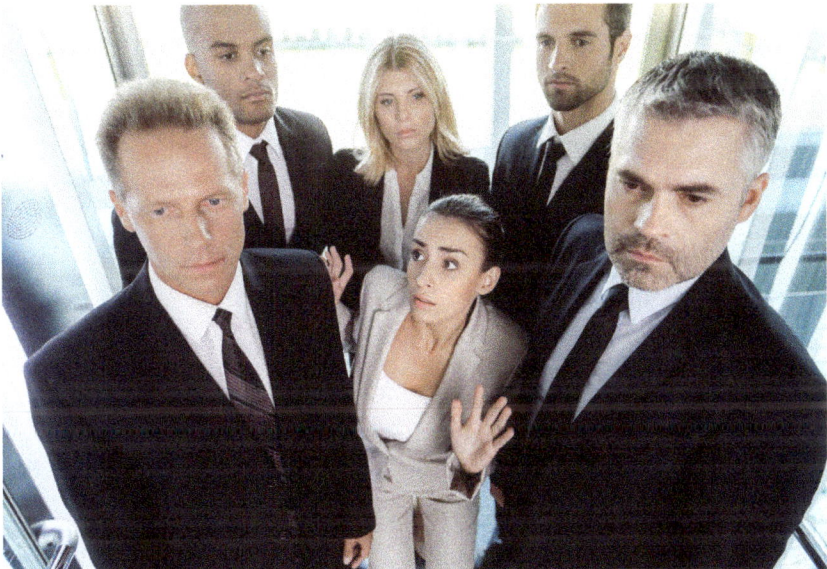

shutterstock/g-stockstudio

To 'Air' is Human

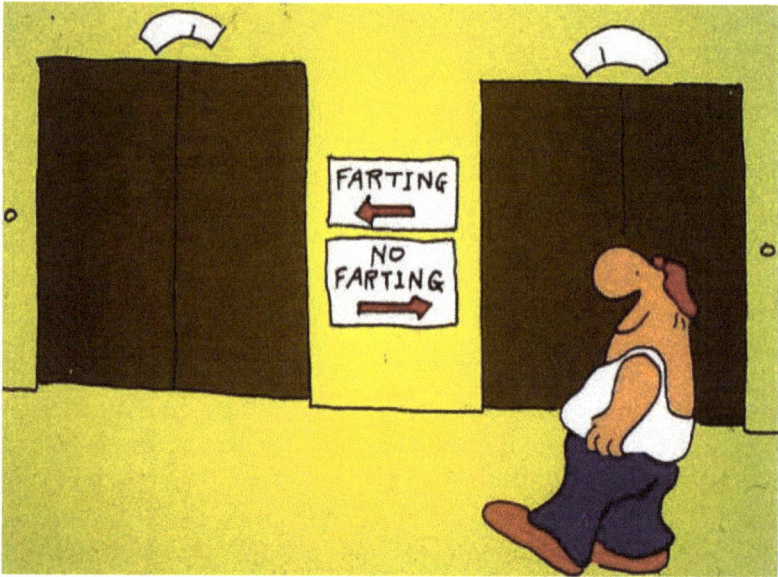

Eructation (Burp, Belch) (see Aerophagia, Gastroesophageal Reflux Disease)

Commonly called a burp or belch the words are now synonymous with the medical term eructation. The English language, as all living languages, continues to evolve. Today the words are interchangeable but they were not always synonymous. In older times, a burp was considered an involuntary release of gas from the stomach. Encouraged and admired in infants and young children, tolerated in most cultures and societies if not in mixed company, and frowned upon by the female spouse, it was recognized as an involuntary act of nature.

The belch however took on a more sinister demeanor being considered a voluntary and thus controllable outburst of gastric gasses. Although considered a talent worthy of development by adolescent males and those who remain in that mindset through their adult years, most of society frowns upon the activity.

Burping or belching may be a symptom of a hiatal hernia, GERD, or of lower esophageal sphincter dysfunction. The other dysfunction that is often associated with GERD and can lead to burping and belching is a motility disorder of the esophagus known as transient relaxation of the lower esophageal sphincter. As you can imagine, the lower esophageal sphincter (LES) isn't supposed to be tightly closed all of the time. The lower esophageal sphincter needs to relax every time you swallow to allow the material ingested to enter the stomach. It also needs to relax whenever you need to burp, belch or vomit to allow for material to exit as well. The condition of transient relaxation of the LES is where the relaxation occurs for unknown reasons at an abnormal time, often without warning. It is much as if a security gate that is only supposed to open for authorized traffic opens on its own at random times.

To 'Air' is Human

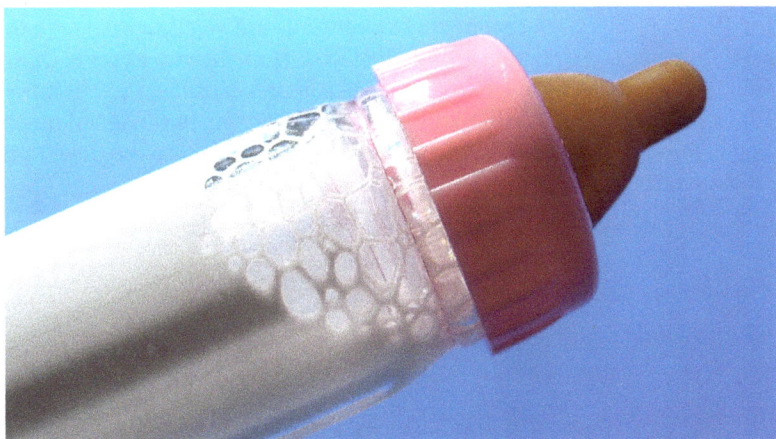

Baby bottles are a common source of aerophagia, air swallowing. Burping the baby after the feeding helps to release the swallowed air. shutterstock/JohannaGoodyear

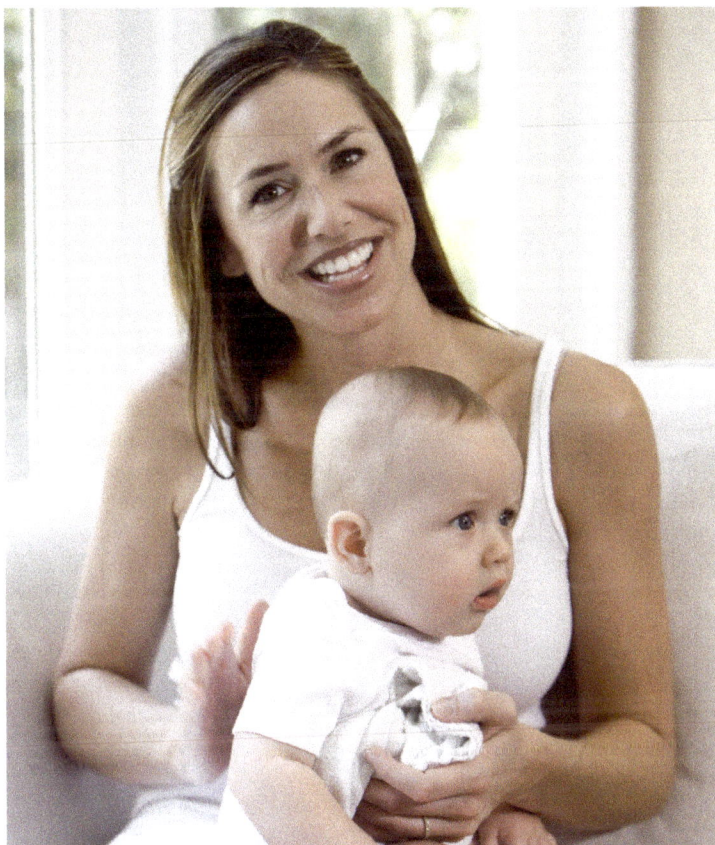

Burping the baby after the feeding helps to release the swallowed air. shutterstock/GoldenPixels

To 'Air' is Human

Air swallowing is a universal event in humans and is also known as aerophagia. We do it with every one of the on average two thousand swallows we take every day, ingesting approximately five ml (1 teaspoonful) of air with every swallow. Air is seventy-eight percent nitrogen, which is a poorly absorbed gas. If it is not released in a burp, it will contribute to bloating and distension. The volume of air swallowed is impressive, but is only a small percentage of what the digestive process can generate in terms of gas production.

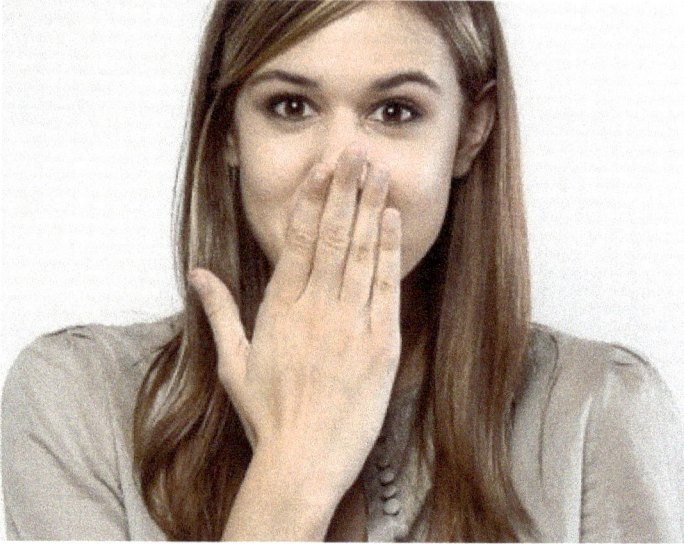

4.bp.blogspot.com Creative Commons License

Aerophagia is the swallowing of air, allowing it to enter the digestive tract, and it occurs naturally and without thinking in every individual. There is a variation of aerophagia in which the behavior becomes a purposeful, and at times obsessive-compulsive, behavior. More often, when excessive spontaneous aerophagia is occurring it is a subconscious or unconscious behavior, much like a nervous tic. The volume of air swallowed in these conditions can be impressive, and a plain x-ray of the abdomen may demonstrate that the entire digestive tract is filled with air from esophagus to rectum.

The important fact is that seventy-eight percent of air is nitrogen and the gastrointestinal tract poorly absorbs the nitrogen, unlike the oxygen and carbon dioxide. Once the nitrogen is swallowed it has only two ways to get out of the digestive tract. Coming up as a burp or belch is its closest exit, but it has to overcome the lower esophageal sphincter, the upper esophageal sphincter and the oncoming rush with peristalsis and gravity of more food, fluid, drink, saliva, and yes even more air being swallowed.

A hidden source of swallowed air is the air content present within many foods. Many fruits contain a great deal more air than you would have imagined. If you take an apple and press all of the juice out you would have all of the air removed.

To 'Air' is Human

When you add the volume of the juice and the pressed fruit together you will find that it was only sixty percent of the volume of the original fruit. In other words, of the entire fruit that you ate forty percent was air.

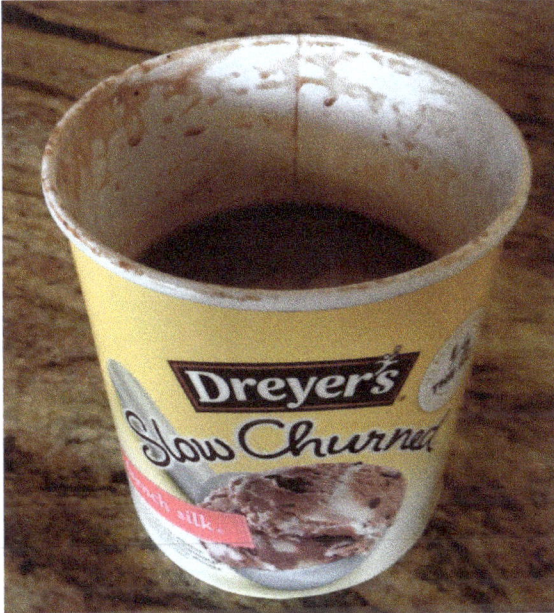

Overrun is the term used to describe air that is added into the finished food product to expand its volume as well as for texture. Air content of ice cream ranges from three percent to fifty percent and has a significant influence on texture, taste, and the value of the product purchased since ice cream is typically sold by volume, not weight. Photo by Lizabeth Weiss.

We have been in love with ice cream for thousands of years. All ice creams are not prepared in an identical manner. There is another important factor that leads to differences besides the ingredients such as cream or milk fat content, flavorings, sweeteners, stabilizers, emulsifiers, lactose, whey, casein, etcetera. It may be surprising to learn that the two largest ingredients in ice cream by volume are water (between fifty-five percent and sixty-four percent) and air (between three percent and fifty percent).

The same proposition is true for bread and most baked goods. The baking process often uses baking powder or yeast. When the dough rises you are seeing the additional volume of gasses such as carbon dioxide being produced by the yeast fermentation process. While we are on the subject of yeast, microbes of this type including *Candida albicans* are a normal constituent of the gut microbiome. Just like one sees with the rising of dough, the yeast organisms ferment carbohydrates and starches resulting in the release of gas. Excess yeast may lead to increase gaseousness. One of the thoughts as to why beer is known for producing intestinal gas are the residual yeast and carbohydrates, in addition to the nitrogen and carbon dioxide gasses already added to the beverage.

To 'Air' is Human

Many foods are whipped with air to increase their volume, which adds to the smoothness and creaminess of the product. It also adds to the bottom line of profitability to the manufacturer, as you are paying for a product typically sold by volume. As long as they don't push it to the detriment of flavor and texture the more air added to a product increases its volume and profitability.

Carbonated beverages are very popular worldwide. In the United States sales of carbonated beverages exceed twenty billion dollars per year, four times the sales volume of dairy products. The majority consumed today already comes carbonated with large amounts of carbon dioxide forced into solution under high pressure. As the pressure seal of the can or bottle is released the carbon dioxide forms bubbles and comes out of the solution, giving a pleasant tickling sensation on the palate, and a full at times bloated feeling in the stomach and gut.

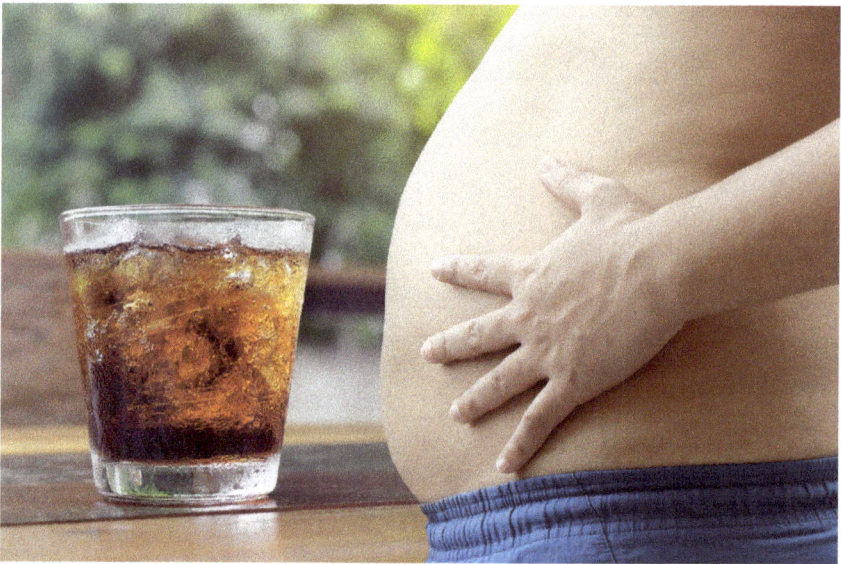

shutterstock/sisacorn

Nitrogen is poorly soluble in liquids, and the high density of bubbles contributes to a smooth creamy mouth feel. Most beers are saturated with a combination of 30% carbon dioxide and 70% nitrogen. The head serves both an aesthetic purpose, as well as accomplishing the dispersal of the beer aroma. You can get an idea of how high the nitrogen content is by looking at the size of the head created. A significant percentage of the volume of your drink is the head, and a friendly bartender will discard some of the head to give you more drink for your money, as well as to encourage a larger gratuity.

Beer drinkers are famous for the burping and belching generated. The added nitrogen gives them an edge up in competitive burping and belching contests since it is not as rapidly absorbed and eliminated via the lungs as is carbon dioxide. As mentioned earlier in this section, yeast microbes including *Candida albicans* are a normal constituent of the gut microbiome.

Just like one sees with the rising of dough, the yeast organisms ferment carbohydrates and starches resulting in the release of gas. Excess yeast may lead to increase gaseousness. One of the thoughts as to why beer is known for producing intestinal gas are the residual yeast and carbohydrates, in addition to the nitrogen and carbon dioxide gasses already added to the beverage. Nitrogen is also used in iced coffee beverages, providing a head of bubbles very similar to that of beer. The same is true of chewing tobacco and even smoking tobacco whether as cigar, pipe, cigarette, or electronic smokeless cigarette. Do you want to hold a conversation while you are eating, go ahead but it will cause even more air swallowing, as will drinking from a straw or tilting your head back to drink from a bottle or can. Rush through your meals and you swallow more air. See entry on aerophagia for more details

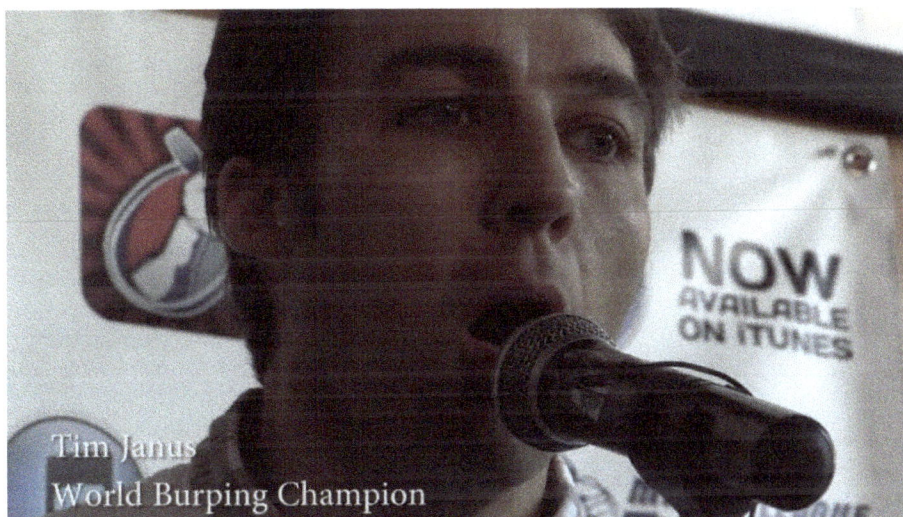

Longest burp at 18.1 seconds. youtu.be/gU3jBonhsrQ.

The World Burping Federation located in Geneva Switzerland holds the annual World Burping Championships. The *Guinness Book of World Records* has a listing for the loudest burp on record. The record holder is Paul Hunn of the United Kingdom. His burp was recorded with a car horn equivalent rating of 109.9 decibels. The longest burp, by Tim Janus, has been recorded at 18.1 seconds. To achieve this record he consumed approximately two gallons of Diet Coke and Mountain Dew. Imagine what would have happened if he swallowed a few Mentos tablets at the time of the competition.

Fart

The word fart is the correct word to use in the English language, and indeed is one of its oldest words. The alternative terms used, such as flatus and flatulence are not original English words as they have been borrowed from the Latin. There is controversy as to the derivation of the word fart. It is thought to have Indo-European roots in the Germanic language word farzen. One thought is that it originated as an onomatopoeia, a word that phonetically imitates the sound of the event it describes. Another thought is that it was related to the term for partridge, as the bird makes a similar sound when it is disturbed in its natural habitat and takes flight.

Farts are ubiquitous, all living creatures generate gas from the cellular respiration, and humans are no exception. The microorganisms in your colonic flora produce microscopic nanofarts and microfarts, which collect into larger bubbles of gas in the bowel. They are intermixed with the atmospheric air swallowed throughout the day and particularly at meals, when chewing gum, when chewing tobacco, or when smoking tobacco or other recreational products.

Aerophagia is universal, and we swallow on average three to five milliliters (one teaspoonful) of air with every swallow. Even when we are not eating or drinking, we regularly swallow the saliva we produce. The average human swallows over two thousand times a day. Chewing gum, hard candies, and use of chewing or smoking tobacco or other recreational products increase the volume of air swallowed. Drinking through a straw, directly from a can or bottle, or talking while eating, will also increase the amount of air swallowed.

Another common source of swallowed air is within the foods we eat. An apple is forty percent air by volume, and bread is over sixty percent air by volume. If you compress an apple or a loaf of bread, you will see that they a sizeable portion of their total volume is air. Whipped foods, soufflés, and baked goods, all have high air content. Have you ever forgotten to put an ice cream container back in the freezer. Ice cream is typically forty percent air by volume and when it melts the air escapes, and the full container is no longer full. By the way, the ice cream industry knows that adding air, known in the industry as overage, enhances the mouth feels texture of the ice cream. They also know that it adds up to forty percent to the profit margin, because ice cream is sold by volume, not by weight.

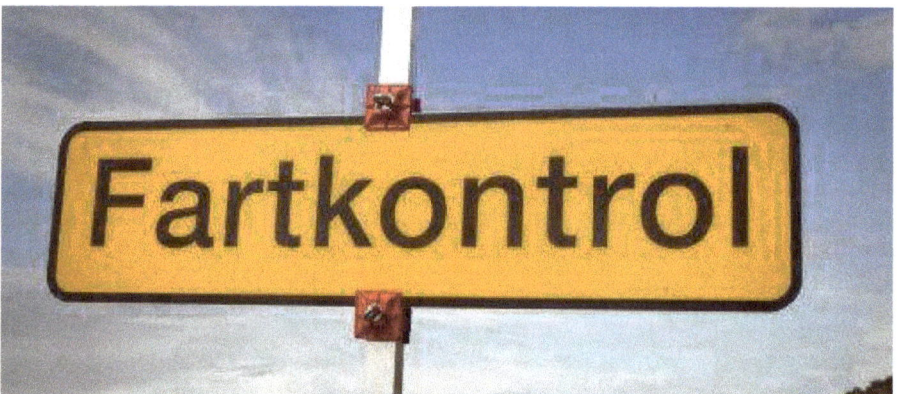

onpasture.com Creative Commons License

To 'Air' is Human

Besides the swallowed air, additional gasses are produced during the enzymatic digestive processes, as well as the neutralization of gastric hydrochloric acid and pancreatic and duodenal bicarbonate. The result is that a large volume of gasses transit the bowel and may be eliminated as a fart. Fortunately, the vast majority of the gasses produced are absorbed by the gut and then into the bloodstream through diffusion into a solution. The gasses leave the blood when they arrive at the alveoli of the lungs where they are exhaled. The chemical component gasses have very different properties of diffusion through the bowel wall and into the bloodstream.

Carbon dioxide readily diffuses and enters solution and is readily exhaled. It is the largest component of the volume of gas generated in the proximal intestinal tract. It is a major contributor to the temporary distension and discomfort that commonly occurs after a meal. Carbonation is also utilized as a common beverage enhancer and adds to the volume of carbon dioxide gas in the stomach. Carbon dioxide is the most rapidly absorbed component of intestinal gas and is the easiest to eliminate by simply exhaling it in the breath. As very little remains in the bowel, it is only a minor component of a fart.

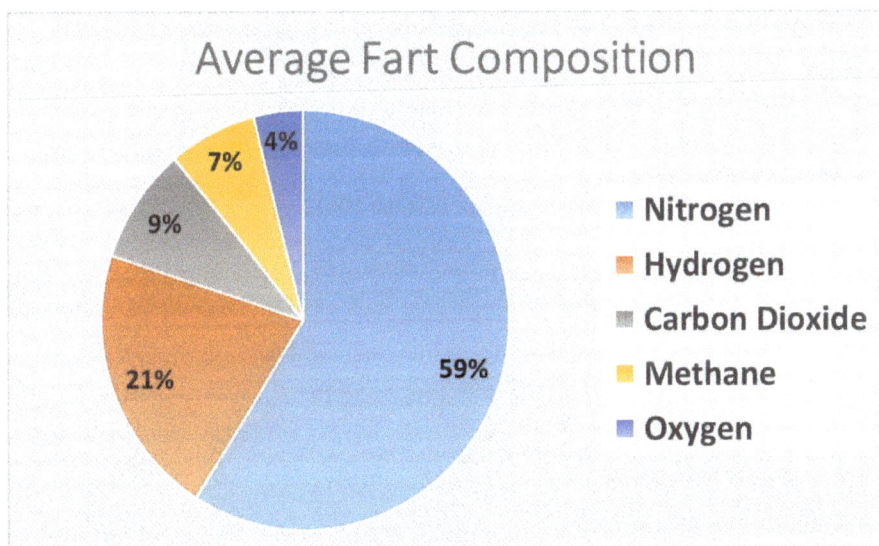

Average Fart Composition

Nitrogen — 59%
Hydrogen — 21%
Carbon Dioxide — 9%
Methane — 7%
Oxygen — 4%

Creative Commons License

The volume of gasses in the gastrointestinal tract is dependent on many factors. The volume of gas produced is determined by the amount and nature of foods ingested, and the body's ability to synthesize and utilize specific enzymes for the various food types. The nature and quantity of the bacteria in the gut flora influences the nature of intestinal gas both by their active metabolism and by their ability to aid or hinder the digestive enzymes and processes.

One of the most common causes of excess gaseousness is the deficiency of the enzyme lactase. Lactase hydrolyses the complex disaccharide dairy sugar lactose into the readily absorbable monosaccharide sugars glucose and galactose. With insufficient lactase, the sugar molecule is not metabolized by the digestive system but is instead metabolized by the gut flora, also known as the microbiome. Lactose deficiency results in gas production and may also give rise to cramps and diarrhea. Another food sugar that can cause excess gaseousness is commonly seen in fruit and is thus known as fructose. The human digestive system can handle only a limited quantity of fructose at a time. If the fructose intake exceeds this capacity the gut flora ferment this sugar, with the release of gas, and often cramps and diarrhea.

That the microbes within our digestive tracts ferment foods that we have not fully digested is to our advantage, which is why the microbiome is considered essential to our good health. We can absorb some of the nutrients the microbes release in the fermentation process, including vitamins and bioactive molecules.
We even use microbe fermentation in the preparation of many foods. When you add yeast to flour and watch, the dough rise you see the release of gasses from the fermentation process. The spongy character of bread and cakes, and why they are sixty percent air, is the result of the gas production of the yeast fungus. The characteristic holes in Swiss cheese are the result of microbial gas production. The entire production of wines, beer, and other alcohol beverages are based on microbial fermentation. In a parallel universe, we are ingesting the waste product of microbial fermentation.

Before you believe that a delicious baked good dependent on yeast farts loses some of its culinary appeals, please read on. A French pastry delicacy is known as Pets de Nonne, also called Pets de Sœurs and translated as nun's farts. They are a dessert puff pastry dating from medieval times and made from butter, milk, flour, sugar, eggs and sometimes honey is added. They are traditionally pan-fried in lard and then baked. Their lightness inspired their name in French, pets de nonne and Pets de Sœurs.

Another baked good named for its association with the fart is Pumpernickel (German: Devil's Fart) bread. It is a heavy dark brown bread traditionally made with coarsely ground rye flour and whole rye berries. It has been long associated with the Westphalia region of Germany for over 500 years. Like most rye breads, it is traditionally made with an acidic sourdough starter, which inhibits the rye amylase enzymes. The name is associated with the coarse bread-giving rise to flatulence.

Beans are known as the musical fruit because of the gas they produce in all humans. The reason for this is that legumes contain complex sugars known as raffinose, verbascose, and stachyose. Humans and other animals lack the enzyme, called alpha-galactosidase, needed to metabolize these complex sugars into absorbable simple sugars. Without the enzyme, the complex sugars are fermented by the gut microbiome producing gas. Alpha-galactosidase is now commercially available as a dietary enzyme supplement to reduce the gas production associated with particular foods such as legumes. Another enzyme that humans do not possess is cellulase, without which we cannot digest the cellulose found in most plants and grasses. Herbivorous animals do have those enzymes, which is why they can subsist on grazing of grasses and forage.

Another factor in gas production is the speed of gastrointestinal transit. Drugs, hormones, food products, and illness may influence this. The absorptive capacity and health of the mucosal lining, and the physical length of the individual's gastrointestinal tract also play a role. The often-quoted figure of twelve farts per day is a reasonable approximation of the average number of farts passed, but there is a very wide range of what is considered normal. Besides the numerical quantity of farts passed per day is the question of what is considered an average volume of gas passed. If you are familiar with physics, a series of natural laws were defined that express the relationship between temperature, pressure, and volume. The relationship between temperature and pressure is direct, i.e. the higher the temperature, the larger the volume of space a gas would occupy.

The expansion to a larger volume of occupied space may result in intestinal bloating, discomfort, and increased burping and farting. The relationship with pressure is indirect, i.e. the greater the pressure, the smaller the volume. We would rarely experience a change in intestinal gas volume based on temperature. On the contrary, we will often experience significant changes in volume due to pressure. Increases in pressure reduce the volume of gas, which is not a problem when it comes to the gut and our symptoms of gas. It can become a major problem when the pressure decreases and the gas volume increases.

The atmospheric pressure changes as we go higher or lower from sea level. The effects on intestinal gas are seen in scuba divers, pilots, airplane passengers, mountain climbers, living at higher elevations, and even taking an elevator to the top of a skyscraper. When the pressure change is rapid, for example, a scuba diver returning to the surface, or an astronaut on the ascent to orbit, the consequences can be dramatic and life threatening and are known as barotrauma. Most gasses that are commercially available (oxygen, helium, air, etc.) are compressed and contained in hardened metal canisters that can withstand very high pressure. Compression of the gas allows for significant savings of space, for example allowing scuba divers to have the equivalent of a roomful of air within a single tank. The intestinal tract is flexible and expandable to a degree, more like a balloon than a metal container. As such changes in the surrounding atmospheric pressure can result in significant volume changes, which in the extreme of barotrauma may lead to perforation and rupture.

The fart would not be as notorious as it is if it were not for its aroma. Over ninety-nine percent of the gasses in a fart are odorless. While a number of individuals may have methane present in their farts, methane is odorless. If you smell a natural gas (methane) leak, it is not the methane you smell, but an odorant gas added by the gas company as a safety precaution to give notice of danger. The majority of the aroma from a fart comes from hydrogen sulfide, skatole, indole, and aromatic fatty acids, the majority coming from the digestion of animal fats.

To 'Air' is Human

While vegetarians may fart more than carnivores, the aroma is not nearly as pungent or offensive.

Aerophagia is universal, and we swallow on average 3-5 cc (teaspoonful) of air with every swallow. Added into the mixture are the gasses produced during the enzymatic digestive processes as well as the neutralization of gastric hydrochloric acid and pancreatic and duodenal bicarbonate. The result is a large volume of gasses transiting the bowel that may be eliminated as a fart. Fortunately the vast majority of the gasses produced are absorbed by the gut, then into the bloodstream through diffusion dissolving into solution. They are finally released when they reach the alveoli of the lungs and are exhaled. The component gasses have very different properties of diffusion through the bowel wall and into the bloodstream.

Carbon dioxide readily diffuses, enters solution, and is readily exhaled. It is the largest volume of gas generated and is the major contributor to distension and postprandial (after meal) discomfort. The good news is it is the easiest to eliminate from the bowel because of its rapid diffusion into the bloodstream. Carbon dioxide is only a minor contributor to flatulence.

The volume of gasses in the gastrointestinal tract is dependent on the quantity and nature of foods ingested, and the body's ability to synthesize and utilize specific enzymes for the various food types. The nature and number of microorganisms in the gut flora also play a major role. It may also be affected by the speed of gastrointestinal transit, which likewise may be influenced by drugs, hormones, food product, illness, absorptive capacity, and the physical length of the individual's gastrointestinal tract.

The often-quoted figure of 11.5 farts per day is a reasonable approximation of the average number of farts passed, but there is a very wide range of what is considered normal. There are so many variables that what is reasonable for an individual can only be determined over a longer period than a single day.

Fart, Art

The fart has been the subject of numerous works of art over the ages. It has been represented in virtually all of the artistic media including literature, music, paintings, sculpture, cinema, photography, etcetera. It has been the material for live and stage performances for thousands of years, and of course is notorious for personal and up-close entertainment.

The following images are just a few of the visual representations over the years. A thorough review of the fart through the arts is found in the unique companion volume to this book, entitled *Artsy Fartsy, Cultural History of the Fart.*

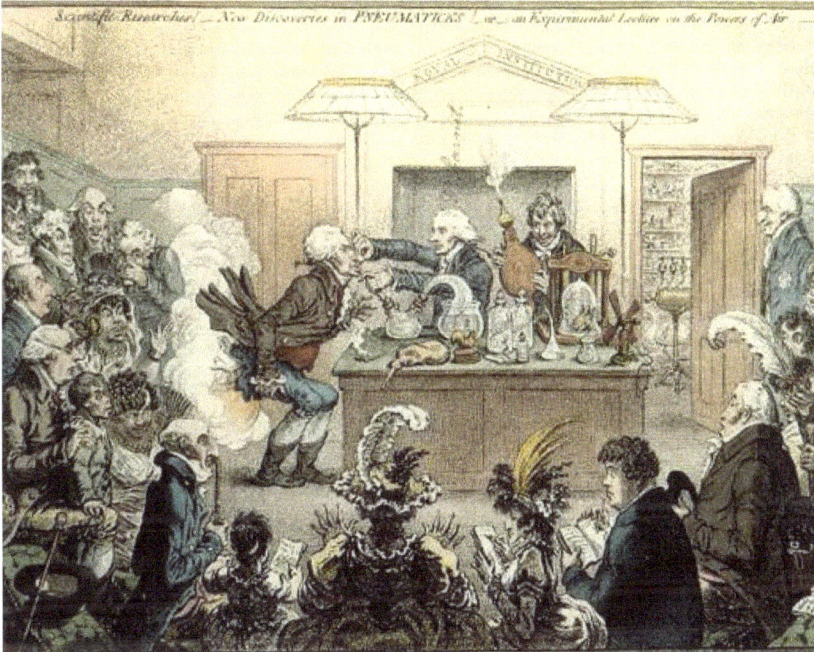

James Gillray, Public Domain

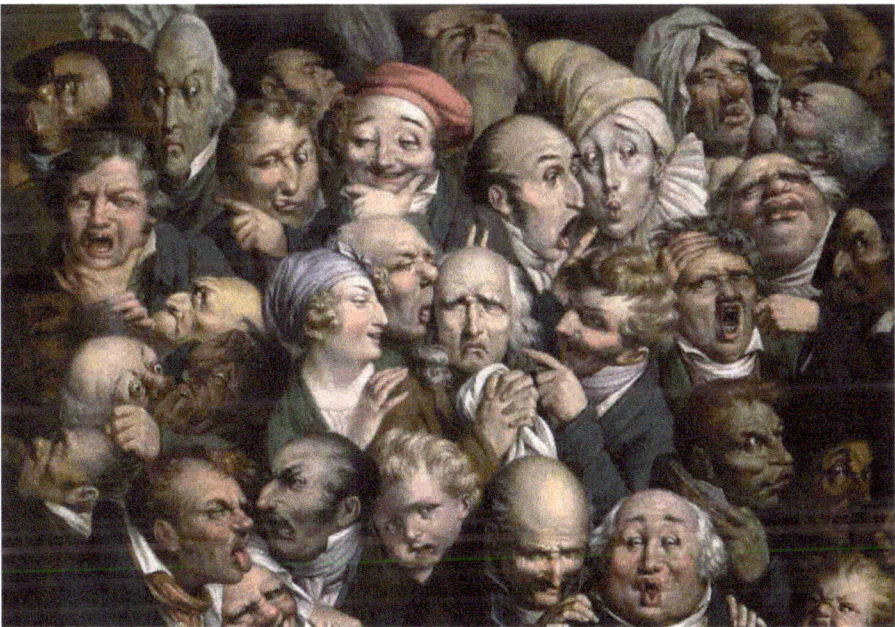

Louis-Léopold Boilly *Thirty-Six Faces of Expression*. Public Domain

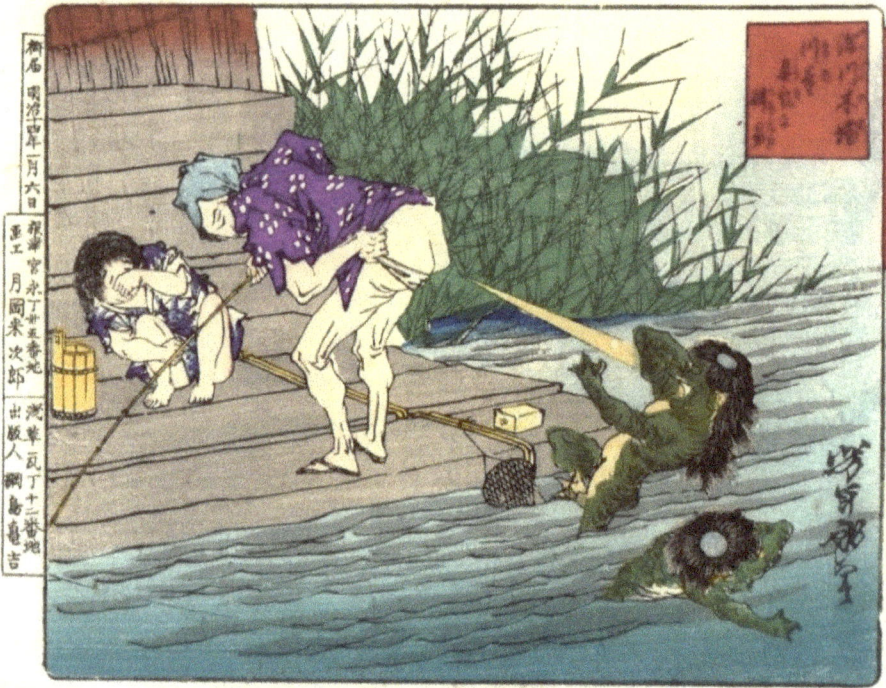

Public Domain

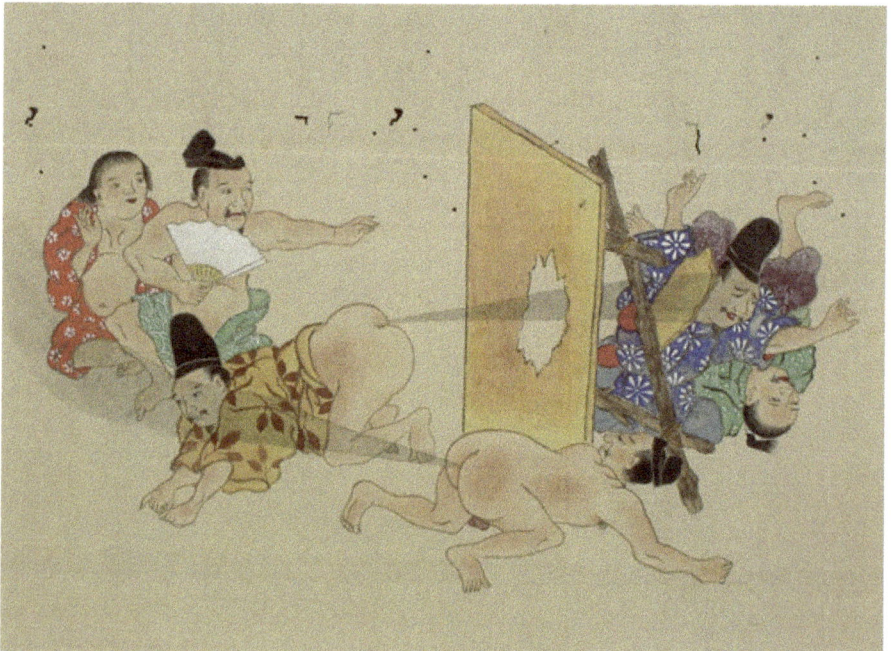

Utagawa Kuniyoshi, Public Domain

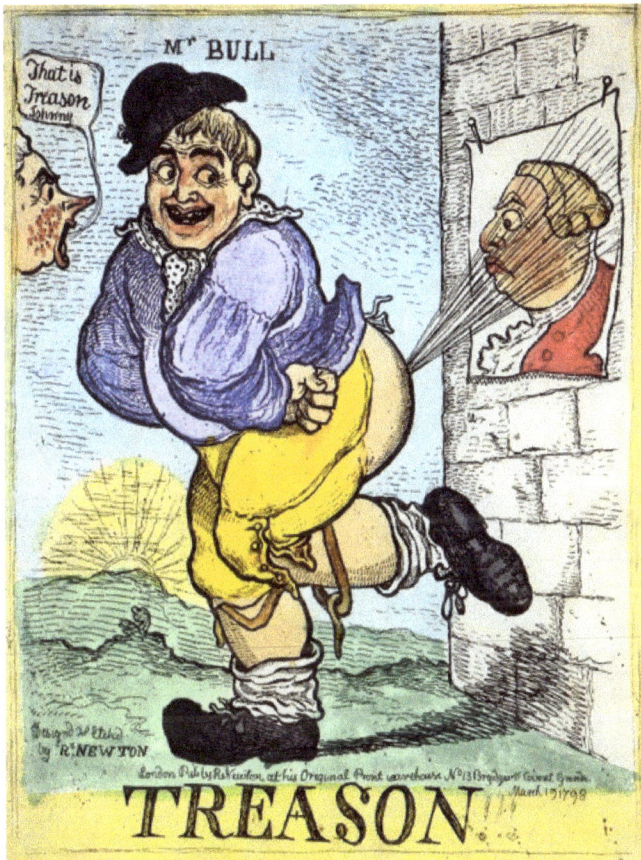

Richard Newton, Public Domain

Fart, Diffusion

The word Fart in northern European languages including German and the Scandinavian languages means speed. In you go by a school or hospital you may go by a no farting zone. Or you might receive a police citation for exceeding the fart limit! The sense of smell requires that molecules from the source material travel to the nasopharynx and touch the olfactory nerve receptors. The detection of a fart by odor requires the direct contact of the odorant molecule and the cilia of the nerve cell. Most people do not realize that a fart actually contains odorants as well as transmissible microbes.

It is possible to become ill and acquire a pathogenic infection from a fart, similar to what can occur with a cough or sneeze. Coughing and sneezing release a large plume of aerosolized droplets impregnated with microbial pathogens. A single sneeze can disperse up to 40,000 aerosol droplets, which can transmit pathogens and disease. The sneeze is a much more effective dispersant of infectious material than a cough, speaking, or squeaking a fart.

To 'Air' is Human

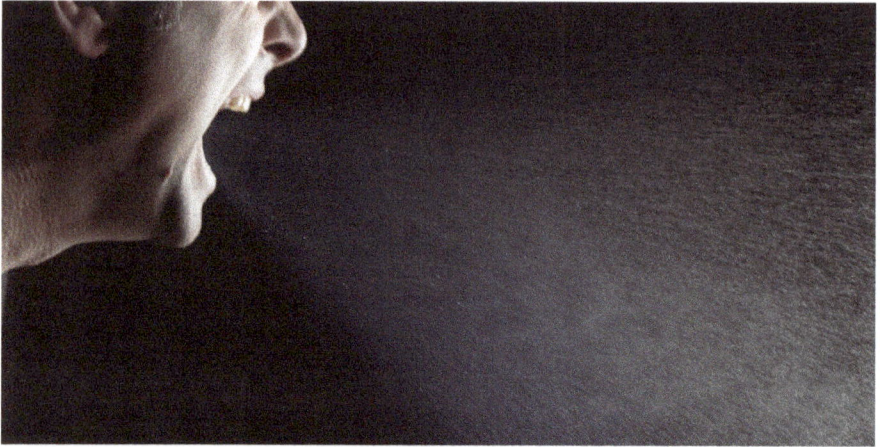

shutterstock/JamesKlotz

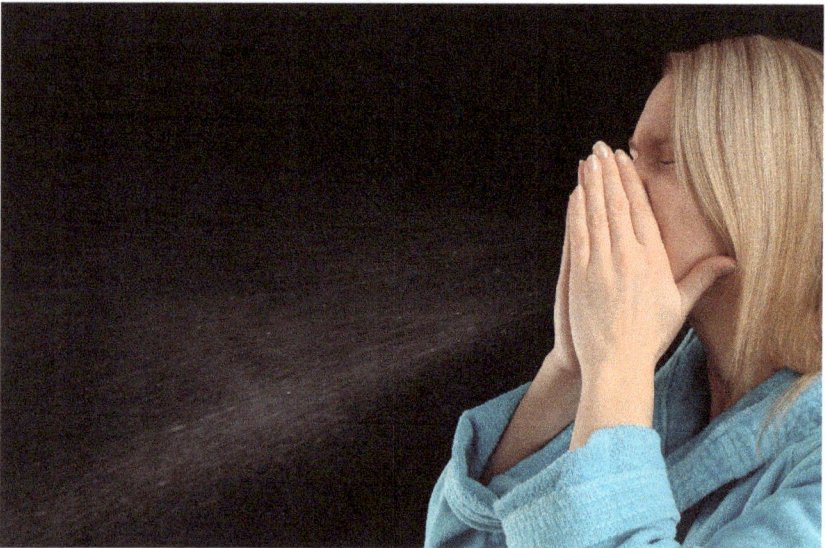

Sneezes reach a velocity of up to 500 miles per hour (750 km/hr.) Some sneezes are so loud the volume may give the impression that they have broken the sound barrier! shutterstock/RioPatuca

A sneeze, or sternutation, is a powerful rapid expulsion of air from the lungs through the nose and mouth. The average velocity of a sneeze is 42 meters/second), equivalent to approximately 95 mph. The average speed of a cough was 15.3 m/s and the average velocity of the breath of ordinary speech is 4.07 m/s. The sneeze and cough can quickly reach a velocity of over 100 miles per hour (150 kilometers per hour) and has been recorded at speeds up to 500 miles per hour (950 km/hour). These discharges will spread contaminants throughout a large size room. The flushing of a toilet will aerosolize fecal microbes that would cover a room with dimensions of twenty feet by twenty feet in a matter of seconds.

To 'Air' is Human

The mechanism of increasing intra-abdominal pressure for a fart is similar to generating intra-thoracic pressure for a sneeze. The size of the exit orifice is a major determinant of velocity. No one has voluntarily gotten close enough to a fart blast to measure its ejection velocity or count the vapor droplets. The brave soul who does so may not get a Nobel Prize, but would certainly be worthy of nomination for an IgNobel Prize.

Farts have been recorded with the speed of aroma travel at a conservative 10 miles per hour. It was not clear if this was from an individual wearing clothing at the time. Science or a dedicated researcher somewhere will one day answer the question about fart speed. Perhaps a luxury watch company will sponsor a competition for the *Guinness Book of World Records* which has a number of fart categories already entered into the competitive arena, but somehow missed out on the exciting competition of fart speed!

Back in the 1946 a spoof recording of the International Crepitation Contest was created, and it is still commercially available today. It was produced by recording engineers for the Canadian Broadcasting Corporation and was supposedly held on February 31, 1946 as the World Championship Crepitation Contest. The fictitious location of the Maple Leaf Auditorium at Thunderblow, Canada between competitors Paul Boomer and Lord Windesmear completed the scene for the blow-by-blow description of the announcer.

Fart, Etymology

English is the richest language on the planet, with more words by far than any other. This richness is due to the significant influence of its history of occupation by foreigners, especially during the days of the Roman Empire. Unlike other conquerors, the Romans did not impose their own language, in this case Latin, on the inhabitants of the British Isles. The population adapted their native tongue to include words borrowed from the occupiers and foreign influences. This led to the rapid expansion of the English vocabulary, including many different words that are synonyms.

The word fart is the correct word to use in the English language, and indeed is one of its oldest words. The alternative terms used, such as flatus and flatulence are not originally English words as they have been borrowed from the Latin. In Latin these words have the general meaning of a wind or a blowing.

There is controversy as to the derivation of the word fart. It is thought to have Indo-European roots in the Germanic language word farzen. The word fart may have originated as an onomatopoeia, a word that phonetically imitates the sound of the event it describes. Another thought is that it was related to the term for partridge, as the bird makes a similar sound when it is disturbed in its natural habitat and takes flight. How it made that transition may be an enlightening example of the evolution of words and language.

To 'Air' is Human

The Indo-European word *perd* means fart, and this led to the Latin word *pedere* the verb form of fart, and *peditum* the noun form of fart. The Indo-European *perd* led to the Greek word for fart πέρδομαι *perdomai*. It is also cognate with Sanskrit *pardate*, Avestan *pərəðaiti*, Italian *fare un peto*, French "péter", Russian пердеть (perdet') and Polish "pierd". The related Greek word *perdix* referred to a type of bird that made an explosive fart-like sound when it was flushed from the brush when startled. While being incorporated from Greek to Old French it became *perdriz*, then Middle English *partrich*, and finally Modern English *partridge*. The final step would be to complete the circuitous history and modify it to the name *fartridge*!

The word fart is also found in other languages, but there it often has a different and unrelated meaning. In the Scandinavian languages, it usually denotes speed or motion. In Danish and Norwegian, it is often used in combination with other words that obscures the meaning even more. For example in Danish a *fartcertifikate* means a trade certificate. In Norwegian, a *fart plan* means a schedule. The Norwegian phrase *stå på fartin* pronounced as stop-a–fartin means ready to leave. Likewise, the phrase *farts måler* pronounced as fart smeller refers to a speedometer. In Swedish, a speed bump is called a *farthinder*. *Fartlek* is speed training by running at alternate intervals of fast and slow paces.

Likewise if you travel on a Scandinavian marine vessel, you may see the control of engine speed labeled as *half fart* and *full fart* for half speed and full speed respectively. Fart kontrol zones are speed zones. In Germany, a similar word *fahrt* means a journey, trip, tour, or passage. It is often seen in signs that say e*infahrt* (sounds like in-fart) and *ausfahrt* (sounds like out-fart) denoting entrance and exit respectively.

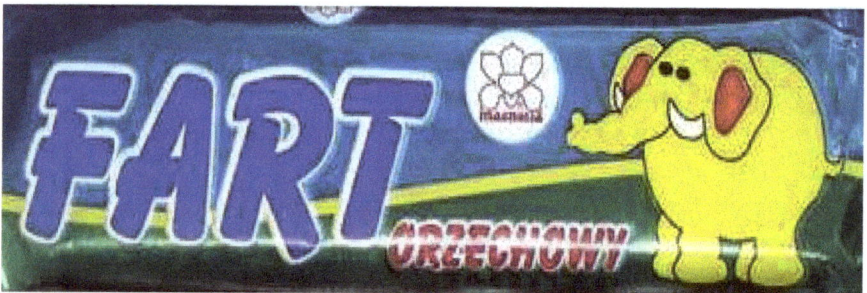

In Spanish and Portuguese *fart* means an excess of anything, especially food. One of the richest desserts they offer is called a *farte*, which means a fruit tarte in Spain, and usually a sugar almond or cream cake in Portugal. In Italy, the word *farto* means mattress. In Hungary, *fartaj* means buttocks. In Poland, if you want to buy a local favorite candy bar with a name that that means lucky, you will be looking for a *Fart* bar.

Several languages have a number of different words for variations on a theme for which there is only one word in English. The word snow is one example where we have a singular word, but the Inuit, Eskimo, Aleut, Sami and other languages of the native people of the Arctic and northern latitudes may have hundreds of words. When it comes to the word fart, the English language is very limited with just the singular word. I will not leap to the conclusion that the language that has the most words for fart needed to do so for necessity. Their population may or may not have the world's highest rate of fart production, but they certainly have the most descriptive fart words.

The Russian words for fart include *perdyozh* (first act of breaking wind), *perdun* (perpetrator and outcome), *perdil'nik* (place from where it comes), *Perun* (ancient God of wind), *bzdun* (silent fart), *bzdyukha* (silent fart as well as a stupid jerk). Some of the Russian verbs for the action of farting are particularly colorful. *Perdet'* (to fart with or without sound), *bzdet'* (to fart silently), *pereperdet* (to fart repeatedly), and my favorite word *nabzdet'sya* (to fart silently to one's complete and utter satisfaction!).

The word fart is one of the oldest words in the English language. One of the most influential dictionaries in the long history of the language is Samuel Johnson's *A Dictionary of the English Language* published in 1755. An important innovation in his dictionary was the use of quotations from literature to illustrate the usage of the word defined.

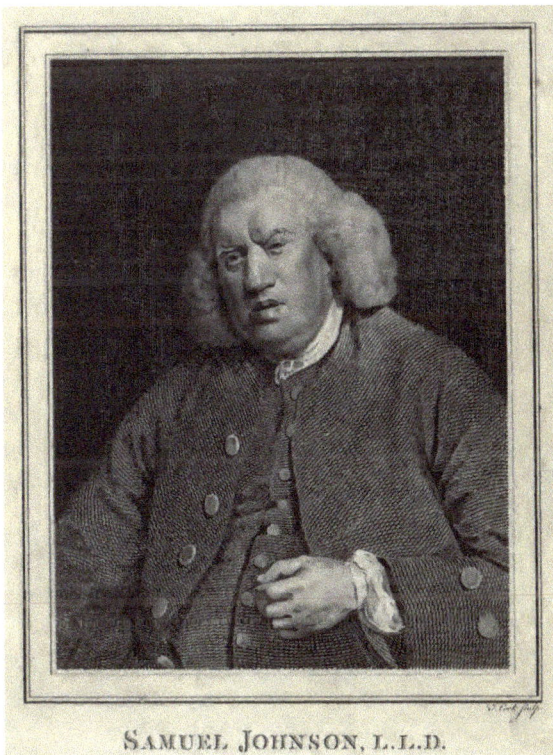

SAMUEL JOHNSON, L.L.D.
Public Domain

To 'Air' is Human

The word fart is proper English and was in use for hundreds of years before relatively recent polite and civil society considered it taboo. Without an alternative term, euphemisms were created and used. The number of terms that were synonymous with fart numbers in the many hundreds. The companion volume *Artsy Fartsy: Cultural History of the Fart* has an extensive inventory of such phraseology.

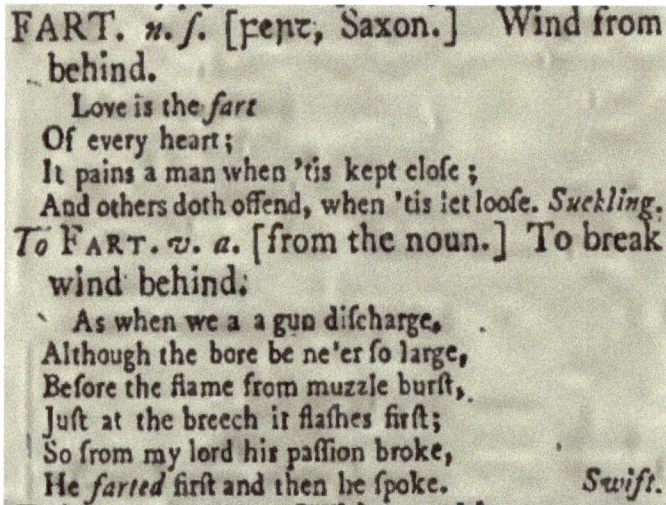

FART. *n. f.* [feɲꞇ, Saxon.] Wind from behind.

> Love is the *fart*
> Of every heart;
> It pains a man when 'tis kept clofe;
> And others doth offend, when 'tis let loofe. *Suckling.*

To FART. *v. a.* [from the noun.] To break wind behind.

> As when we a a gun difcharge,
> Although the bore be ne'er fo large,
> Before the flame from muzzle burft,
> Juft at the breech it flafhes firft;
> So from my lord his paffion broke,
> He *farted* firft and then he fpoke. *Swift.*

Public Domain

The origins of these phrases and their acceptance into the cultural lexicon, are often obscured. Sometimes new words are added directly by an author creatively using a newly invented word in a literary work. I am fond of a new word coined by David Gilmour, an entrepreneur, and philanthropist. He described a word that combines the sense of anticipation and subsequent disappointment, when the experience is not as satisfying as expected. The word he created 'anticipointment' is a portmanteau that should stand the test of time.

I am tempted to add to new words in the lexicon as well. I am using the author's prerogative to place the word in print below, and although I have not heard them elsewhere before, someone may well have created them before me. The word is fartigenic, or its alternative, fartogenic. Fartigenic is a portmanteau combining the word fart, with the Latin root suffix -genic of Genesis and creation fame. The term describes a substance, which induces the creation of a fart. Refried beans and chili con carne would be good examples of fartigenic foods.

The colloquialisms, idioms, and synonyms that for better or for worse, are part of the lexicon can be found in a number of resources including the unique companion volume to this book *Artsy Fartsy, Cultural History of the Fart.* This volume provides an informative and entertaining overview of the fart through human history and culture, including works of literature, music, and the arts.

To 'Air' is Human

Fart, Flammable

The individual gasses that make intestinal gas flammable (inflammable and flammable are synonyms and interchangeable words, their antonym nonflammable means the exact opposite) and explosive are hydrogen, methane, and oxygen. Hydrogen is a chemical element the symbol H and atomic number 1. It is the lightest element and in its single atom form it is by far the most abundant element in the universe, comprising approximately 75% of its total mass. In the earth's atmosphere as the diatomic H2 molecule, it is a colorless, odorless, tasteless, non-toxic, highly explosive gas. Most of the hydrogen on Earth is in molecules such as water and organic compounds because hydrogen readily forms covalent bonds.

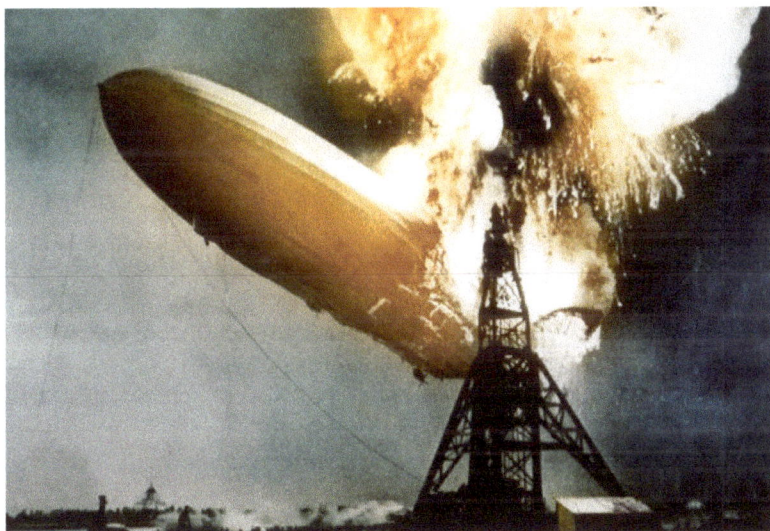

Public Domain

Hydrogen is lighter than air and lighter than helium. Unfortunately, it is also explosively flammable. Hydrogen fires are less destructive to immediate surroundings because of the buoyancy of H_2, which causes the heat of combustion to be released upwards as it ascends in the atmosphere. On May 6, 1937, the hydrogen-filled German airship Hindenburg burst into flames while attempting to land at Lakehurst, New Jersey. In little more than 30 seconds, the largest object ever to soar through the air was incinerated.

In 1766, Henry Cavendish was the first to identify hydrogen gas. In 1783 Antoine Lavoisier gave the element the name hydrogen (Greek ὕδρω hydro water and γενῆς genes creator) when he and Laplace confirmed Cavendish's finding that water is produced when hydrogen is burned. Methane is produced in the human intestinal tract by microbial organisms. Methanogens are microorganisms of the Kingdom Archaea, not bacteria as previously thought. They produce methane as a metabolic byproduct in anaerobic conditions when oxygen is not present.

To 'Air' is Human

Methanogens have been found in a variety of extreme environments, and can thrive and reproduce in boiling water as well as in ice cores taken miles down in arctic glaciers. They are common in wetlands, where they produce marsh gas, and in the digestive tracts of animals and humans where they generate the methane content of flatulence as well as the ruminant belch. It was discovered by Carl Scheele Sweden in 1773, but his publisher delayed publication for two years. The delay in publication inadvertently allowed British clergyman Joseph Priestley, who independently discovered it a year later, to be given priority as its discoverer because his work was published first.

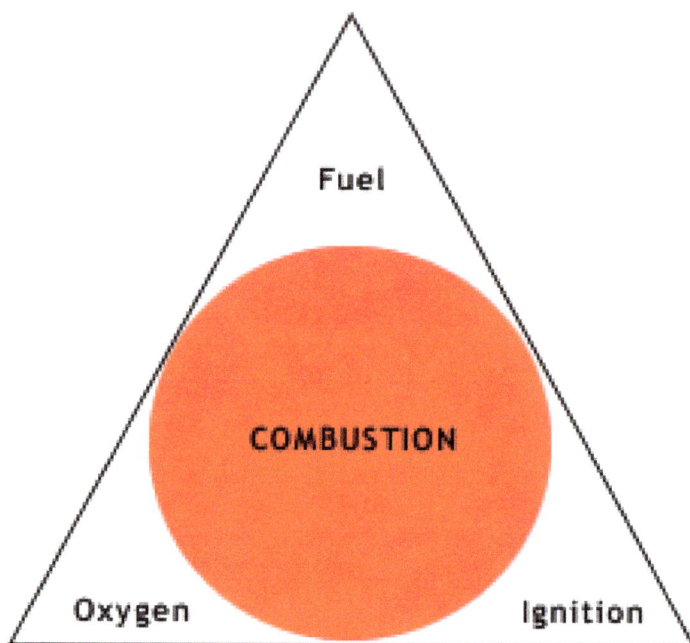

Oxygen is a chemical element with symbol O and atomic number 8 that firms dioxygen a colorless odorless and tasteless gas. It was mistakenly named Oxygen (the Greek ὀξύς (oxys) "acid", and γόνος (gonos) "producer"), by Antoine Lavoisier because he incorrectly thought that all acids required oxygen. Acids actually require the element hydrogen, not oxygen.

Oxygen is a highly reactive element that forms compounds with most elements except the noble gases. Oxygen is a strong oxidizing agent, and only fluorine has greater electronegativity. Oxygen is the third most abundant element in the universe, after hydrogen and helium. On the surface of the Earth, it is the most abundant element making up half of the earth's crust and nearly twenty-one percent of the air.

Intestinal gas that contains hydrogen or methane, in addition to oxygen, is potentially combustible. Electrical cautery devices used during routine colon and intestinal surgery can potentially ignite these gasses. With the advent of colonoscopy electro-cautery loop snares to remove colon polyps was developed. A few cases of fatal colonic explosions occurred before the danger of explosive intestinal gas was recognized as a risk of the procedure. The bowel preparation solution was found to increase hydrogen and methane gasses and raised the risk of explosion. The bowel preparation has been changed, and carbon dioxide is often used to inflate the colon to reduce the risk of explosion even further.

Now that you know intestinal gasses are flammable see if the numbers from the following Internet survey surprise you with how many people already knew this from personal experiments Hydrogen and Methane are combustible gasses. In the presence of oxygen and an ignition source, you have a potent flammable commodity. When methane burns, it has a characteristic blue flame that you may see in a pilot light if you have a gas stove or furnace. Adolescent males and those who remain as adolescents intellectually have a fondness for demonstrating their dragon-like ability to be human flamethrowers by igniting their farts. The lighting of farts is not a recommended activity, and severe injury has resulted from the successful ignition of flammable gasses near exposed sensitive anatomy.

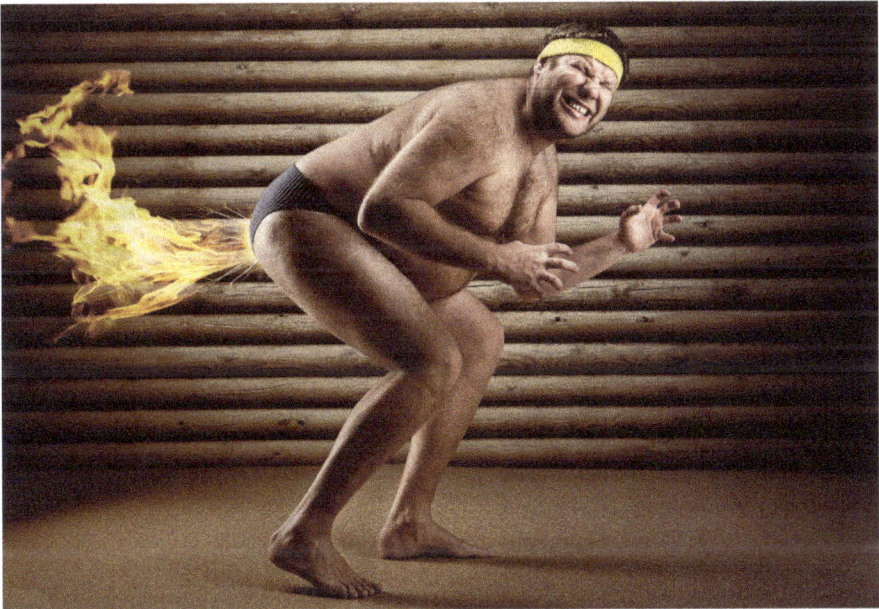

shutterstock/Nomad_Soul

One of the more unusual injuries from a lit fart was second and third degree burns on the buttocks and a broken arm. The stout gentlemen was sitting on the toilet defecating and farting extensively for some time. Being overweight his buttocks formed a firm seal around the toilet seat, retaining all of the gasses in the enclosed space of the toilet bowl. He was smoking at the time and made a little space under his cheeks to innocently toss the lit cigarette into the toilet bowl. It promptly ignited blowing him off the seat, shattering the porcelain toilet bowl, and causing extensive burn injuries to his buttocks. His wife called the paramedics, and as he was being carried down the stairwell to the waiting ambulance he told them what caused the explosion. They laughed so hard they dropped the gurney thus breaking his arm.

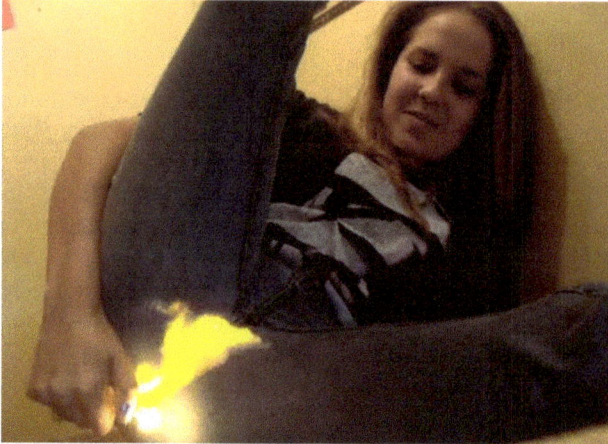

Moment of ignition of a fart, video is at youtu.be/Zt9rvaijpPY

Hydrogen and methane are the two flammable gasses that may be found in a fart making them flammable. Lighting a fart to see if one produces these gasses is a dangerous activity. Significant burns to the anogenital area have occurred, especially when ignited without a clothing barrier. The popular television show *Mythbusters* filmed an episode confirming that many farts are indeed flammable. It appears that the network found the episode too provocative and, perhaps for liability concerns that children watching might attempt their own demonstrations, decided to not 'air' the episode.

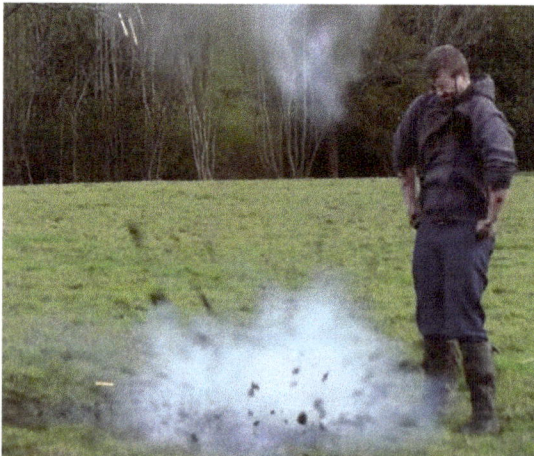

Lighting a match to a pile of cow dung is not a sign of higher intelligence. The methane and hydrogen generated by the microbes active in the manure pile may accumulate to explosive levels. youtu.be/bZI1eeV88lQ

To 'Air' is Human

On occasion dung and excrement can be more than just flammable, it can be explosive. The microorganisms that produce hydrogen and methane that lead to ignitable farts continue their activity while sitting in a pile. For those foolish enough to light a match in a pile of cow dung to see what happens up close and personal the link to the video above should be convincing.

Now that you know intestinal gasses are flammable see if the numbers from the following Internet survey surprise you with how many people already knew this from personal experiments.

Women: Have you ever considered lighting one of your pass intestinal gas?

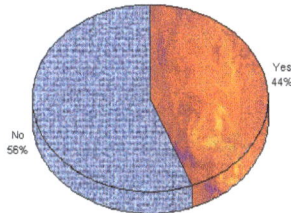

Almost half of the women surveyed indicate that they have considered an attempt to ignite their release of intestinal gas. They may not have done it or tried it, but they have thought about it.

Women: Have you ever attempted lighting one of your passages of intestinal gas?

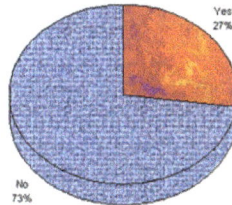

About a quarter of the women surveyed have attempted to ignited their passed intestinal gas.

Women: When you attempted to light your passed intestinal gas, did it ignite?

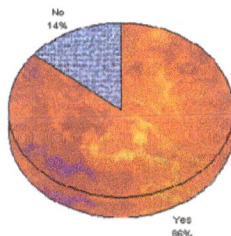

The large majority of women that have made the attempt were successful in confirming that the gas was flammable. The other fourteen percent may not have tried to ignite enough gas, or their diet and gut flora did not generate a flammable mixture of gasses. It appears that most women in the survey passed intestinal gas that burned with a blue flame due to the methane. Those who produced hydrogen had intestinal gas that burned with a yellow flame. Yellow flame was the second most common flame color.

Women: If you have lit your pass intestinal gas have you ever gotten burned?

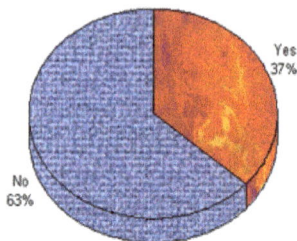

Yes
37%

No
63%

Women: If you lit your own pass intestinal gas and been burned was the of burn of your body, hair, or pants:

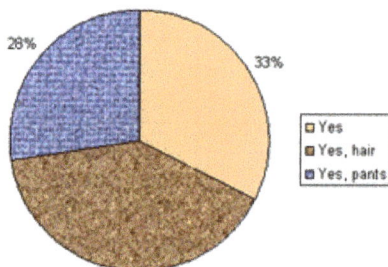

28%

33%

☐ Yes
☐ Yes, hair
☐ Yes, pants

Lighting pass intestinal gas can be very dangerous. About a third of the women that admit lighting their intestinal gas admit getting some type of burn. About half of these burns consist of just singing of hair. Twenty-eight percent of these burns consist of burning a hole in one's underwear, and thirty-three percent are unfortunate enough to burn their skin.

Women: Have you ever lit another person's intestinal gas?

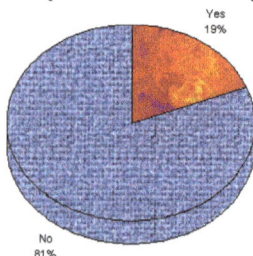

Yes
19%

No
81%

About one-fifth of the women surveyed were brave or foolish enough to light another person's intestinal gas. Most of these experiences were with friends or spouses. About half of the women surveyed admit seeing someone light a fart.

Spontaneous Human Combustion

As explosive and flammable farts are a well-recognized phenomenon, a theory has developed that they may also be responsible for spontaneous human combustion. A rare and bizarre event, spontaneous human combustion has been a proposed explanation of cases where a human body is consumed by flame without an external source of ignition. Typically the body is incinerated but the surrounding area has not been damaged by fire. Once a body begins to burn the tissue can continue to fuel the flames with a wick effect drawing on melted fat and other tissues.

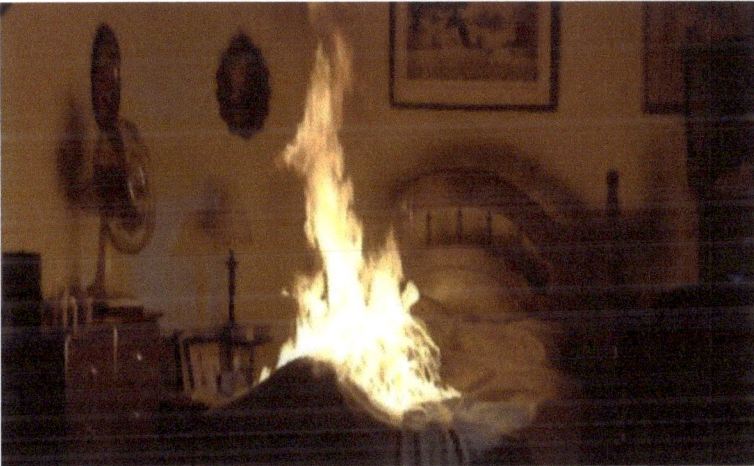

img.gawkerassets.com

Although the external source could not be identified, there are several potential explanations. Combustible fuel is undoubtedly present, perhaps as the gases methane and hydrogen, flammable clothing and alcohol, as well as body fat. Human fat is similar to the animal fats that were used in tallow candles. The external ignition source may have been a cigarette or spark of static electricity. Curious rural phenomena with similar spontaneous combustion effects include swamp gas, St. Elmo's fire, ball lightning, gamma ray discharges, and others.

Static electricity is an imbalance of electric charges between objects. As the imbalance is discharged with the transfer of electrons between the objects, most people can feel, see and hear the spark of the static shock. Lightning is a static discharge, different only in its intensity. A spark, which is responsible for the majority of industrial fires and explosions, occurs between objects at different electric potentials.

The energy released in a static electricity discharge may vary over a wide range and the charge buildup increases as the humidity decreases. As little as 0.2

milli joules is the ignition energy for methane, and a miniscule 0.017 mJ is the ignition energy for hydrogen. The low spark energy is often below the threshold of auditory, visual, or sensory perception of humans and may the ignition that results appears to be spontaneous.

The ignition of the flammable gasses of hydrogen and methane often present in fart may thus appear to be a spontaneous occurrence. Of course, there may have been a more obvious source such as a lit cigarette that was consumed in the event never to be found. There is a saying in medicine that is used as analogy for the search for a disease that will explain the symptoms. When you hear hoof beats, look for a horse, but be prepared for a zebra.

In spontaneous human combustion, the most likely explanation is an accidental fire from a cigarette. The cigarette may ignite the clothing and then the wicking effect continues to burn fueled by human tissue and fat until the body fire has exhausted itself. To be a bit more creative one can imagine a large fart with hydrogen and methane attracted the pet dog to come over and investigate the noise and smell. Close contact of the pet may have released a static spark and the rest is history. When in doubt, the standard excuse is to simply blame the poor dog.

Fart, Frequency

The fact is that all living creatures created gas from the cellular respiration, which is ubiquitous through life forms. The bacteria in your colonic flora generate microscopic nanofarts and microfarts, which collect into larger bubbles of gas in the bowel. They are intermixed with the atmospheric air swallowed throughout the day and particularly at meals, when chewing gum, chewing tobacco, or smoking tobacco or other recreational products.

Aerophagia is universal, and we swallow on average 3-5 cc (teaspoonful) of air with every swallow. Now add into the mixture the gasses produced during the enzymatic digestive processes as well as the neutralization of gastric hydrochloric acid and pancreatic and duodenal bicarbonate. You now have a virtual windstorm of voluminous gasses transiting the bowel.

Fortunately, the vast majority of the gasses produced are absorbed by the gut. They then enter into the bloodstream through diffusion, finally being exhaled when they reach the alveoli of the lungs. The component gasses have very different properties of diffusion through the bowel wall and into the bloodstream. Carbon dioxide readily diffuses and enters solution and is exhaled. Carbon dioxide is the largest volume of gas generated, and is a major contributor to distension and postprandial (after meal) discomfort. It is also the gas most readily absorbed and eliminated from the bowel. Carbon dioxide is thus only a minor contributor to flatulence.

Nitrogen is the largest volume component of atmospheric air, and as would be expected, represents an identically high proportion of the gasses swallowed

To 'Air' is Human

through aerophagia. Once in the body the carbon dioxide of the air is absorbed and eliminated as discussed above. The nitrogen however, is a very poorly absorbed gas, and will either come back up as a burp or come out the other end as a fart.

The oxygen in the air, representing nearly 21% of the air gasses swallowed during aerophagia, is absorbed slowly, as the gut is not nearly as efficient as the lungs for respiration. As the carbon dioxide and oxygen are absorbed the percent of the gastrointestinal tract air that is nitrogen increases. As soon as the digestive process begins, the hydrochloric acid of the stomach is neutralized by bicarbonate of the duodenum and pancreas. Large volumes of carbon dioxide gas are generated, as are smaller quantities of hydrogen, methane and other aromatic gasses.

The amount of gas in the gastrointestinal tract is dependent on the quantity and nature of foods ingested, and the body's ability to synthesize and utilize specific enzymes for the various food types. It is also dependent on the nature and number of the microorganisms in the gut flora, and the speed of gastrointestinal transit. Gastrointestinal transit may be influenced by drugs, hormones, food product, illness, the absorptive capacity of the mucosal lining, and the physical length of the individual's gastrointestinal tract.

The question of what is the average number of farts per day is similar to the question if what is an average price for a typical used car. To answer that question you would need more information, such as which year, make, model, condition, diesel or gas or electric or hybrid, mileage, etcetera. The quoted figure of 11.5 farts per day is a reasonable approximation. It came from a very small sample size of male medical students, but normal has a very wide range depending on the variables. The female medical students were too smart to participate in the study, so as far as science knows, women do not fart.

Later suggestions that they fart, but less than the guys, is just as suspect. The differences in the physical attributes of the male and female of a species represent their sexual dimorphism. The theory of sexual selection advanced by Charles Darwin in 1871 is closely related to sexual dimorphism. On average, adult humans males are four percent taller and eight percent heavier than females. In a number of other species, it is the female that is larger, occasionally dramatically so.

The triple wart sea devil, an anglerfish, exhibits extreme sexual dimorphism. The male becomes little more than a stunted sperm-producing body permanently attached to the female. It lives a parasitic existence off of the females hard work and effort in providing livelihood and producing the next generation of offspring. Some human males appear to have evolved their behavioral patterns from the anglerfish modus operandi.

In most mammals, humans included, the males are larger in size, mass, and caloric intake. In most species is the make that is diminutive in size, sometimes dramatically so. It would only make sense that makes would generate more gas, but how do the two compare if the caloric intake and composition were identical. Since there are no identically comparable cases studies would have to be average large populations of each gender and minimize the variables as much as possible.

As curious as we may be to know the answer to this question vital to gender politics and security, no studies are planned or anticipated. There have been reports of extreme flatulence in the medical literature of what may be considered the upper limits of the normal range, up to one hundred and fifty farts in a twenty-four hour period. There are probably more accurate reports of what is the upper limit of spousal tolerance in divorce court proceedings and depositions.

So for general health we talk about achieving our target heart rate during exercise. Is there an equivalent for a target fart rate? For harmonious relationships, ideal would be below the quoted figure of 11.5 farts per day, that way you could reasonably attest that you fart less than average. You could also argue that the twenty-three you passed were each only a half-fart so you still are within the normal range.

As we age, we produce less digestive enzymes, and there is an argument to be made that there should be an adjustment and tolerance allowed for 'old farts'. The sheer number of variables allow many explanations for why you fart much less than expected for your given circumstances. But perhaps the best excuse is that you did not do anything, it's the billions of nanofarting and microfarting microorganisms that are to blame. If you are told to pick on someone closer to your own size you could blame the dog and claim it is a talented ventrilo-farter.

Trying to arrive at a definition of what constitutes a discrete individual fart is a challenge worthy of drafting and approving a United Nations resolution. Is a staccato stutter, often very small farts completed in rapid succession, to count as one single fart or as ten? Is one large long loud fart the equivalent of four small farts over thirty seconds. Should a loud eardrum shattering tuba blast count the same as a faint and dainty toot? Perhaps the nebulous definition should allow the creator of the wonder poetic license.

Fart, Global Warming

Global warming due to greenhouse gas production from human activity is mainly due to deforestation, the combustion of fossil fuels, livestock enteric fermentation and manure management, and landfill emissions. In terms of biomass bacteria would be the main contributors to global warming by their methane production. A ruminant (Latin *ruminare* - to chew over again) is a mammal that digests plants in a multi compartment stomach through bacterial fermentation. It regurgitates the semi-digested mass, called cud, and chews it again and repeats the swallow. The process of re-chewing the cud is called "ruminating". There are about 150 species of ruminants, which include both domestic and wild species. Ruminating mammals include cattle, goats, sheep, giraffes, yaks, deer, camels, llamas, and antelope.

To 'Air' is Human

Other contenders nominated have been termites, which have over 2000 species and are prolific methane producers (initial reports suggested that they produce 40% of global methane), livestock such as cows, sheep, and pigs, and lastly dinosaurs, which are no longer around to defend their reputations.

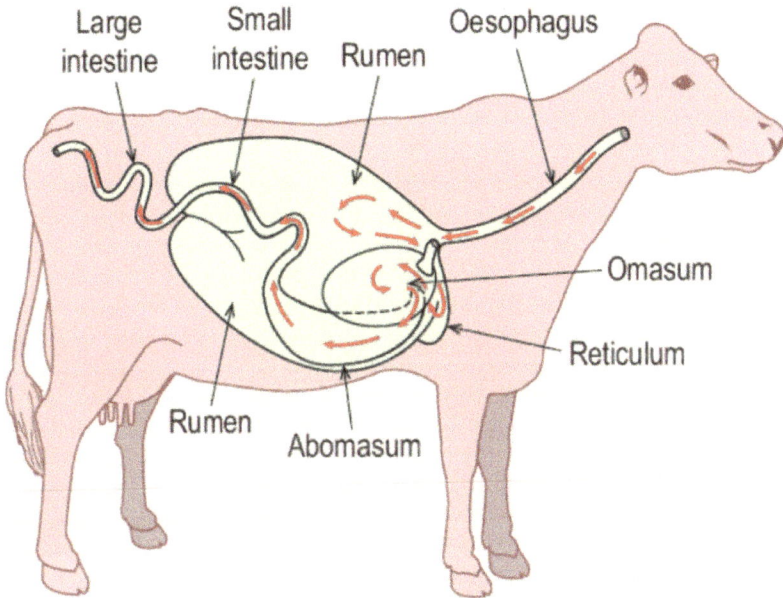

Creative Commons License

Ruminant bacterial fermentation is a significant contributor to global methane production, which is over twenty times as potent greenhouse gas. To incentivize efforts to reduce livestock methane production a number of countries have proposed taxes on the release of greenhouse gasses. University of Alberta, Canada, Professor Stephen Moore is examining the genes from ruminant stomachs with the goal of developing a cow breed which burps less to reduce methane in the greenhouse gases responsible for global warming. A different approach is being undertaken by Professor of Animal Nutrition Winfried Drochner at the University of Hohenheim, Stuttgart, Germany. A fist-sized plant-based pill bolus combined with a special diet and strict feeding times reduces the methane produced by cows. "Our aim is to increase the wellbeing of the cow, to reduce the greenhouse gases produced and to increase agricultural production all at once. It is an effective way of fighting global warming. We could use the energy to boost the cow's metabolism, the fist-sized tablets mean that microbiotic substances can slowly dissolve in the cow's stomach over several months," said Professor Drochner.

Another method being used to reduce methane emissions is reducing the grass and low efficiency foods the livestock are receiving that require excessive fermentation. Replacing the feed with a diet higher in energy and rich in edible oils can reduce methane production by up to 25%. New Hampshire-based Stonyfield Farm reduced emissions from their cows an average of 12 percent by adding alfalfa, flax or hemp to livestock feed. 'If every U.S. dairy farmer reduced emissions by 12 per cent it would be equal to about half a million cars being taken off the road,' said Nancy Hirshberg, Vice-President of Stonyfield's Natural Resources department. It took extensive scientific experimentation to collect the intestinal gasses of herds of cattle before it was discovered that the methane production was coming from the other end of the cows and other ruminants. It is the burps and belches from the multi compartment ruminant stomach that is the primary source of methane.

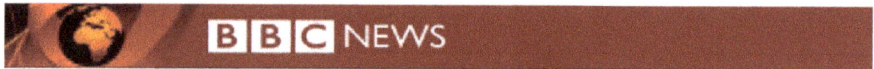

BBC NEWS

FLATULENCE TAX

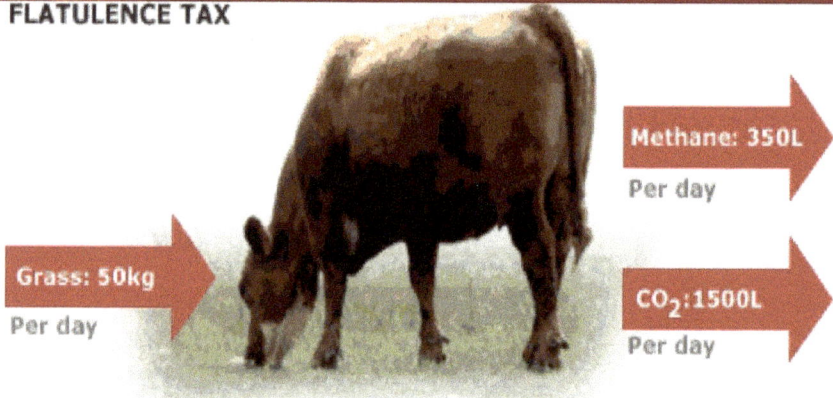

Grass: 50kg Per day

Methane: 350L Per day

CO_2:1500L Per day

	COW	SHEEP
Example herd size	500	3,000
Methane produced*	63,875,000	21,900,000
CO2 produced*	273,750,000	82,125,000
Tax per litre	$0.046	$0.0003
Tax per farmer	$300	$300

*- Litres per year

In spite of it being labeled as a flatulence tax, the predominant source of global warming from ruminants comes from fermentation in their multi compartment stomachs. It should really be called a burping and belching tax, but that is not as newsworthy.

Kangaroos are herbivores and as marsupial their burps and farts contain little or no methane, a potent greenhouse gas. It appears that the reduced methane emissions are due to the microbes in the kangaroos' gut flora. Australian researchers hope that introducing a similar gut flora to other methane producing herbivores such as cattle and sheep will contribute to a reduction in greenhouse gasses and the resultant global warming. Methane can cause about 20 times as much atmospheric warming as an equivalent volume of carbon dioxide.

Kangaroos, like cattle and sheep, are ruminants that re-chew their cud with the assistance of the gut flora to digest the and metabolize their cellulose based grazing diet. In the foregut the meal is broken down by fermentation with carbon dioxide and hydrogen released. In cows and other ruminants, microbes called methanogens transform these gases into methane. But in the kangaroos' guts the same hydrogen and carbon dioxide may be utilized by bacteria called acetogens to produce acetate, a volatile fatty acid.

These microbes compete with methanogens to use the carbon dioxide and hydrogen, so the more acetogens the less methane production. The odds are in generally in favor of methanogens, since the process of methane production is generally more energy efficient than producing acetate. One of the acetogen microbes, *Blautia coccoides,* is in the gut flora of cows as well as in kangaroos. Further research is being undertaken to understand why the organism is more successful in competing with the methanogens in kangaroos than in other herbivores.

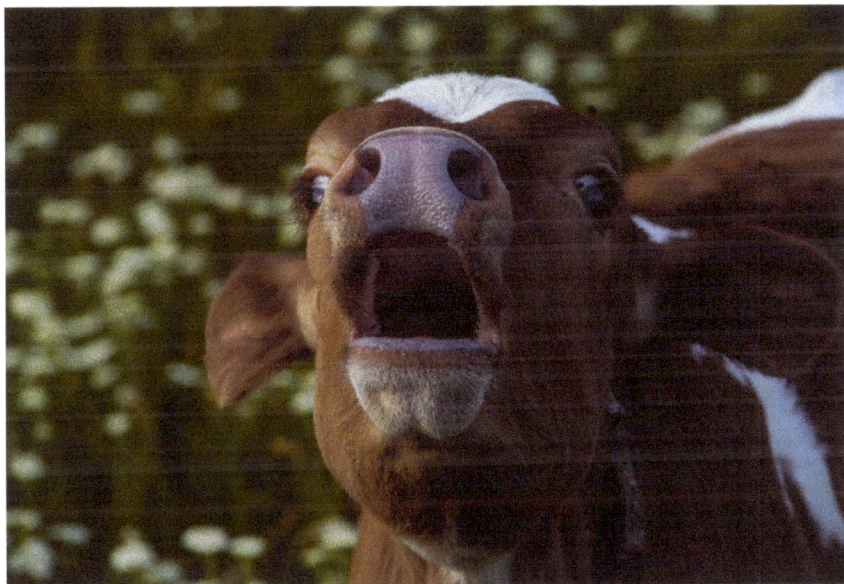

It is the burps and belches from the multi compartment ruminant stomach that is the primary source of methane. shutterstock/AlisaBurkova

Carbon dioxide, methane, nitrous oxide (N_2O) and three groups of fluorinated gases (sulfur hexafluoride (SF_6), hydro fluorocarbons (HFCs), and per fluorocarbons (PFCs) are the major greenhouse gases impacted by human activity. These are regulated under the Kyoto Protocol an international treaty that was adopted in 2005. Nitrogen dioxide (NO_2) warms the atmosphere 310 times more than carbon dioxide and methane 21 times more than carbon dioxide. Although CFCs are greenhouse gases, regulations were initiated because CFCs' cause ozone depletion, not because of their contribution to global warming. Ozone depletion itself has a relatively minor effect on greenhouse warming.

To 'Air' is Human

Dinosaurs are no longer around to defend themselves and have been accused of contributing to global warming. We do not know if they were ruminants and contributed by belching up gasses as well, but there should be no doubt that they were big time farters. Their nickname "thunder lizards" may have more to do with their farts than their footsteps. For more information about fart contributions to global warming see entries on methane and carbon dioxide.

Fart, History & Culture (Art, Music, Literature)

Artsy Fartsy: Cultural History of the Fart is a fascinating and factually correct review of the common fart through human culture and history. The cough, sneeze, hiccup, stomach rumble, burp, belch, and other bodily sounds simply cannot compete with the notoriety of the fart. Whether encountered live and in person or through the medium of literature, television, film, art, or music it may leave a powerful and lingering memory.

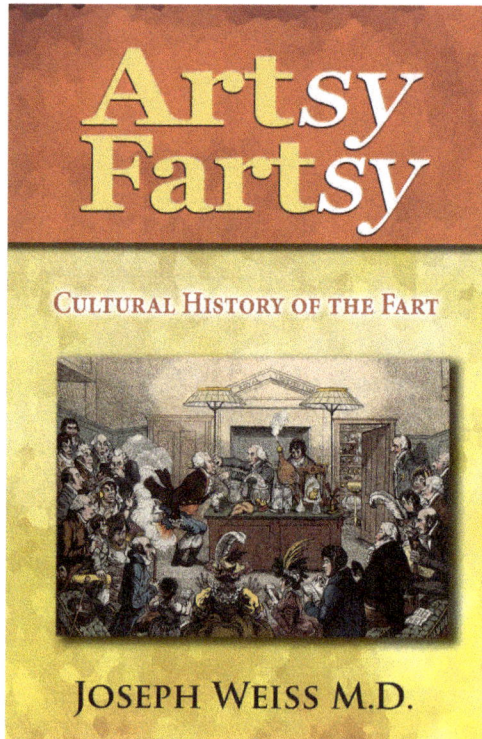

The history of the fart in culture and society is a seldom told but fascinating tale. The very same fart that has triggered wars and the deaths of thousands of innocents (see entry on Flavius Josephus) has also led to the laughter and entertainment of millions worldwide (see entry on Joseph Pujol and Cinematic Arts). Even today the response to a fart can reach from the extremes of triggering violence to inducing spasms of uncontrollable laughter.

To 'Air' is Human

The intent of *Artsy Fartsy: Cultural History of the Fart* is to demonstrate that the ubiquitous fart has a more illustrious story to share than just lowbrow humor. The societal standards and cultural acceptance of this normal physiologic event have evolved over the years, and it is currently popular as a point of humor even in sophisticated circles. *Artsy Fartsy*, is a chronological survey of some of the high and low points in the cultural history of this ubiquitous but inherently controversial activity. Rather than an exhaustive and long-winded discourse, this volume is meant to introduce the reader to the colorful and extremely varied response to the fart over the course of human history.

The book provides an entertaining overview of the fart in human culture and history, not an extensively referenced academic treatise. The number of references to farts in the arts, especially over the recent years, is so numerous that a complete list is not practical or possible. The good news for those wanting more in depth information about any author, artist, or topic of interest is the powerful reference resource of the Internet.

I expect that many will be surprised that the fart was a subject near to the hearts and minds of many illustrious and enlightened notables over the course of thousands of years of human history. The cultural mores of Western society have evolved and the fart has become a normal physiological event that has become more tolerated, although not yet universally accepted.

Fart Non-Human

Blue Whale

The Blue Whale is the largest animal on Earth, up to 100 feet (30 meters) long and 170 tons. The blue whale is a mammal that ingests and digests up to 8 tons of plankton per day. The wale digestive tract generates large quantities of gas and when the blue whale releases a fart the bubble expands as it rises to the surface. The decreasing atmospheric pressure as it continues to rise contributes to its expansion as described in physics by Boyle's Law. When it just reaches the surface of the ocean the fart bubble is so huge it could easily enclose and asphyxiate a large horse.

Cat

Cats fart just like dogs, but they are wiser and more discreet. Because of they are generally more diminutive in size than dogs they are not as easily identified or innocently blamed as the source of the fart. The alpha-galactosidase enzyme has also been marketed as a veterinary product with the brand name Curtail. It has been offered as a solution for dogs and cats that have farted one time too many.

Cow, Sheep, & Ruminant

A ruminant (Latin *ruminare* - to chew over again) is a mammal that digests plants in a multi compartment stomach through bacterial fermentation. It regurgitates the semi-digested mass, called cud, and chews it again and repeats the swallow. The process of re-chewing the cud is called "ruminating". There are about 150 species of ruminants, which include both domestic and wild species. Ruminating mammals include cattle, goats, sheep, giraffes, yaks, deer, camels, llamas, and antelope. Ruminant bacterial fermentation is a significant contributor to global methane production, which is over twenty times as potent greenhouse gas. Please see the entries on Global Warming and Methane for more details about ruminant gas production.

Dinosaur

Dinosaurs are no longer around to defend themselves and have been accused of contributing to global warming. We do not know if they were ruminants and contributed by belching up gasses as well, but there should be no doubt that they were big time farters. Their nickname "thunder lizards" may have more to do with their farts than their footsteps.

The hulking sauropods were widespread about 150 million years ago, and methane-producing microbes aided the sauropods' digestion by fermenting their plant food. Dave Wilkinson of Liverpool John Moores University, Graeme Ruxton from the University of St Andrews, and methane expert Euan Nisbet at the University of London studied the implications. Wilkinson, Ruxton, and Nisbet calculated global methane emissions from sauropods to have been approximately 520 million tons per year. By comparison modern livestock ruminant animals produce methane emission of up to 100 million tons per year.

There is a common public misperception that petroleum is predominantly derived from the organic remains of the great dinosaurs. Rather than the enormous dinosaurs, it was microscopic bacteria that produced the petroleum reserves if our time period. Single-celled bacteria evolved in the earth's oceans about three billion years ago, and were the dominant life form on the planet until about 600 million years ago. In fact, if dominant is qualified as largest by biomass, bacteria retain that distinction today.

As microscopic as the individual bacteria may be, the bacterial colonies known as "mats" were of enormous proportions. They had masses of millions of tons compared to the hundred tons for the largest dinosaur, the sauropods. As these massive colonies died off and decayed they subsided to the bottom of the sea and were covered by layers of accumulating sediments. Over millions of years these layers of sediment thousands of feet underground were compressed under tremendous pressure and temperature, and developed into the liquid hydrocarbons we recognize as petroleum.

The vast majority of the world's coal deposits date back to the Carboniferous period, about 300 million years ago. The first dinosaurs would not make their grand entrance in the evolutionary timetable until 75 million years later. During the Carboniferous period the earth was heavily forested. With the death and decomposition of these trees and plant life buried under great pressure and temperature under heavy layers of sediment, they were transformed into solid coal rather than liquid petroleum. As the search for petroleum and coal preserves often entails drilling and excavation of deep layers of sediment, it is not uncommon for fossils of dinosaurs and other prehistoric forms of life to be uncovered. The discovery of a theropod dinosaur during fossil fuel exploration in China has been given the appropriate name Gasosaurus. It looks as though Dino's story may have come full circle.

Dog

Dogs are just like any other organism, they do fart. Some breeds fart more than others especially the short snouted English bulldog and similar breeds are serious air swallowers and farters. Several hundred years ago lap dogs were specifically bred to be small enough for a lady to keep with her at all times and if intestinal gas ruffled her undergarments it would not ruffle her composure as she would simply excuse her dog for the emission

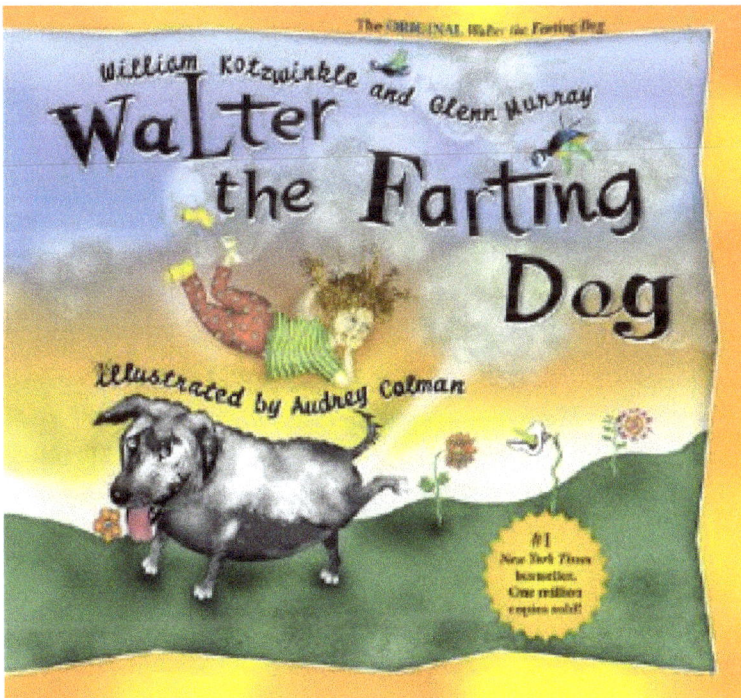

Walter the Farting Dog by William Kotzwinkle & Glenn Murray.

Hippopotamus

The hippopotamus (Greek hippos-horse and potamus-river) is considered by many experts to be the most dangerous animal in Africa (excluding the malaria carrying mosquito) having killed many more people than lions have. The hippo is extremely aggressive with its huge canine teeth and sharp incisors, unpredictable and fearless of humans. Most deaths occur when the victim gets between the hippo and deep water or between a mother and her calf.

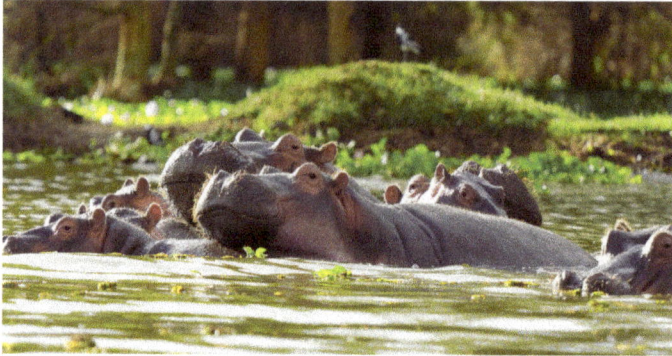

Hippopatamus shutterstock/IvanMateev

Hippos weigh up to 8000 pounds, gallop at 18 M.P.H., sleep or lounge around on riverbanks and in the water most of the day, and graze on the grasslands at night. Their skin secretes a sticky pinkish oil that helps protect them from the sun. They defecate generous amounts of excrement into the rivers and ponds in which they wallow all day, punctuated by voluminous farts. They also participate in marking territory by what the hippo experts refer to as "dung showering." They blow feces mixed with urine over a large area around their watering hole, twirling their relatively short tails like fans to distribute the aromatic spray.

Horse

The well-known phenomenon of horse farts have been exploited on television with an episode of the comedy series Seinfeld entitled the Rye. Cramer feeds the horse a beef and pasta meal pulling a hansom carriage in Central Park in New York City. It makes the horse so extremely flatulent so that Cramer and the passengers in the carriage cannot bear the gas exposure.

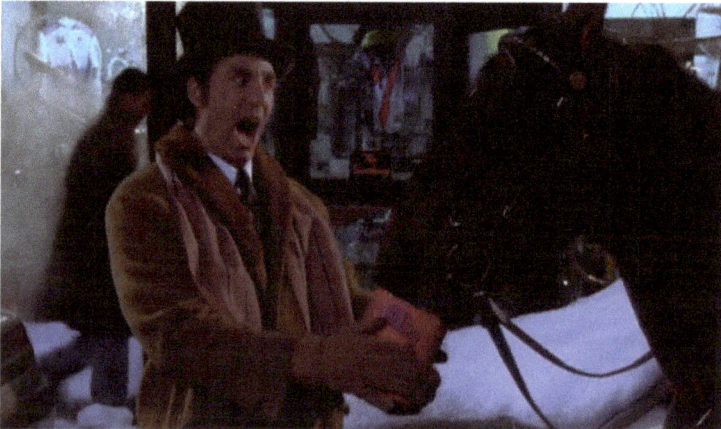

mapsaboutnothing.wordpress.com

To 'Air' is Human

A similar equine theme took place in a prime and extremely expensive Super Bowl advertisement for Budweiser beer. A man and a young woman are in a romantic horse drawn carriage. He presents her with a lit candle and reaches down to pull up some bottles of Budweiser beer. As he is out of the way getting the beer the horses tail lifts and the candle explodes in a ball of flame singeing her features. When he resurfaces he smells smoke and asks if she smells a barbeque.

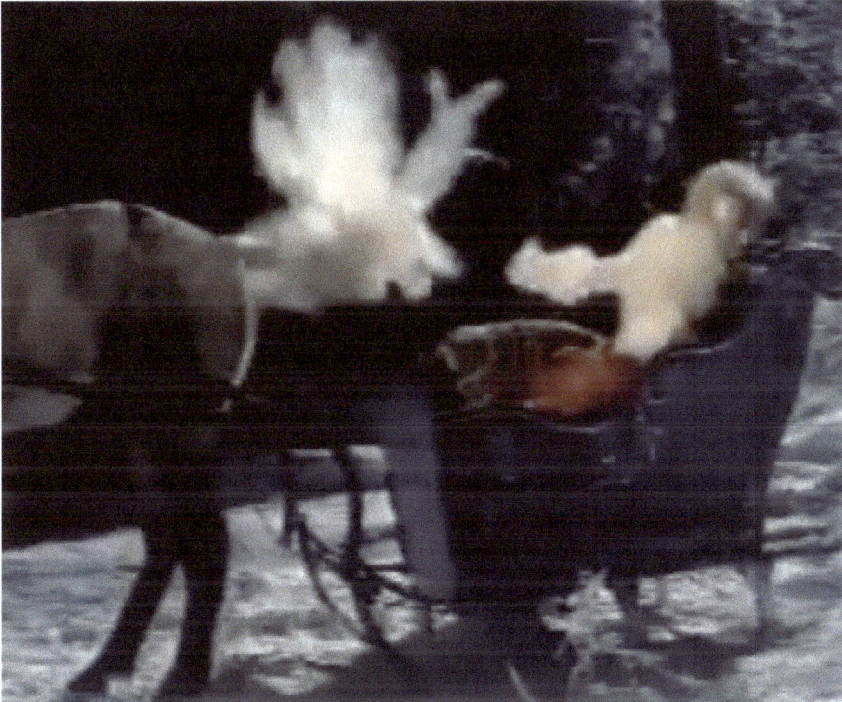

critbritlit.blogspot.com Creative Commons License

Ronald Wilson Reagan (1911 – 2004) was the fortieth President of the United Sates. I heard an apocryphal story from a normally reliable source that served in a high position in the administration of former president Ronald Reagan. Then again the source was a politician, which should automatically double the suspicion that this story was just the continued passage of excessive hot air.

Her Majesty, Queen Elizabeth II was visiting the presidential ranch, Rancho Cielo, in the Santa Ynez Mountains of California. The ranch is at a high elevation (Rancho Cielo is Spanish for Sky Ranch) and as both the president and queen are horse aficionados they went for a ride on the ranch trails. At higher altitude, as you may recall from Boyle's Law of the physics of gasses, the atmospheric pressure is less than at sea level and the volume of gasses expands. The horse's intestinal tracts likewise experienced expanding gasses and being natural animals they release it at will, even if they are in the presence of a Royal Queen and President

To 'Air' is Human

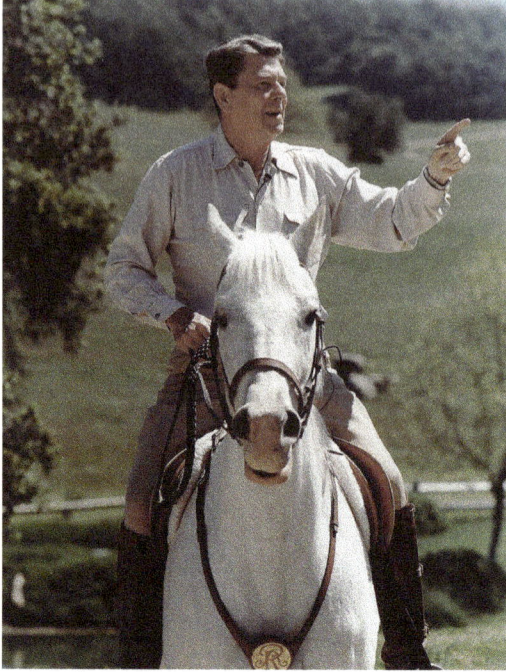

US President Ronald Reagan riding a white horse. 2004 Pete Souza official White House photographer
Public Domain

Along the trail the Queen's horse in particular became increasingly flatulent with noisy and pungent emissions. At one point the aroma became particularly strong and the Queen said to Mr. Reagan. "Mr. President I really must apologize for the terrible aroma." Some observers thought that perhaps President Reagans Alzheimer Disease was beginning to take hold, but much more likely it was his quick wit that rose to the occasion. Mr. Regan responded, "Your Majesty, you needn't have apologized at all. In fact, if you hadn't said anything, I would have thought it was the horses!"

Kangaroo

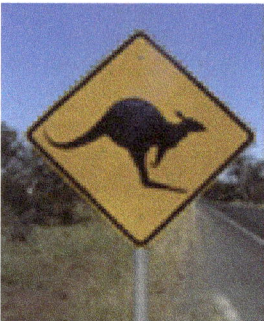

img1-azcdn.newser.com Creative Commons License

To 'Air' is Human

Kangaroos are herbivores and as marsupial their burps and farts contain little or no methane, a potent greenhouse gas. It appears that the reduced methane emissions are due to the microbes in the kangaroos' gut flora. Australian researchers hope that introducing a similar gut flora to other methane producing herbivores such as cattle and sheep will contribute to a reduction in greenhouse gasses and the resultant global warming. Methane can cause about 20 times as much atmospheric warming as an equivalent volume of carbon dioxide.

Kangaroos, like cattle and sheep, are ruminants that re-chew their cud with the assistance of the gut flora to digest the and metabolize their cellulose based grazing diet. In the foregut the meal is broken down by fermentation with carbon dioxide and hydrogen released. In cows and other ruminants, microbes called methanogens transform these gases into methane. But in the kangaroos' guts the same hydrogen and carbon dioxide may be utilized by bacteria called acetogens to produce acetate, a volatile fatty acid.

These microbes compete with methanogens to use the carbon dioxide and hydrogen, so the more acetogens the less methane production. The odds are in generally in favor of methanogens, since the process of methane production is generally more energy efficient than producing acetate. One of the acetogen microbes, *Blautia coccoides,* is in the gut flora of cows as well as in kangaroos. Further research is being undertaken to understand why the organism is more successful in competing with the methanogens in kangaroos than in other herbivores.

Microbe

Microbes including bacteria, Archaea, fungi, viruses, protists, and parasites are a major component of the gastrointestinal tract flora, also known as the gut microbiome. These organisms play a major role in the metabolism of the diet, and thus play a direct role in intestinal gas production. Although the organism's microfarts may seem to be inconsequential, the trillions of their numbers make them major contributors to the intestinal gasses of all larger organisms. The methane production that used to be blamed on bacteria is actually generated by the non-bacterial microbes from the Kingdom Archaea.

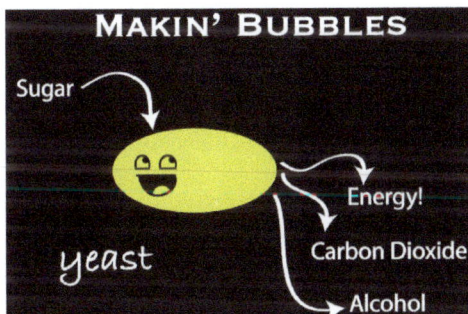

MAKIN' BUBBLES

Sugar

yeast

Energy!

Carbon Dioxide

Alcohol

domesticlabrat.files.wordpress.com Creative Commons License

To 'Air' is Human

The gastrointestinal tract flora, is influenced by many environmental factors. These include diet, water purity, antibiotic exposure, chemicals, pesticides, and exposure the microbiome of others. The gastrointestinal tract of the newborn is sterile at birth, but rapidly becomes colonized by microbes that are swallowed. Infants born via a normal vaginal delivery have a markedly different microbiome than those delivered by Cesarean section. Those born by Cesarean section have a higher incidence of allergies, asthma, and immune disorders.

Plant

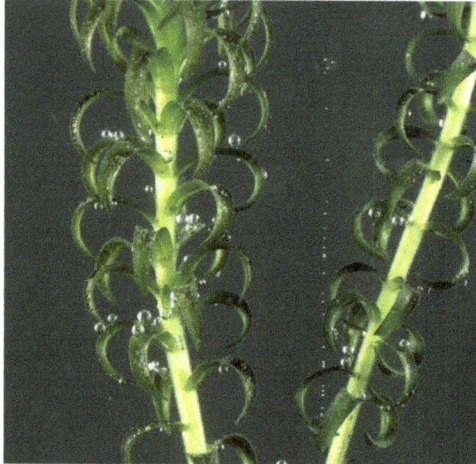

Plant placed underwater to demonstrate the production and release of oxygen gas bubbles
www.pinterest.com Creative Commons License

Plant life also contributes to gas production, but one of the most important gasses the produce as far as humans are concerned is oxygen. Although not described as a fart, the plant release of gas is analogous to a fart as it is a gas waste product of their metabolism. It just so happens that their waste product of oxygen is one humans and other animals , which we require for life.

Plants are also critically important in taking carbon dioxide out of the atmosphere as well as fixing nitrogen into products the other life forms can access and utilize. With plant death the decay of decomposing organic matter adds gasses that can contribute to global warming.

Stinkbug

The stinkbug is an agricultural pest which has caused significant losses of fruit and vegetable crops in numerous countries including the United States. They invade human domestic dwellings during cold winter months. When they find a comfortable habitat they release an aggregation pheromone to attract other stinkbugs, which huddle closely together. The pheromone does not have an unpleasant aroma. They lay about 400 eggs which hatch in less than a week. One home found to be harboring 26,000 stinkbugs. They do not damage the house structure and they do not bite humans. The stink glands are located on the underside of the thorax, between the first and second pair of legs, and on the dorsal surface of the abdomen. Although the stink glands are associated with the insect's abdomen they are not an intestinal gas, although some incorrectly believe this is the source of odor.

The odor from the stink gland is due to its release of chemicals including the aldehydes trans-2-decenal and trans-2-Octenal, both of which have a pungent odor similar to cilantro and coriander. Most people find the aroma offensive but others do not, perhaps due to a genetic basis. Some species also release a cyanide compounds with a rancid almond scent. The odor is a defense mechanism and the insect can control the quantity ejected as well as whether just one or both glands are activated. Stinkbugs are commonly eaten in Laos, where the extremely strong odor s believe to enhance the flavor. The insects are crushed and mixed with seasoning including chilies and herbs creating a paste known as cheo.

Termite

Termites are major producers of methane and because of the enormous size of the termite population and biomass they are thought to be significant contributors to global warming producing over twenty-five percent of the world total methane production. Of interest, termites trapped in the sap of a tree have often been frozen in time as the sap turns to amber over the ages.

The tiny bubble of gas at the tail end of the termite entrapped in amber has been analyzed and is indeed methane produced thousands of years ago from the bacterial fermentation of the wood termites ingest. The termite gut microbiome flora generates tiny bacterial nanofarts, which coalesce into the termite microfarts that have been captured in amber eons ago.

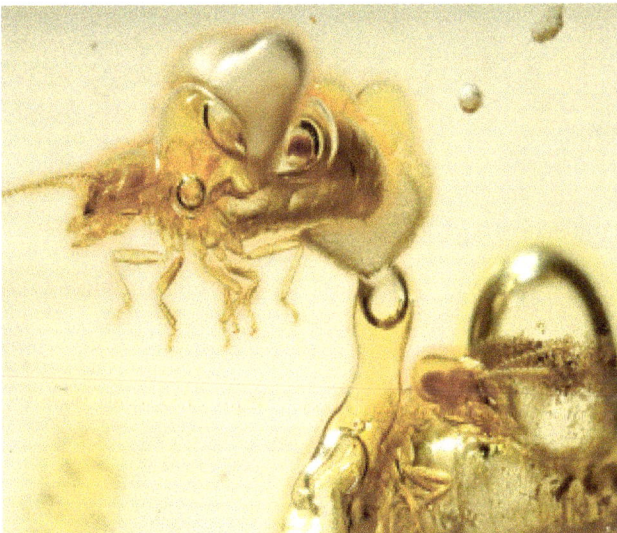

Termite farts trapped in amber have been analyzed for gas composition and indeed it is methane.
1.bp.blogspot.com Creative Commons License

To 'Air' is Human

Fart, Smell (Aroma, Olfaction)

Olfaction, also known as olfactics is the scientific term for the sense of smell. Olfaction occurs when odorant molecules bind to specific sites known as the olfactory receptors. The olfactory receptors are specialized sensory cells in the nasal cavity of vertebrates. Invertebrates, such as insects, typically house their olfactory sense organ on their antennae. In the snake the olfactants are acquired by the tongue, which taking advantage of its forked anatomy deposits them on the olfactory cells on the respective sides of the nasal cavity. The difference in concentration of the olfactants on each side of the nasal cavity allows the receptors to discriminate and localize the source of the scent, much like binocular vision allows depth perception. Because humans and other animals have two nostrils, each with separate inputs to the brain, it is possible for them to have perceptual rivalry in the olfactory sense akin to binocular vision.

Many vertebrates, including most mammals and reptiles, have two distinct olfactory systems. The main olfactory system identifies general odorants while the accessory olfactory system is used mainly to detect pheromones. For air-breathing animals the main olfactory system detects volatile aerosolized chemicals, and the accessory olfactory system detects chemicals usually in the fluid phase. Olfaction, along with taste, is a form of chemoreception. Although taste and smell are separate sensory systems in land animals, water-dwelling organisms often have one chemical sense.

Odors are also commonly called scents, and these terms can refer to both pleasant and unpleasant stimuli. The terms fragrance and aroma are used primarily by the food and cosmetic industry to describe a pleasant odor, often referred to as a perfume or bouquet. In contrast malodor, stench, reek, and stink are used specifically to describe unpleasant odor. The sense of smell gives rise to the perception of odors, mediated by the olfactory nerve. The olfactory receptor (OR) cells are neurons present in the olfactory epithelium, a small patch of tissue in back of the nasal cavity. There are millions of olfactory receptor neurons, each neuron has hair-like projections known as cilia. The cilia has receptor proteins that are in direct contact with air and bind directly with the odorant chemicals and molecules initiating a neuron mediated electric signal. Volatile small molecule odorants, non-volatile proteins, and non-volatile hydrocarbons may all produce olfactory responses and sensations. Much like some animal species are able to visualize ultraviolet or infrared beyond the spectrum visible to humans a number can smell carbon dioxide and other odorants that are not detectable and thus considered odorless based on human sensitivity.

Olfaction, taste, and trigeminal receptors with a property known as chemesthesis together contribute to flavor. The human tongues us able to distinguish five distinct qualities of taste, salt, sweet, acidic, bitter, and umami. The nose and olfactory sense of smell has a much greater sense of discrimination can distinguish among hundreds of substances, even in extremely minute quantities. The olfactory sense of smell takes place during inhalation, while the olfactory contribution to flavor occurs during exhalation. The olfactory system is unique among the human senses in that the neural pathway bypasses the thalamus and provides neural input directly to the forebrain. In human females the sense of olfaction is strongest around the time of ovulation, significantly stronger than during other phases of the menstrual cycle and stronger than the sense in males. The association of heightened olfactory sensitivity in association with ovulation has raised speculation about pheromone activity in humans but it has yet to be scientifically confirmed.

Scent hounds as a group can smell one- to ten-million times more acutely than a human, and bloodhounds , which have the keenest sense of smell of any dogs, have noses ten- to one-hundred-million times more sensitive than a human's. They were bred for the specific purpose of tracking humans, and can detect a scent trail a few days old. The second-most-sensitive nose is possessed by the Basset Hound, which was bred to track and hunt rabbits and other small animals. The silvertip grizzly bear found in parts of North America, have a sense of smell seven times stronger than that of the bloodhound. This keen sense of smell is essential for its skill in locating food underground. Bears can detect the scent of food from up to 18 miles away.

Olfaction, the sense of smell, is a form of chemoreception that in humans occurs when odorant molecules bind to olfactory receptors. The stimulation of olfactory and taste receptors is through a process known as chemesthesis. Cloning of olfactory receptor proteins and identifying that odor molecules bind to specific receptors led to the 2004 Nobel Prize award to Linda B. Buck and Richard Axel.

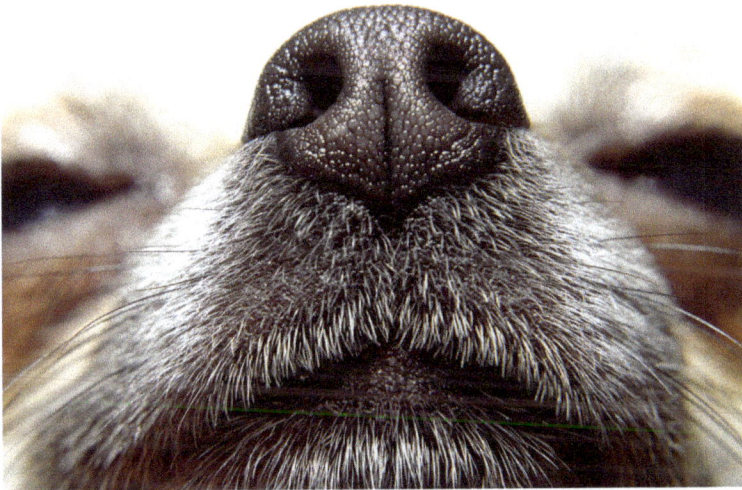

shutterstock/bimka

Females have greater olfactory sensitivity than males, particularly at the time of ovulation. More than pheromones is involved and females can detect by olfaction potential mates that have a genetic diversity that would be beneficial for their offspring. Odor information is retained in long-term memory and the olfactory system is anatomically associated with the regions of the brain associated with emotion. It has been long recognized that odors can trigger memories and emotions from remote times.

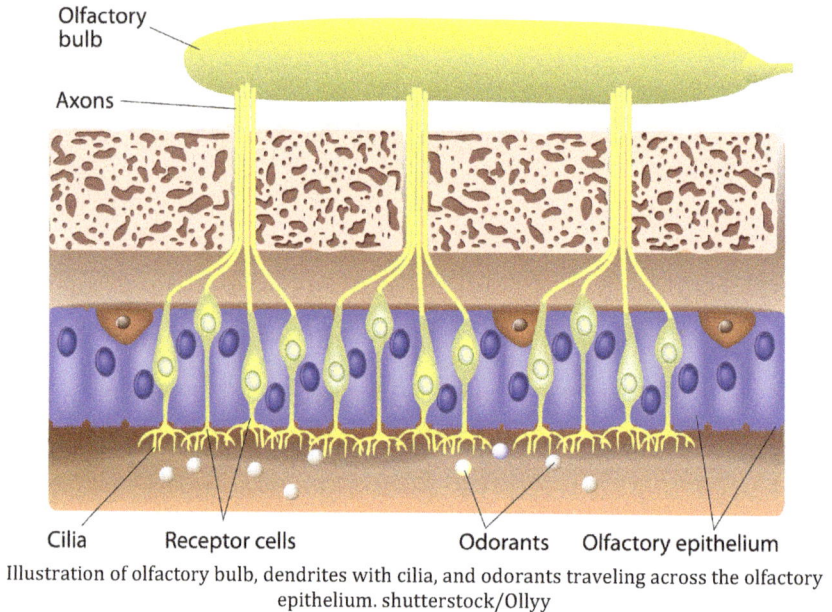

Illustration of olfactory bulb, dendrites with cilia, and odorants traveling across the olfactory epithelium. shutterstock/Ollyy

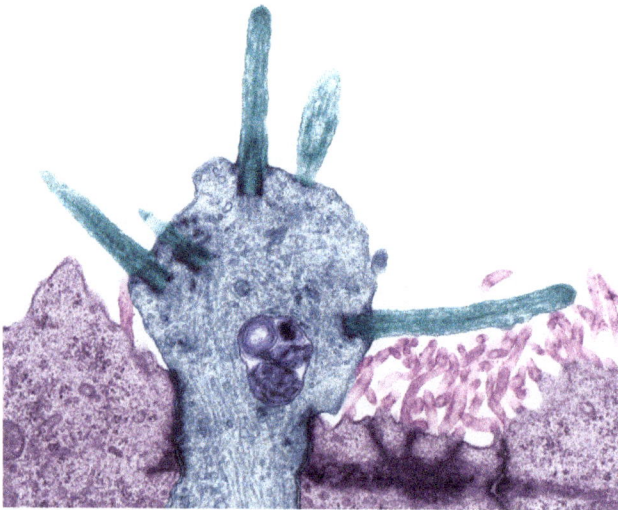

The sense of olfaction is the most sensitive of all human senses. The nose can identify the single scented molecule hiding amongst two billion unscented ones. To use a visual analogy, paint one single square sheet of a toilet paper roll the

color red. Now wrap that unlimited length roll of toilet paper around the twenty five thousand mile long equator of the planet earth, and go around a second time, a third, a fourth, and a full fifth time.

Your nose can instantaneously identify the single red square of a one hundred and twenty five thousand mile roll of toilet paper. Are you impressed with our sense of smell? Just like wealth and beauty there is always someone who has more to keep us from being number one. Human's olfactory epithelium is less than ten of the surface area of dog, which also has one hundred times more receptors per square centimeter.

Bloodhounds have olfactory receptors up to one hundred million times the sensitivies of humans and are trained to track a human trail several days old. North American grizzly bears have the keenest sense if smell seven times greater than the bloodhound.

Salmon utilize their keen sense of smell in ocean waters to locate the stream from which they hatchlings years earlier to return to spawn. A mosquito smelling the "odorless" carbon dioxide that mammals exhale to locate their next blood meal illustrates the olfactory sensitivity located on their antennae.

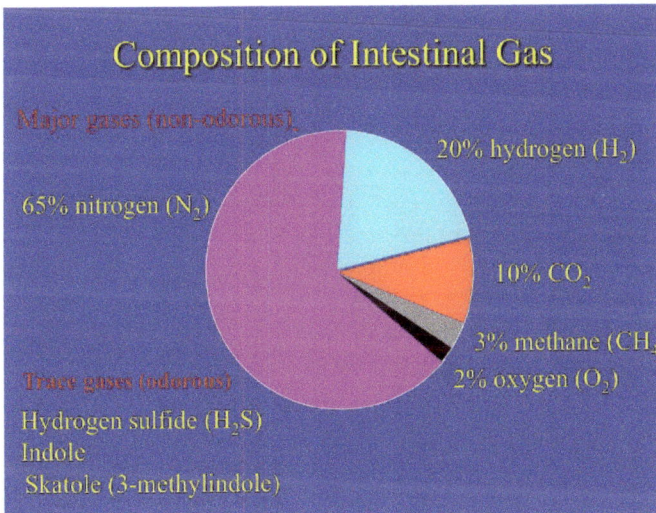

Composition of Intestinal Gas

Major gases (non-odorous):

65% nitrogen (N_2)

20% hydrogen (H_2)

10% CO_2

3% methane (CH_4)

2% oxygen (O_2)

Trace gases (odorous):
Hydrogen sulfide (H_2S)
Indole
Skatole (3-methylindole)

The vast majority of the gasses in intestinal farts, with Nitrogen, Hydrogen, Carbon Dioxide, Methane, and oxygen contributing 99.9% by volume are odorless. So what on earth is in that other tiny but overwhelming fraction of 1%? Indole skatole, thiol, sulfhydryl, mercaptan, and aromatic fatty acids are the major culprits. The aromas generated by farts are normally considered unattractive or offensive. There is a surprising percentage of the presumably normal population (predominantly males) who profess enjoyment and pleasure with the olfactory stimulation generated by their own farts, but not those of others.

To 'Air' is Human

Indole

Indole is an organic compound known as an aromatic heterocyclic because it consists of a six-membered benzene ring fused to a five-membered nitrogen-containing pyrrole ring. Indole is often used as a component of fragrances and is used in the production of a number of pharmaceutical products. The amino acid tryptophan is the precursor of the neurotransmitter serotonin and is an example of an indole derivative.

Tryptophan is one of the twenty-two amino acids, and is also considered an essential amino acid. Essential amino acids are those amino acids that cannot be synthesized by humans, and therefore must be obtained through the diet. Because of its importance as an essential amino acid, tryptophan is a common constituent of most protein foods and supplements. A diet rich in tryptophan can contribute to the fecal aroma of intestinal gas.

Indole occurs naturally in human feces and contributes to the characteristic fecal odor. Surprisingly, at very low concentrations it has a flowery smell and is a constituent of many perfumes. The name indole was created from the words indigo and oleum. Indole was first isolated by the dye industry in treatment of the deep blue indigo dye with oleum. It takes several million jasmine blossoms to make one pound of natural jasmine oil, which is two-point-five percent indole. It is priced over one thousand times as much as synthetic jasmine, which takes advantage of the commercial production of indole.

Skatole

Skatole (from the Greek το σχατος = feces), or methylindole, is a mildly toxic organic compound belonging to the indole family. It is the primary source of the odor of feces and is produced from the breakdown of the important amino acid tryptophan, the precursor of the neurotransmitter serotonin. Surprisingly, in low concentrations skatole has a very pleasant flowery smell and is found in orange blossoms, jasmine, and other flowers and essential oils. It is used as a fragrance in many perfumes.

Skatole is attractive to males of various species of bees, who gather the chemical to synthesize pheromones. It is also an attractant to gravid (pregnant) mosquitos. The U. S. military has used skatole as a non-lethal malodorant weapon. The German physician Ludwig Brieger, who also identified cadaverine and putrescence, discovered skatole in 1877. His neighbors were probably not pleased with the smell coming from his laboratory as the names he gave his discoveries were derived from their source material.

Skatole also plays a major role in the aroma of pork obtained from mature male pigs (boars). After puberty, under the influence of the male hormone androstenone, the gut microbiome of the male pig generates skatole. This odorant is deposited in the fat and muscle giving it an offensive smell and taste known as taint. Because it cannot be sold at market, male pigs are typically castrated at a young age or slaughtered before puberty. The male of the human species, under similar hormonal influence is also a larger producer of skatole contributing to the enhanced offensive potency of male farts after puberty.

Of particular interest to some scientists is that androstenone, and its effect on skatole, appear to have a pheromone like effect on the human female. Much like color-blindness, there appear to be some odors that cannot be smelled by all people. Initial studies suggested that about thirty percent of human females could not sense androstenone. Further studies revealed that the majority of the non-scenters could be trained to identify it, yet there remained a small proportion of less than five percent who could not perceive the scent. The ability to sense androstenone was found to be genetic and the gene responsible was identified.

The sense of smell in the human female is intimately tied to the menstrual cycle. The height of olfactory sensitivity peaks at the time of ovulation. The androstenone and skatole scents are perceived to be less offensive or more attractive at the time of ovulation. The androstenone skatole connection also explains why the feces and flatus of males is considered more powerful or offensive than that of females.

Diet also plays a role in that the ingestion of more meat and fat also leads to more skatole production than a diet with higher fiber content. This is partly due to the diet containing more tryptophan, the amino acid precursor of skatole, as well as the diet induced change in the microbiome. Androstenone also occurs naturally in some plants, including celery, parsnip, and truffle. The celery has long had a reputation as an aphrodisiac dating from Greek and Roman times.

Thiol, Sulfhydryl, Mercaptans

The sulfur hydrogen functional group may also be referred to as a thiol group or a sulfhydryl group. Thiols are also referred to as mercaptans. The term mercaptan (Latin mercurium captans 'capturing mercury') is used because the thiolate group bonds so strongly with mercury compounds. Hydrogen sulfide is known for its characteristic odor of smelling like rotten eggs. Surprisingly women tend to produce more hydrogen sulfide then men. Diet certainly plays a role as cruciferous vegetables such as broccoli, cabbage, cauliflower, and Brussels sprouts are common offenders. Dried fruits such as apricots are often treated with sulfur products that create odiferous gasses. Red meat, beer, garlic, and aromatic spices are other significant contributors. The offensive smell of sulfur products led to religions ascribing an association between the devil and sulfur.

Hydrogen sulfide is a toxic substance in high concentrations yet very valuable and beneficial on a cellular level when present in minute quantities. The human nose is exceptionally sensitive to this toxin and can identify in in minute concentrations, such as in a fart. When present in very high concentrations the olfactory cells are overwhelmed and can no longer sense it. This has led to a sever hazard for farmers and workers in animal waste manure pits and sewage treatment facilities. A worker collapses on exposure to the high concentration of hydrogen sulfide and fellow workers coming to their aid are likewise stricken because there was no olfactory warning. With a toxic potency equivalent to cyanide workers in such hazardous occupations are urged to use self-contained breathing apparatus to avoid exposure.

Volatile thiols have distinctive and strong garlic like odor. The spray of skunks consists mainly of s and derivatives. These compounds are detected by the human nose at concentrations as low as ten parts per billion. Human sweat contains methyl-sulfanylhexan (MSH), found in higher concentrations in females, and has a fruity onion-like odor. Not all thiols have unpleasant odors. The aroma of roasted coffee is due to thiols as is the characteristic scent of grapefruit. Dimethyl sulfide has an aroma that is often described as sweet. Natural gas distributors were required by law to add odorants such as thiols to odorless natural after a tragic school explosion in New London, Texas, in 1937.

Most natural odorant additives used today contain mixtures of mercaptans and sulfides. T-butyl mercaptan is often utilized as the main odorant constituent. The characteristic and pungently offensive odor of animal flesh decay is caused by putrescence and cadaverine. Putrescence and cadaverine are the breakdown products of the amino acids ornithine and lysine, respectively. Cadaverine and putrescence were also used as odorant additives for natural before improved odorants became commercially available.

Methanethiol

Methanethiol (methyl mercaptan) is a flammable, colorless with a powerful smell like rotten cabbage or decomposing vegetables. It is a natural substance found in certain foods such as some nuts and cheese, and is released from decaying organic matter. Methanethiol is also a byproduct produced by the metabolism of asparagus. The change in the odor of urine may be apparent within thirty minutes of eating asparagus. It is one of the main chemicals responsible for bad breath and the smell of feces and flatus.

Natural gas and propane are colorless and odorless, and an undetected leak can lead to tragic consequences. To serve as a odorous marker that a leak is occurring small amount of methyl mercaptan or ethyl mercaptan may be added as an odorant. The addition of an odorant is often required by law to prevent the danger of natural leaks going undetected.

Fatty Acids

A fatty acid is a saturated or unsaturated carboxylic acid with a long aliphatic tail or chain. Fatty acids with carbon–carbon double bonds are known as unsaturated, and those without as saturated. Fatty acids are derived from triglycerides or phospholipids, and when unattached to other molecules are described as "free". Fatty acids are an important cellular fuel and yield large quantities of ATP when metabolized. Many cell types can use either glucose or fatty acids for this purpose. Heart and skeletal muscle prefer fatty acids although most cells can use glucose interchangeably. The brain has the ability to use fatty acids, glucose, or ketone bodies as a fuel.

Fatty acids that must be obtained via the diet because humans cannot synthesize them are called essential fatty acids. Fatty acid chains are categorized by their length. Short-chain fatty acids (SCFA) have aliphatic tails of fewer than six carbons. Medium-chain fatty acids (MCFA) have tails of six to twelve carbons and can form medium-chain triglycerides. Long-chain fatty acids (LCFA) have tails of thirteen to twenty-one carbons, while very long chain fatty acids (VLCFA) are longer than twenty-two carbons.

Short- and medium-chain fatty acids are absorbed by the intestines directly into the blood stream. Long-chain fatty acids are absorbed into the cells of the intestinal villi and converted into a triglyceride cholesterol compound known as a chylomicron. These enter lymphatic capillaries called lacteals and are transported via the thoracic duct of the lymphatic system, eventually entering the circulatory system via the left subclavian vein. Fatty acids enter and chylomicrons in the blood circulation may be processed in the liver and subsequently circulate as very low-density lipoproteins (VLDL), low-density lipoproteins (LDL), and high-density lipoproteins.

Aromatic Amino Acids

Aromatic amino acids are amino acids that include an aromatic ring. Examples include phenylalanine, tryptophan, histidine, and tyrosine. Phenylalanine, histidine, and tryptophan are essential amino acids in that animals cannot synthesize them and they must be obtained from the diet. Tyrosine is semi-essential in that it can be synthesized but only if phenylalanine is ingested. The disorder phenylketonuria occurs when there is an absence of the enzyme phenylalanine hydroxylase, which is required for tyrosine synthesis.

All plants and microorganisms synthesize their aromatic amino acids, unlike animals, which obtain them through their diet. Animals have lost these energy intensive metabolic pathways, since they obtain aromatic amino acids through their diet. Herbicides and antibiotics inhibiting enzymes involved in aromatic acid synthesis, are toxic to plants and microorganisms dependent on this pathway, but not to animals which do not utilize these enzymes.

Volatile Organic Compounds

The term volatile refers to the ability of a substance to evaporate or readily vaporize at room temperature. Most instances of vaporization refer to evaporation where a liquid becomes a gas, such as liquid water boiling into gaseous steam and water vapor. Some solids vaporize from the solid state directly without entering an intermediate liquid phase, a process is known as sublimation. One example would be dry ice, frozen carbon dioxide, which leaves the solid state and is immediately transformed into a gas.

To 'Air' is Human

Vaporization also has another form that is not evaporation, but is the scattering or diffusing of molecules or particles through the air. The particles have so little mass that they can remain airborne for extended periods of time, and become airborne again upon being disturbed or moved even by a gentle gust of air. This is frequently noticed when a bright beam of light enters a darkened room and the dust particles circulating in the air become visible.

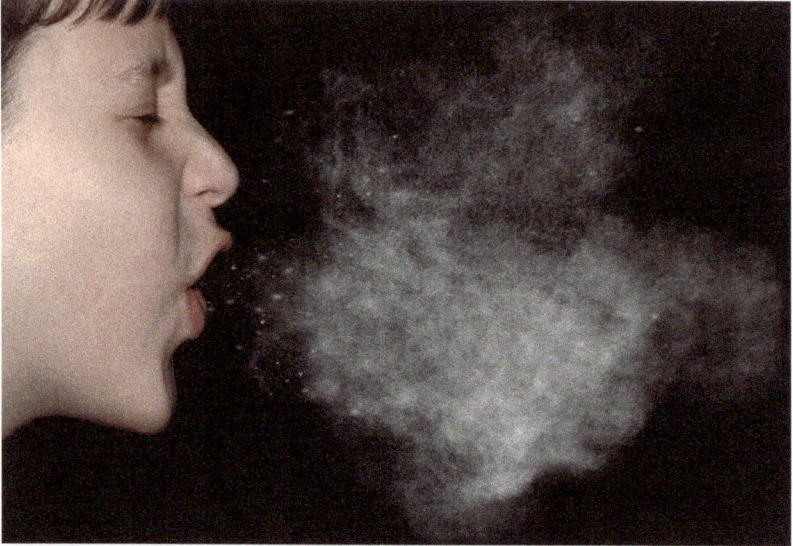

Mold, spores, pollens, viruses, bacteria, fecal matter of mites, volatile organic compounds and others can circulate and spread through large open spaces. Allergies, acquiring viral or bacterial infections from the sneeze or cough of others even hours earlier, occur because of this aerosolization. The ability to detect the aroma of certain compounds, and volatile organic compounds are the result of this form of vaporization as well as they can vaporize at room temperatures.

A list of the volatile organic compounds found in strawberries includes approximately two dozen chemicals including methyl butyrate, octyl acetate, hexanol, and others. Since these compounds are volatile they may vaporize and if they reach your olfactory receptors you may detect them and identify them as coming from a strawberry.

Fart, Social Standards (see Fart Survey)

The Ontario Ministry of Health embarked on a o public education campaign to curb tobacco usage. A common theme used by smokers to avoid the stigma of nicotine addiction was to describe their habit as a social smoker. The public education campaign focused on the denial as being analogous to describing oneself as a social farter than enjoyed farting while in the company of others.

Fart, Sound (Acoustics, Auditory)

The physics involved in the generation of the sound of a fart is very complex. Variables of the colonic and anal components, as well as the surrounding environment when it is released are multiple. Within the colon and rectum this includes the pressure, volume, temperature, moisture content, chemical nature of the gasses within the colon, and whether it is being released concomitantly with any liquid, semisolid, or solid material.

"Yes, that was very loud, but I said
I wanted to hear your HEART!"

Within the anal canal it includes the anatomy of the sphincter including whether it is symmetrical or irregular such as with fissures, hemorrhoids, anal tags, etc.,

To 'Air' is Human

sphincter tone and pressure, elasticity and degree of relaxation, and the velocity and physical nature of the expelled material. In the immediate post expulsion state, factors include the atmospheric pressure, temperature, and volumetric constraints such as whether by clothing, sitting on a cushion, under a blanket, or voluntary social considerations.

The physics of and fluid dynamics allow calculations with the understanding and application of natural laws. If you have taken a course in physics you may recall with great fondness Laplace's Law, Boyle's Law, Charles' Law, Avogadro's Law, Gay-Lussac's Law that were integrated into what is called the Ideal Law. This summarizes the close interrelationship between the pressure, volume, and temperature of gasses. To understand the physics of farts you need to incorporate the additional principles of physics and engineering called the "choked" compressible flow effect. The character that becomes choked or limited is the velocity, although after release the term choked makes take on an entirely different meaning.

The velocity of the material increases as it is passed through a constriction. You may have experienced this if you have used a garden hose and notice that as the opening at the nozzle tip becomes smaller the velocity increases. You may also have noticed that the frequency of the sound generated also changes both by constricting the nozzle orifice or rotating the faucet leading to the garden hose. This involves recognition that the Ventura effect causes the static pressure, and therefore the density of the gasses, to decrease once released from the anus.

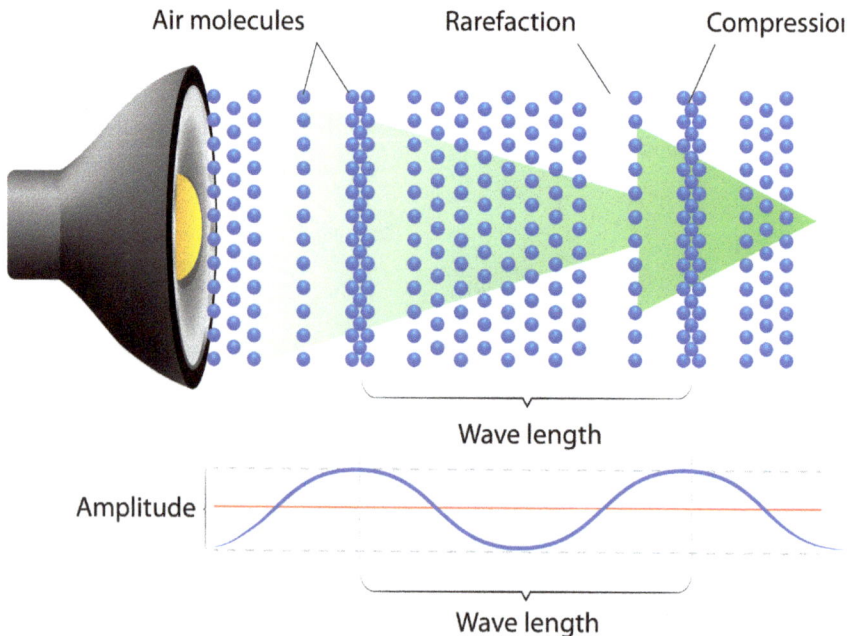

Air molecules   Rarefaction   Compressioı

Wave length

Amplitude

Wave length

To 'Air' is Human

If the material passed includes a liquid component, a different type of choked flow can occur. In unusual circumstances dependent on the vapor pressure and temperature of the liquid, the liquid may partially flash into bubbles of vapor that collapse in a process called cavitation. When this occurs in a closed system of pipes such as plumbing fixtures the effect can be very noisy and sufficiently violent as to cause physical damage to valves, pipes, and associated equipment. Thankfully, humans are not a closed system but the noise and reverberations they generate may be comparable.

In general the more tone the anal sphincter is the tighter it can hold on to the gasses to create a greater pressure gradient. The greater the pressure gradient the louder the potential sound will be. If the opposite occurs the less noise is generated. As an example it is said that if you blow air slowly into a trumpet without puckering your lips to generate an air pressure gradient the air will just flow through the instrument without "trumpeting".

The anal sphincter tone changes with age becoming more lax. This is also the case after childbirth, and any activities that stretch the anal opening on a regular basis, such as passing large stools with constipation, or engaging in anal receptive intercourse. With the loss of sphincter tone farts may escape involuntarily, but they also tend to be quitter as the larger the opening of the orifice the slower the velocity.

With so many variables it should come as no surprise that the sounds generated are equally variable. As the famous Greek philosopher Heraclitus (c. 535 BCE-475 BCE) said, "You could not step twice into the same river; for other waters are ever flowing on to you." It would be fair to say that no two farts are identical, much like snowflakes, although somehow pure white innocent snowflakes do not seem to be the right analogy.

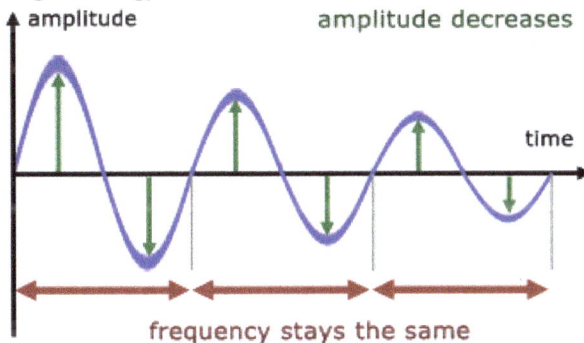

At the time that a fart is about to be released the variables under the control of a talented and experienced professional farter include the velocity of its release, the tension and symmetry of the sphincter, and the selection of the environmental nature of the location of its liberation. Yes there is a significant amount of science behind the fart, but there is also an 'art to the fart'. As to the teleological question, is there an advantage to audible fart sounds, there are several theories. One is that the fart sounds are an auditory warning that noxious gasses being released and to seek shelter or at least distance to protect oneself.

A second theory suggests that these are actually primitive mating calls, especially attempt of adolescent males to attract the female of the species. And the third is so that people with anosmia, the loss of the sense of smell, can participate in the experience of a fart as well.

Using the principles of speed of travel of various phenomena you may recall that you can calculate the distance of a lightning strike. The speed of light is 186,282 miles per second; the speed of sound is 768 miles per hour in dry air at 68 degrees Fahrenheit at sea level. Obviously the light will reach you first and you will see the flash, but no sound as it is lagging behind. The more distant you are from where the lightning struck, he greater the time lag. If you see the flash of lightening count the number of seconds before you hear the thunder. Now simply divide the number of seconds of lag time by the number 5 to adjust for the differences in speed of light and sound, and voila, you have a good approximation of the distance in miles that you are from where the lightning struck.

The lightning flash of a fart is a very special event discussed in greater detail in the section on combustible farts containing hydrogen and methane, and the section on spontaneous human combustion. Can one use science to compare the speeds of sound and smell transmission? The answer is an unequivocal yes, but circumstances are rarely optimal. The speed of sound of a fart is the same as the speed of sound of a lightning strike, is 768 miles per hour in dry air at 68 degrees Fahrenheit at sea level. The speed of smell diffusion has been measured at 10 feet per second (6.8 mph) in an unventilated room with no circulating airflow.

Using the sound of the fart as a shotgun start for the stopwatch, count how many seconds it is until you smell the fart. To simplify calculations the fart sound is about 100 times faster than the fart smell. For a crude approximation simply take the number of seconds from the fart sound until the smell arrives as the number of feet you are distant to its source. Any circulation of air in the room, clothing that the fart has to pass through, and direction of the jet exhaust blast with which it is released can either accelerate or delay its arrival at your nose. This formula is at its most accurate in identifying the source of the fart if there are no more than two people in the room. The adage he who smelt it dealt it is usually accurate unless the other party was in a compromised position with his own nose closer to the anus of the emanation.

The pressure generated by the abdominal muscles can be infinitely adjusted by the individual (the Valhalla maneuver generates this pressure with a bearing down motion with the breath held) and will affect the velocity and sound of a fart. Leaning to one side to deform the anal canal into an irregular shape to allow them to escape with less velocity is a technique learned by experience even one does not recognize the principles of physics underlying its utility. Sitting on a cushion to muffle the sound and absorb the aroma is a common technique.

With practice, some individuals have developed the remarkable musical ability to play their own human wind instrument. They have performed in public to great acclaim like Joseph Pool, known as Le Ptomaine on the Moulin Rouge of Paris (see chapter?). The sound of farts can be a source of entertainment and humor or offense and embarrassment, but it is a natural phenomenon that follows the laws of nature.

Scientific papers entitled "Sounds produced by herring (*Clupeid harangues*) bubble release" by Magnus Wahlberg and Haman Westerberg in the journal *Aquatic Living Resources* (2003, 16.271-275), and "Pacific and Atlantic Herring Produce Burst Pulse Sounds" by Ben Wilson, Robert S. Batty and Lawrence M. Dill in *Biology Letters* (2003, 271.S95-S97) confirm that herring communicate distress signals to the rest of the school of fish by farting. The papers are demonstrate scholarly research and have spectrographic confirmation of the high frequency sound bursts up to 22 kilohertz with visual confirmation of a stream of bubbles from the anus.

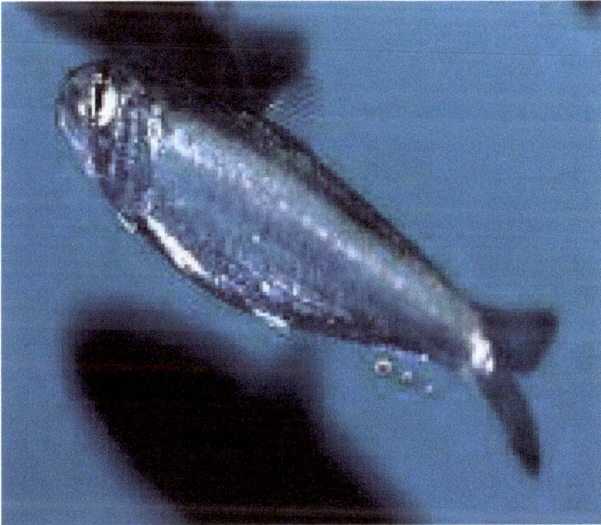

Herring communicate danger by high frequency sounds generated from bubbles escaping their anus described as F.R.T. fast repetitive ticks in published scientific papers first reported in 2003. Creative Commons License

Herring travel in enormous schools of fish that number in the billions. During the height of the cold war during the 1980's U.S. and NATO forces believed they had detected by sonar a unique sound pattern that was the signature of a new secret Soviet nuclear submarine. The new submarine appeared to be making provocative incursions into the territorial waters of Sweden and Norway, which complained forcibly through diplomatic channels. When the sound pattern was detected deep into the territorial waters of a Norwegian Ford the West decided to trap the submarine and blockaded the entrance to the fjord. After days of waiting for the submarine to surrender they finally realized that the sonar sounds they were hearing were not a Soviet submarine but the sounds of a school of herring farting their way into the Norwegian Fjord.

During interviews with the National Geographic Society research team leader Ben Wilson a marine biologist studying pacific herring at the Bam field Marine Science Centre, British Columbia, Canada was quoted saying "We know [herring] have excellent hearing but little about what they actually use it for. It turns out that herring make unusual farting sounds at night." Their collaborator Robert Batty, senior research scientist at the Scottish Association for Marine Science in Oban, Scotland added "In video pictures we can see the bubbles coming out of the anal duct at the same time. It sounds very much like someone blowing a high-pitched raspberry. "They labeled the sounds generated as F.R.T. for fast repetitive tick. They were awarded the 2004 IgNobel Prize in Biology.

There is a phrase called 'holding back the helium' which refers to farting by substituting the name of another , in this case helium. Is there another possible connection between helium and farting? Because gases have different densities, the speed of sound in helium is nearly three times the speed of sound in air. Inhaling a small volume of helium changes the sound of the human voice into a characteristic high resonant frequency sound. The sound generated is similar to the famous cartoon character Daffy Duck.

The opposite effect, with low resonant frequencies more like the Star Wars character Darth Vader, can be obtained by inhaling a dense with higher density such as xenon, sulfur hexafluoride, or tungsten hexafluoride. Helium by far the most readily available typically associated with access through party favor stores to fill helium balloons for parties and entertainment. Helium actually plays a major role in industry and the biomedical sciences and is critical for scientific research in the fields of quantum mechanics, super fluidity, and superconductivity.

Now to the question that is undoubtedly keeping you up at night, what happens to the sound quality of a helium fart. First question is how does the helium get into the digestive tract. Inhaling pure helium will not lead to helium farts because you would die of asphyxiation within minute. This is why even playing with the idea of helium to make your voice sound like a cartoon character is a very foolish and dangerous idea. Those who have done so and died from oxygen deprivation are considered candidates for what is called the Darwin Awards. This is offered, usually posthumously, to those who have improved the human gene pool for future evolution by removing themselves and their obviously substandard intelligence genes from future procreation activities.

So let's say you know better than to breathe in helium, but undertake a swallowing effort to fill your digestive tract with helium to get it to pass as a fart. Not much of an improvement as the helium is such a small molecule that it easily diffuses through most membranes, as you can tell by how quickly the helium escapes from a rubber balloon, and over a period of a few days, even from a metallic balloon.

Which leave only one last logical way to fill the colon with helium, yes go to a party store and ask them to 'fill it up' for you. Now that you have a colon filled with helium you don't want to waste much time, as the helium will once again diffuse through the colonic epithelium. Will you fart like a duck? The answer is yes, but not because of a high frequency sound, but because a duck fart sounds like any old fart. What went wrong with the common impression that it would sound like fingernails scratching a chalkboard? The problem is that the anal opening does not have a structure equivalent to the vocal cords of the human larynx also so appropriately called the voice box.

Phonation, the creation of sound and voice arises from the ability of the vocal cords to open and constrict to exceptionally nuanced degrees, allowing an infinite variety and modulation of frequencies. Humans are not the sole possessors of such a talent as songbirds and other animals can generate sounds in an even greater range of frequencies, often beyond the auditory abilities of our ears to hear the sounds. You are probably familiar to dog whistles that dogs respond to but are outside of our hearing range. It is the ability of the vocal cords to generate the range of frequencies that is impacted by the density of the gasses passed through that makes the voice reach higher frequencies with helium. It also can reach much lower frequencies sounding like Dart Vader from the Star Wars movie franchise id you use a much denser like xenon, sulfur hexafluoride, or tungsten hexafluoride.

The anal opening has hemorrhoid sinusoids, the internal anal sphincter, the external anal sphincter, and the occasional skin tag and in spite of the great control of some individuals like Joseph Pujol the Petomaine, it does not even come close to the resonance and sensitivity of sound creation of the vocal cords. Which is too bad, as a new Star Wars character a very short and squat Farth Vader could have become a cult hero.

Another species creates sounds in a different fashion. Many fish have a swim bladder that is inflated or deflated as needed to maintain buoyancy. Usually expelled exits the mouth but the sand tiger shark, *Carcharias taurus*, discharges it out the anus. The carbon dioxide produced is eliminated via the gills. Methane, hydrogen, and other gasses would typically be released as a fart.

Fart, Speed (Velocity)

The word fart in northern European languages including German and the Scandinavian languages literally means speed. In you go by a school or hospital you may go by a no farting zone. Or you might receive a police citation for exceeding the fart limit!

So a title of fart speed might seem redundant A sneeze, or sternutation, is a powerful rapid expulsion of air from the lungs through the nose and mouth. The average velocity of a sneeze is 42 meters/second) equivalent to approximately 95 mph. A single sneeze can disperse up to 40,000 aerosol droplets, which can transmit pathogens and disease. The sneeze is a much more effective dispersant of infectious material than a cough or peaking. The average velocity of a cough was 15.3 m/s and the average velocity of the breath of normal speech is 4.07 m/s.

Although the mechanism of increasing intra-abdominal pressure is similar to generating intra-thoracic pressure for a sneeze the exit orifice is a major determinant of velocity. No one has voluntarily gotten close enough to a fart blast to measure its ejection velocity or count the vapor droplets. The brave soul who does so may not get a Nobel Prize, but would certainly be worthy of nomination for an IgNobel Prize.

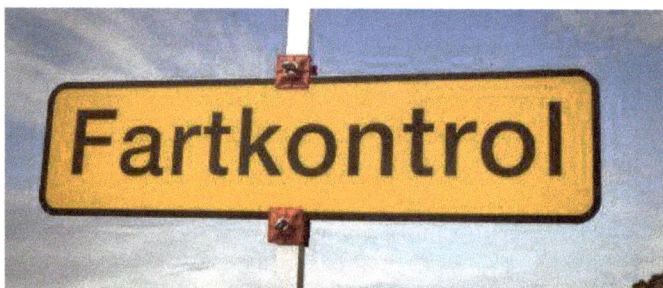

onpasture.com Creative Commons License

Coughing and sneezing release a large plume of aerosolized droplets impregnated with microbial pathogens. The sneeze and cough, which can easily reach a velocity of over 100 miles per hour (150 kilometers per hour) and has been recorded at speeds up to 500 miles per hour (950 km/hour) , will spread throughout a large size room. Even the flushing of a toilet will aerosolize fecal microbes that would cover a room in dimensions of twenty feet by twenty feet in a matter of seconds.

Farts have been recorded with the speed of aroma travel at an extremely conservative 10 miles per hour. It was not clear if this was from an individual wearing clothing at the time. A vigorous blast from a wet fart would probably look like the third photograph humorously labeled as Save the Whale. Perhaps science will one day answer the question about fart speed, or perhaps a watch company will sponsor a competition for the Guinness book of world records which has a number of fart categories already entered into the competitive arena. Another aspect that defines the extent of the reach of a fart besides its initial velocity and volume is the rate of diffusion. This is dependent on physical barriers such as layers of clothing or sitting on a cushion as well as air turbulence and ventilation. Please see entry on fart diffusion for more details.

Back in the 1946 a spoof recording of the International Crepitation Contest was created, and it is still commercially available today. It was apparently produced by some recording engineers for the Canadian Broadcasting Corporation and was

To 'Air' is Human

held on February 31, 1946 as the World Championship Crepitation Contest at the Maple Leaf Auditorium at Thunderblow, Canada between competitors Paul Boomer and Lord Windesmear.

Fart, Survey

The following Internet based survey of over 1300 male participants and an unspecified number of female participants does not qualify as scientifically or statistically valid. However for anecdotal and entertainment purposes it is as good as it gets when it comes to this subject matter.

Number of times women fart per day:

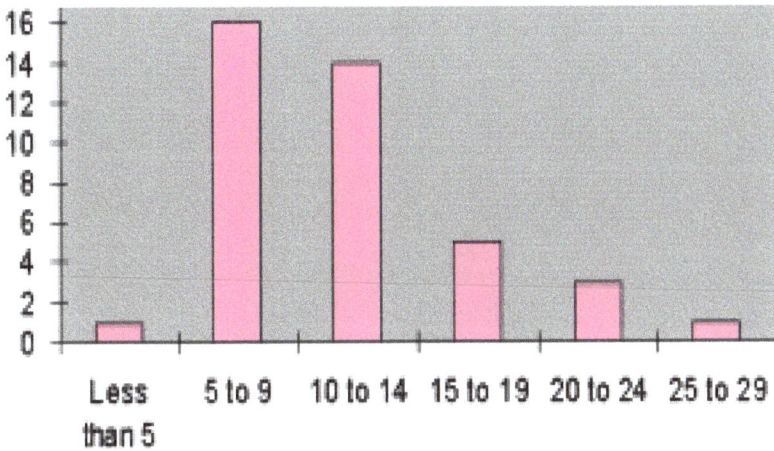

Women fart an average of eight times per day. Fifty percent of the women surveyed fart between five and ten times per day.

Women: Can you fart on command also called "Butt Breathe"?

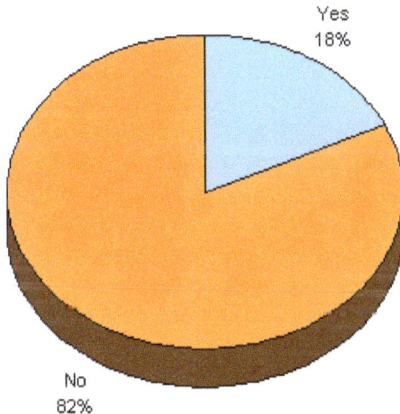

Eighteen percent of the women surveyed can fart on command by sucking air into the colon.

Women: Do you like to fart?

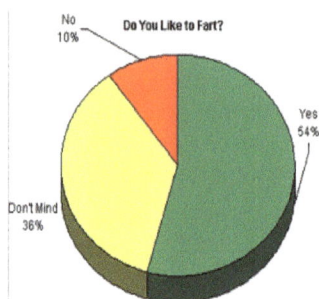

Only half of the women surveyed admit that they like to fart. About one fifth don't mind farting, but don't necessarily like it. Only 10% of women absolutely do not like to fart!

Women: When you were younger did you like to fart in water to make bubbles?

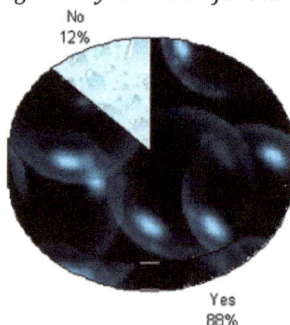

Most women liked to fart in the bathtub or pool to make bubbles.

Number of times men fart per day:

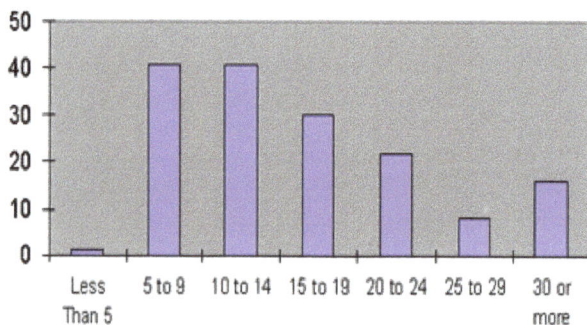

Men fart an average of fourteen times per day. Fifty percent of the men surveyed fart between five and fifteen times per day.

Men: Can you fart on command also called "Butt Breathe"?

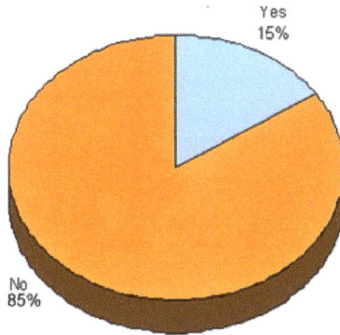

Yes
15%

No
85%

Only fifteen percent of the men surveyed can fart on command by sucking air into the colon. One third of all men did not even know that this is possible.

Men: When you were younger did you like to fart in water to make bubbles?

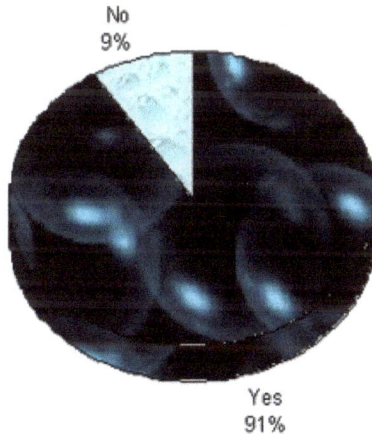

No
9%

Yes
91%

The vast majority of men liked to fart in the bathtub or pool to make bubbles.

Fart, Therapeutic Options

Many individuals have issues with unpleasant fecal odors, and unfortunately it is not as easily remedied as flushing or walking away. The fecal aroma generated by the gut microbiome that smells in defecated feces is the identical aroma that may be discharged with intestinal gas, fecal incontinence, fistula, ostomies, diarrhea, inflammatory bowel disease, after gastric bypass surgery, and a host of other conditions. The numbers of individuals affected is in the millions in the United States alone. Unfortunately, the majority of the general public remains uninformed and impose a social stigma on a medical condition over which they have limited or no control.

Fortunately there are a number of effective therapeutic options available, but too many sufferers are not aware of or have access to them. They range from external appliances and clothing, to external and internal deodorants and suppressants. Of course there are also tongue-in-cheek suggestions ,such as getting a dog to blame as the source of the fart odor. The Merck Manual a few years back suggested working on perfecting one's glare, just glare at someone else as if they were the source.

More direct references to farts has been employed in the advertising campaign of air-freshener company Poo-Pourri. Although the advertising campaign received a nomination as one of the worst ads by a national newspaper, it was a major hit on social media with over thirty million views. For a holiday themed advertisement Santa Claus is farting on the toilet while an attractive model sings a parody of a seasonal tune.

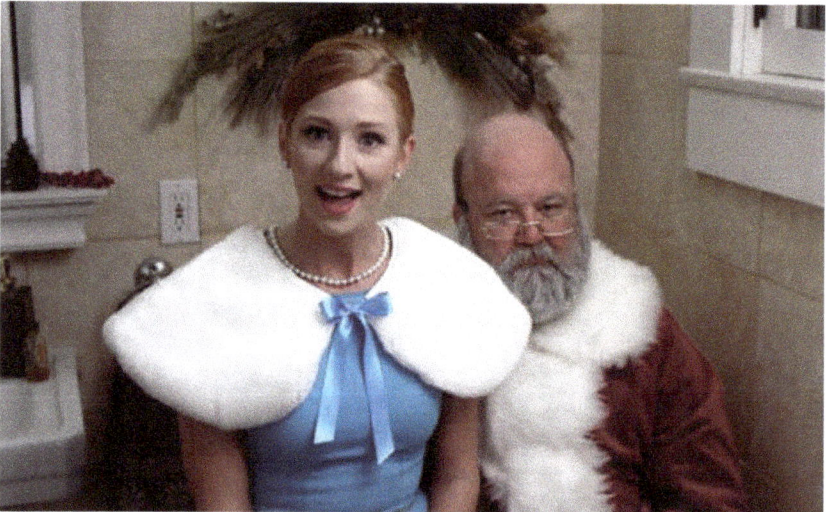

Poo-Pourri Advertising video www.ninjamarkweting.it

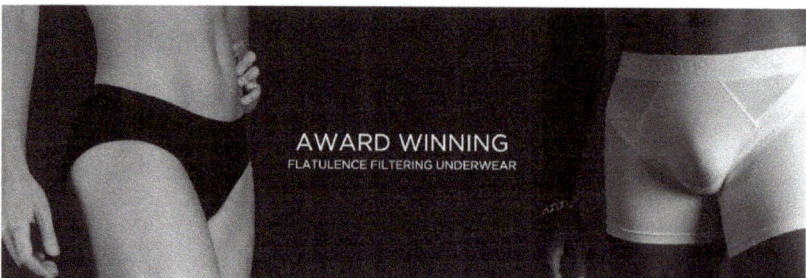

AWARD WINNING
FLATULENCE FILTERING UNDERWEAR

Shreddies advertising campaign for activated charcoal odor adsorbing underwear myshreddies.com

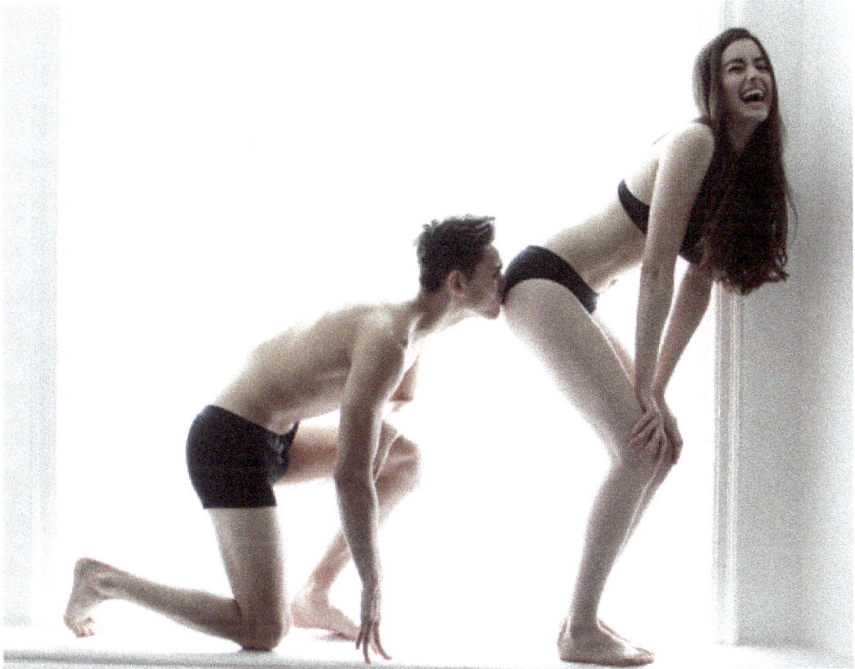

Shreddies advertising campaign for activated charcoal odor adsorbing underwear myshreddies.com

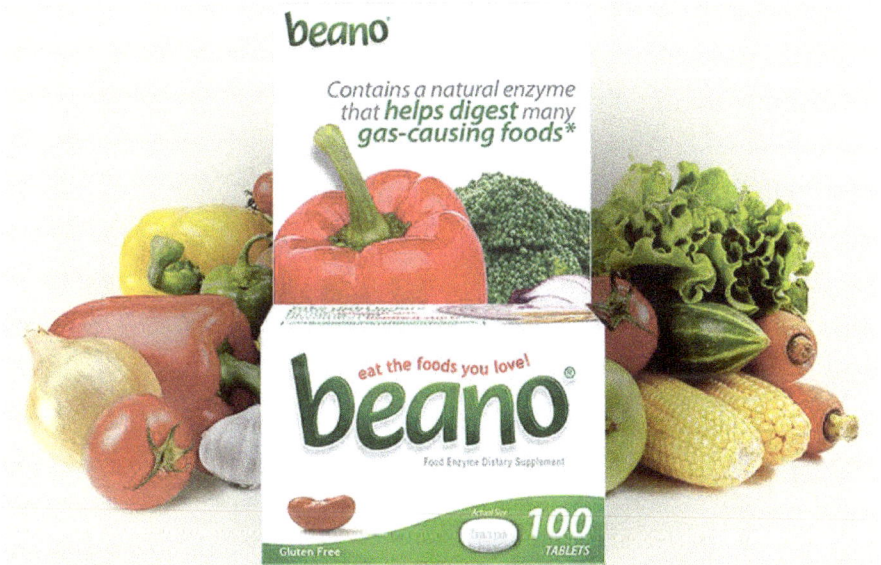

Beano was one of the first products to advertise a product designed to reduce intestinal gas. Its ad first appeared in Vegetarian Times

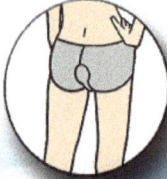
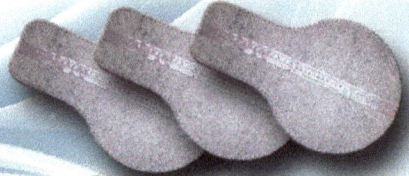

Premium Pad

Flatulence Deodorizer - Premium

Premium pad = Premium results!

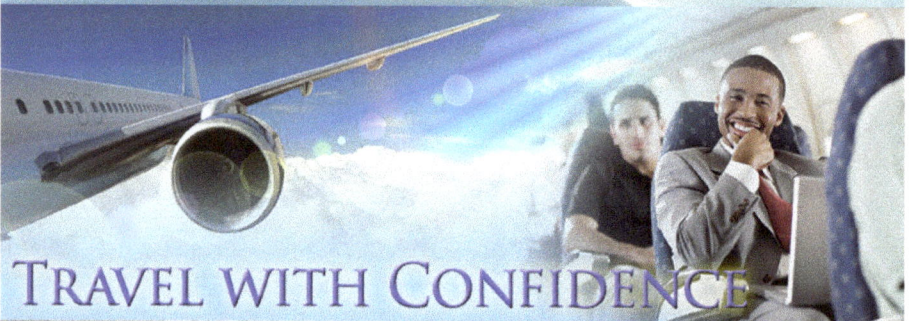

TRAVEL WITH CONFIDENCE

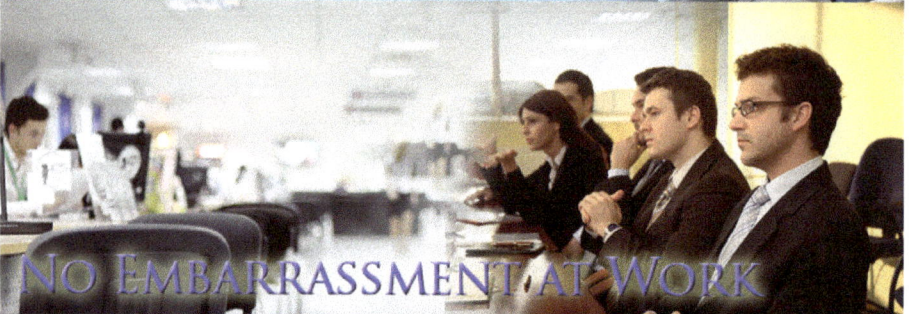

NO EMBARRASSMENT AT WORK

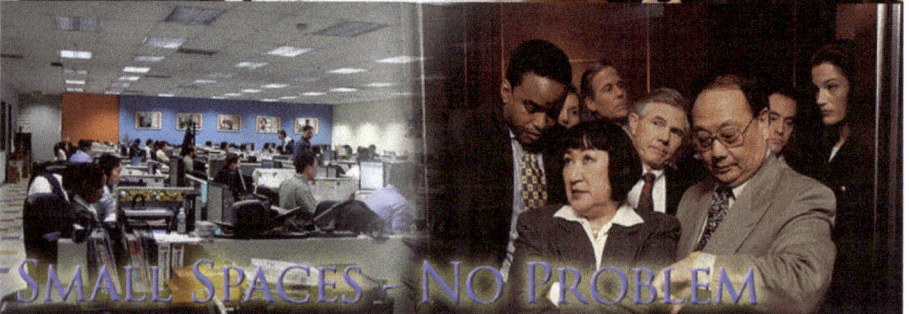

SMALL SPACES - NO PROBLEM

Flat-D advertises and markets a wide variety of activated charcoal products to adsorb the aroma of flatus and other body odors. www.flat-d.com

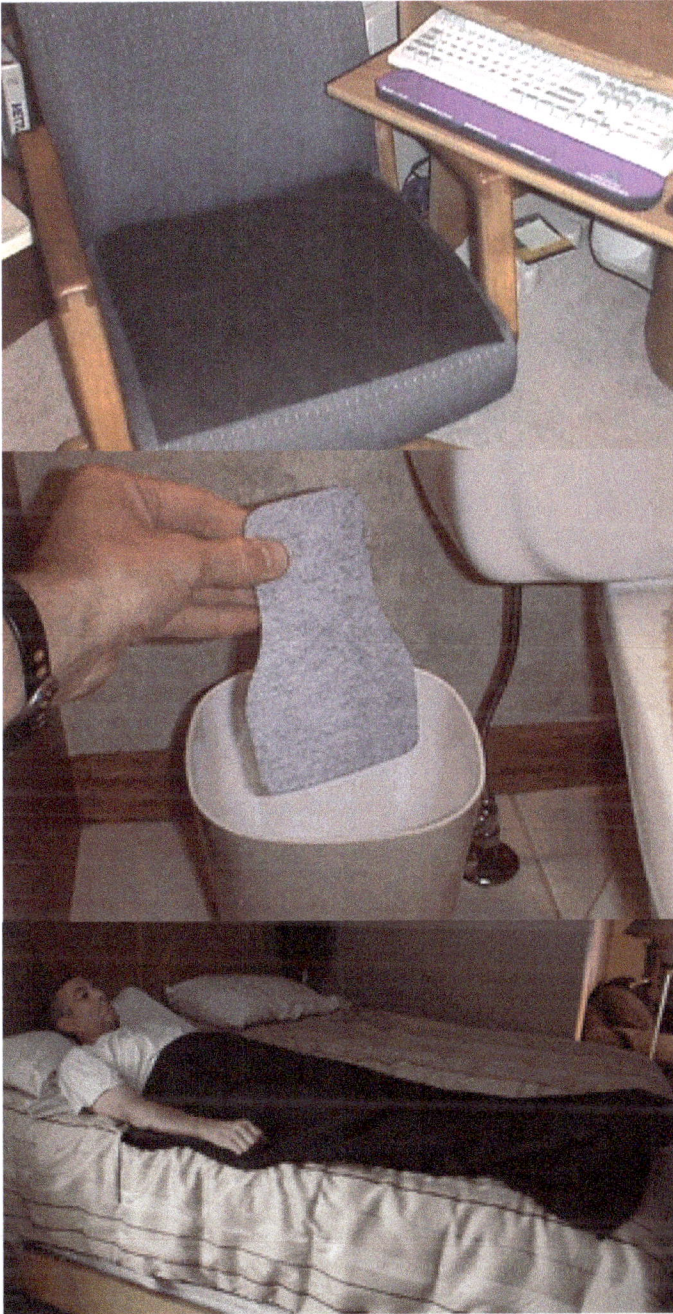

Flat-D advertises and markets a wide variety of activated charcoal products to adsorb the aroma of flatus and other body odors. Activated charcoal seat cushions, liners for underwear and clothing, and sleeping sack are amongst the numerous products they offer. www.flat-d.com

To 'Air' is Human

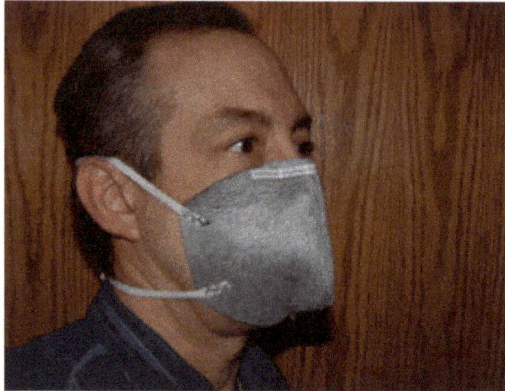

Flat-D offers another approach to protect the individual from offensive odors, by wearing an activated charcoal facemask covering the mouth and nose. www.flat-d.com

Surprisingly where it can provide relief and comfort to many sufferers, some media outlets refuse to place advertisements for products dealing with flatulence and ostomy odors. Deodorants, feminine hygiene douches, tampons, sanitary napkins for menstruation, diapers for adults with incontinence, erectile dysfunction prescriptions, etcetera have been seen by the public and the country still stands. Devrom, an effective internal deodorant that suppresses fecal odor was not allowed to place their advertisement in Reader's Digest or AARP (Association for the Advancement of Retired People) because it contained the word stool and smelt flatulence. Somehow the publications did not see the irony in that their policy did not pass the smell test.

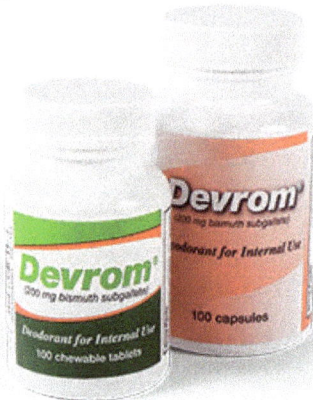

Devrom is an over the counter preparation of bismuth subgallate and has been marketed for over fifty years as an internal deodorant. Bismuth does have antibacterial properties it may change the microbiome by reducing the organisms that contribute to offensive flatulence. Another bismuth product that has been popular in the marketplace is Pepto-Bismol, which is a bismuth subsalicylate. Bismuth subsalicylate is related to aspirin (salicylic acid) and does not appear to provide as significant relief from the unpleasant odors as has been reported with Devrom.

To 'Air' is Human

It has been particularly popular for individuals who have undergone gastric bypass surgery, inflammatory bowel disease, as well as those with ostomies, and others. With advances in surgery, and the ability to preserve sphincters or create artificial sphincters, ostomies are seen less frequently. This is where the intestinal discharge exits the body through an artificial opening, the ostomy, created at surgery. Because the bowel is diverted from the colon less moisture is absorbed and the feces may be semi-formed or liquid.

The more liquid form allows for the more rapid vaporization of volatile organic compounds and gasses that give rise to the feculent odor. In spite of being in otherwise excellent health, many individuals with these issues find themselves socially restricted in their activities because of concern about embarrassment or offending others. Safe and effective products are available, but many individuals are unaware and suffer unnecessarily because of the lack of information and understanding.

Bismuth is a chemical element, number eighty-three on the periodic table, which has long history of being used in preparations designed to treat gastrointestinal complaints. It is a heavy metal with a low level of toxicity. Its various compound have also been used historically to treat syphilis and the severe diarrhea from cholera. Bismuthinite is a mineral consisting of bismuth sulfide (Bi_2S_3) and is an important ore for bismuth.

The mechanism of action is unknown and may be related to its known antimicrobial activity, perhaps inhibiting the microbes that generate some of the more offensive gasses that are usually contain sulfur as well as aromatic and volatile organic compounds. Bismuth also reacts directly with sulfur generating bismuth sulfide, a dark black insoluble compound. This can cause darkening or blackening of the tongue if sulfur is found in high concentrations in the saliva. It will also cause blackening of the stool as it binds with the sulfur that would otherwise give rise to hydrogen sulfide and other offensive sulfur gasses. The dark black color of the stool may be mistaken for melena, a sign of internal bleeding that results from the digestive process on blood cells and hemoglobin. The black coloration is not a health concern and is temporary clearing with cessation of bismuth intake.

Activated carbon is used to treat oral poisonings by binding to and preventing the poison from being absorbed by the gastrointestinal tract. Charcoal biscuits were marketed in the early 19th century as an antidote to flatulence, and are still marketed today for diarrhea, indigestion, flatulence, and as a pet care product. Unfortunately orally ingested charcoal pills are not effective in appreciably reducing intestinal gas. This may be because the adsorptive capacity of the activated charcoal is fully utilized before it finally gets to the colon where its gas adsorbing properties are needed. Fortunately, bismuth products do provide a significant advantage by binding to the sulfur compounds and eliminating them without producing offensive gas.

To 'Air' is Human

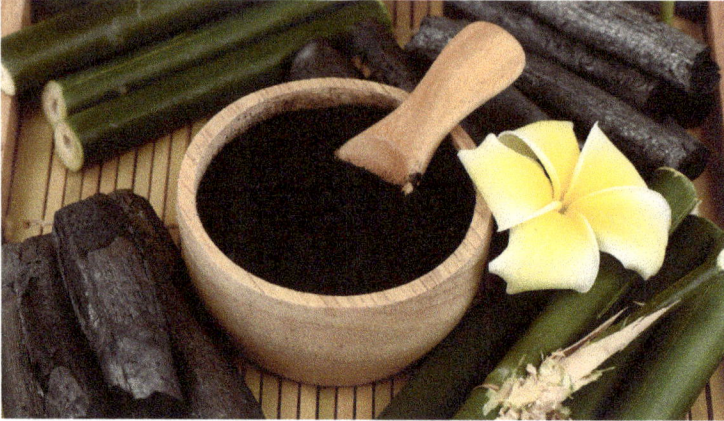

Activated charcoal used as a treatment of aerophagia. shutterstock/wasanajai

Fart, Underwater

It is to be expected that all living creatures that pass gas on land and in the air will do so underwater as well. A large number of humans find this to be a particularly pleasurable activity as confirmed on a large Internet based survey found under the section fart, survey. Of course other animals will release gas underwater as a matter of nature, although they may find it entertaining as well as humans.

For more information about the sounds generated by underwater farts please see entry on fart, sound (Acoustic, auditory).

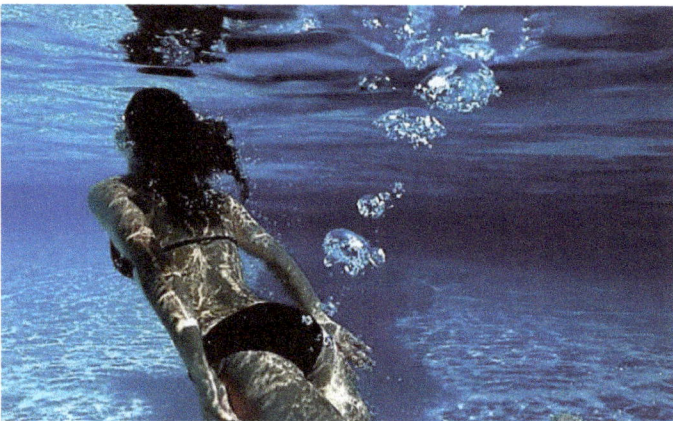

www.home-remedies.br Creative Commons License

The hippopotamus (Greek hippos-horse and potamus-river) is considered by many experts to be the most dangerous animal in Africa (excluding the malaria carrying mosquito) having killed many more people than lions have. The hippo is extremely aggressive with its huge canine teeth and sharp incisors, unpredictable and fearless of humans. Most deaths occur when the victim gets between the hippo and deep water or between a mother and her calf.

To 'Air' is Human

Hippos weigh up to 8000 pounds, gallop at 18 M.P.H., sleep or lounge around on riverbanks and in the water most of the day, and graze on the grasslands at night. Their skin secretes sticky pinkish oil that helps protect them from the sun. They defecate generous amounts of excrement into the rivers and ponds in which they wallow all day, punctuated by voluminous farts.

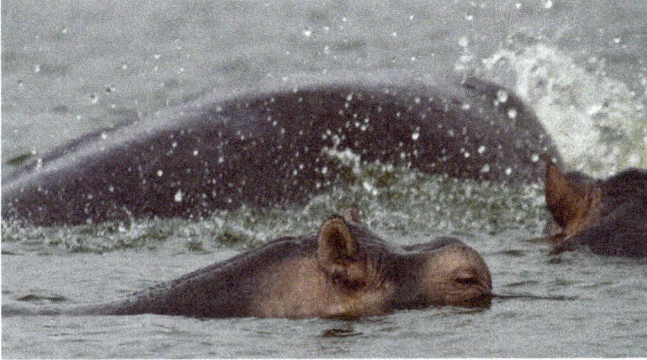

white-voodoo.deviantart.com Creative Commons License

They also participate in marking territory by what the hippo experts refer to as "dung showering." They blow feces mixed with urine over a large area around their watering hole, twirling their relatively short tails like fans to distribute the aromatic spray.

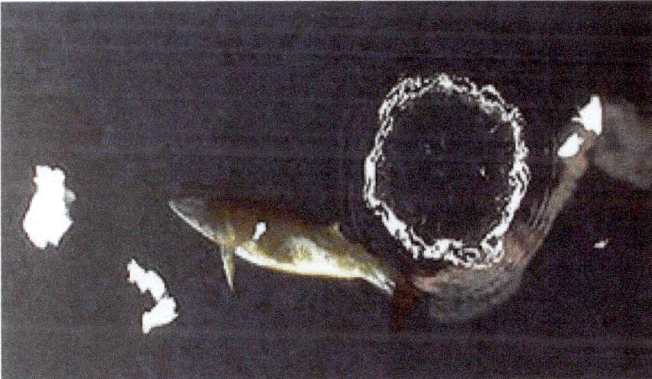

Marine research scientists studying the minke whale population near Antarctica were able to capture a whale fart on film for the first time. The photograph was taken from the bow of the research vessel and the fart subsequently surfaced right under their noses. "We got away from the bow of the ship very quickly ... it does stink," said Nick Gales, a research scientist from the Australian Antarctic Division. However, the skunk like episode did not detract them from completing their mission of collecting DNA from whale dung and attaching satellite tracking devices to the whales to study their migration patterns.

To 'Air' is Human

Many fish have a swim bladder that is inflated or deflated as needed to maintain buoyancy. Usually expelled gas exits the mouth but the sand tiger shark, *Carcharias taurus*, discharges it out the anus. The carbon dioxide produced is eliminated via the gills. Methane, hydrogen, and other gasses would typically be released as a fart. Fisherman knew about herring farts and they were even written about back in 1914 by Swedish author Ludvig Runebergwrote in his masterpiece Bottenhavsfiskare (Bothnian Bay Fishermen). The section below is freely translated from the Swedish.

"In the evening they were rowing away to the barren islands, pulled up the boats, lit a fire and made coffee, opened the dinner box and ate. While they were sitting there a group of fishermen were staring out towards the sea, the sun sinking, the sky turning red, and the waves smoothing, wind dying, moon sailing out, lonely and large, the ducks moving back and forth in trains, and in all this, which no longer looked like the earth but more seemed to be an advection into the sky, a distant boiling was seen on the blank water surface. Thousands and thousands of small blisters glaring into the sea, without it being possible to say wherefrom they came, and only in one small defined place: it was the herring which was approaching them on its migration."

Fart, Vagina

Fart is also a term used for an emission or expulsion of air from the vagina. It may occur during or after sexual intercourse or during other sexual acts, stretching, exercise, getting g up from as chair, etcetera. Puffs or small amounts of air passed into the vaginal cavity during cunnilingus are normally not associated with vaginal fart. However "forcing" or purposely blowing air at force into the vaginal cavity can cause an air embolism which is dangerous for the woman, and if pregnant for the fetus.

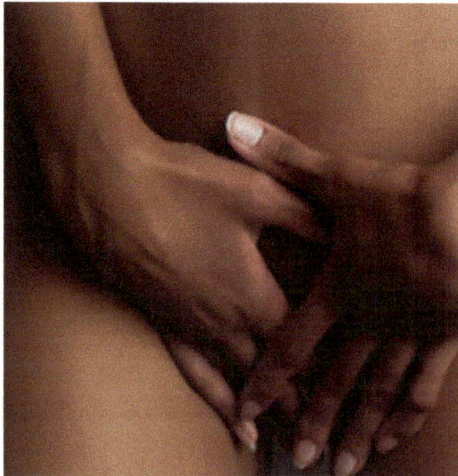

i9.photobucket.com Creative Commons License

To 'Air' is Human

The sound of flatus from the vagina is somewhat comparable to flatulence from the anus but does not have a feculent odor in the normal state. If a feculent odor is present it may be because of a colovaginal fistula, a serious condition involving a tear between the vagina and colon. A colovaginal fistula can result from surgery, childbirth, diseases such as the inflammatory bowel disease Crohn disease and other causes. This condition can lead to urinary tract infection and other complications. Slang terms for vaginal flatulence include *vart*, *queef* and *fanny fart*(mostly British).

Fart, Visual

It may sound hard to visualize a fart, but it is actually fairly simple, it's that the circumstances have to be just right. Yes, in releasing an invisible gas into invisible air you would normally not expect to see it with the limited visual spectrum of the human eye. However if you had vision in the infrared portion of the electromagnetic spectrum it would be very visible. With the advent of infrared photography and thermographic imagery the invisible fart can be visualized.

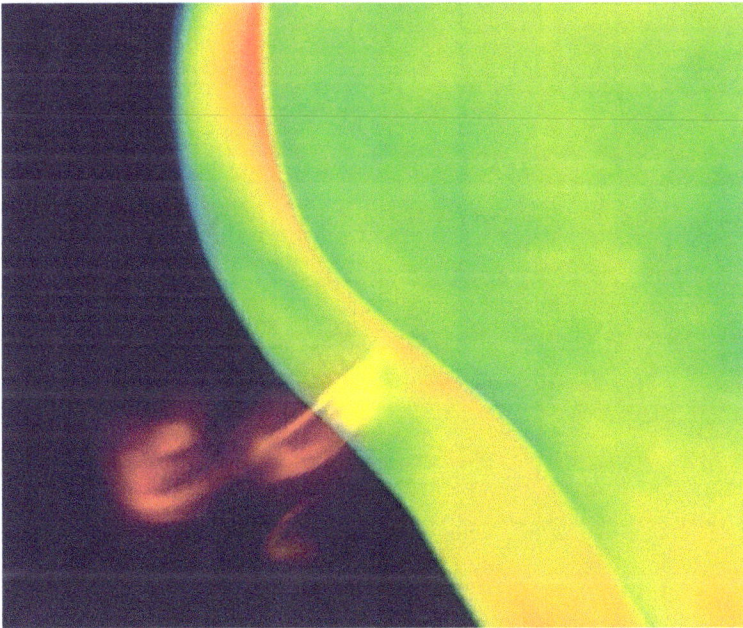

i.telegraph.co.uk

You can also see the fart if the temperature and humidity are just right. If you were in the polar zones, at very high altitude, in frigid weather, or even in a walk-in freezer, dropping a fart from exposed buttocks would look much like the steamy cloud of warm breath on a cold winter day. One should be careful about trying this when it is dangerously frigid as frostbite of this sensitive part of the anatomy may result in a new medical malady, which I hereby name 'frostbutt'.

To 'Air' is Human

Frostbite is a real risk for mountaineers, and for Mount Everest climbers the comforts of base camp at an altitude of 17,590 feet may be the last chance they have for a protected bowel movement without exposing their behinds to the extreme winds and weather approaching the summit. Frozen poop stays permanently frozen and does not decompose at that altitude, so there is a growing collection from earlier expeditions that is of concern. Climbers are having a more challenging timed finding ice that has not been contaminated for melting into drinking water. Drinking contaminated water and developing diarrhea would increase the exposure to frostbite dramatically.

The most visible of the visual farts occur in the bathtub or when immersed in water, like a swimming pool or hot whirlpool tub. If you are sharing the water with someone else the innocent looking telltale bubbles underwater, can deliver a powerful bouquet to the unsuspecting nose. The intensity of the olfactory message of the human sense of smell is modulated by the brain and limbic system. If you are in a bathroom having a bowel movement the fart odor is less noticeable and certainly less alarming then when you are in an elevator, theater, or restaurant and you are aromatically assaulted without forewarning.

Fart, Volume (Quantity)

The fact is that all living creatures created gas from the cellular respiration, which is ubiquitous through life forms. The bacteria in your colonic flora generate microscopic nanofarts and microfarts, which collect into larger bubbles of gas in the bowel. They are intermixed with the atmospheric air swallowed throughout the day and particularly at meals, when chewing gum, and chewing or smoking tobacco or other recreational products. Aerophagia is universal and we swallow on average 3-5 cc (teaspoonful) of air with every swallow. Now add into the mixture the gasses produced during the enzymatic digestive processes as well as the neutralization of gastric hydrochloric acid and pancreatic and duodenal bicarbonate and you have a virtual windstorm of voluminous gasses transiting the bowel.

Fortunately the vast majority of the gasses produced are absorbed by the gut, then into the bloodstream through diffusion and as a solution, finally being exhaled when they reach the alveoli of the lungs and can be exchanged with atmospheric air. The component gasses have very different properties of diffusion through the vowel wall and into the bloodstream. Carbon dioxide readily diffuses and enters solution and is exhaled, such that although it is the largest volume of gas generated by far, and temporarily is a major contributor to distension and postprandial (after meal) discomfort, it is the easiest to eliminate from the bowel and is only a minor contributor to flatulence.

Nitrogen is the largest volume component of atmospheric air, and as would be expected, represents an identically high proportion of the gasses swallowed through aerophagia. Once in the body the carbon dioxide of the air is absorbed and eliminated as discussed above. The nitrogen however is a very poorly absorbed gas, and in essence will either come back up as a burp, or will sooner or later, comes out the other end as a fart.

The oxygen in the air, representing nearly 21% of the air gasses swallowed during aerophagia, is absorbed slowly, as the gut is not nearly as efficient as the lungs for respiration. As the carbon dioxide and oxygen are absorbed the percent of the gastrointestinal tract air that is nitrogen increases. As soon as the digestive process begins, hydrochloric acid of the stomach is neutralized by bicarbonate of the duodenum and pancreas. Large volumes of carbon dioxide gas are generated, as are smaller quantities of hydrogen, methane and other aromatic gasses discussed later. The volume of gasses in the gastrointestinal tract is dependent on the quantity and nature if foods ingested, the body's ability to synthesize and utilize specific enzymes for the various food types, the nature and quantity of the bacteria in the gut flora, the speed of gastrointestinal transit which may be influences by drugs, hormones, food product and illness, the absorptive capacity and health of the mucosal lining, and the physical length of the individuals gastrointestinal tract.

The question of what is the average number of farts per day is similar to the question if what is an average price for a normal used car. What year, make, model, condition, diesel or gas or electric or hybrid, mileage, etc. etc. The quoted figure of 11.5 farts per day is a reasonable approximation from a very small sample size of male medical students, but normal has a very wide range depending on the variables. The female medical students were too smart to participate in the study so a far as science is concerned, women do not fart. Later suggestions that they fart, but less than the guys, is just as suspect.
The differences in the physical attributes between male and female of a species represent their sexual dimorphism. The theory of sexual selection advanced by Charles Darwin in 1871 is closely related to sexual dimorphism. On average adult humans males are on 4% taller and 8% heavier than females. In a number of other species it is the female that is larger, occasionally dramatically so.

The triple wart sea devil, an anglerfish, exhibits extreme sexual dimorphism, with the male becoming little more than a stunted sperm-producing body that lives a parasitic existence off of the females hard work and effort in providing livelihood and producing the next generation of offspring. Some human males appear to have evolved their behavioral patterns from the anglerfish modus operandi.
In most mammals, humans included, the males are larger in size, mass, and caloric intake. In most species is the make that is diminutive in size, sometimes dramatically so. It would only make sense that makes would generate more gas, but how do the two compare if the caloric intake and composition were identical. Since there are no identically comparable cases studies would have to be average large populations of each gender and minimize the variables as much as possible.

As curious as we may be to know the answer to this question vital to gender politics and security, no studies are planned or anticipated. There have been reports of extreme flatulence in the medical literature of what may be considered the upper limits of the normal range, up to 150 in a 24-hour period. There are probably more accurate reports of what is the upper limit of spousal tolerance in divorce court proceedings and depositions. So for general health we talk about achieving our target heart rate during exercise. Is there an equivalent for a target fart rate? For harmonious relationships ideal would be below the quoted figure of 11.5 farts per day, that way you could reasonably attest that you fart less than average. You could also argue that the 23 you passed were each only half fart so you still are within the normal range.

As we age we produce less digestive enzymes and there is an argument to be made that there should be an adjustment and tolerance allowed for 'old farts'. The sheer number of variables allow 101 + explanations for why you fart much less than expected for your given circumstances. But perhaps the best excuse is that you did not do anything, it's the billions of nanofarting and microfarting bacteria that are to blame. If you are told to pick on someone closer to your own size you could blame the dog and claim it is a talented ventrilo-farter. Trying to arrive at a definition of what constitutes a discrete individual fart is a challenge worthy of drafting and approving a United Nations resolution. Is a staccato stutter often small farts completed in rapid succession to count as 1 or ten? Is one large long loud fart the equivalent of four small farts over 30 seconds. Should a loud tuba blast count the same as a faint toot?

Fart, Weight

As a fart is composed of atoms and molecules it has physical properties, including a mass and weight. Since it is composed of gasses and volatile molecules it is very light, yet the weight is measureable. Each fart is unique, much like fingerprints, although don't expect it to be used for personal identification. The total mass of the average fart is 0.0371 grams. For those wishing to lose weight every fart means you weigh just a little bit less. The constituent gasses and mass of the average fart is listed below:

Nitrogen: 0.0263 grams
Hydrogen: 0.0003 grams
Carbon Dioxide: 0.0063 grams
Methane: 0.0018 grams
Oxygen: 0.0016 grams
Odiferous Products: 0.0008 grams

Fiber

Dietary fiber, also referred to as roughage is the indigestible component of plants consumed as food. There are two main types, differentiated by their solubility in water. Soluble fiber, which dissolves in water, is readily fermented in the intestinal tract producing gases and byproducts. It us further divided into viscous fiber and prebiotic fiber. Is commonly found in oat bran, beans, peas, and most fruits.

To 'Air' is Human

Insoluble fiber does not dissolve in water. It is further divided into fiber that is metabolically inert and simply provides added bulk and fluid retention, or prebiotic which is metabolically fermented by the gut flora. The bulk enhancing fibers ease defecation both by adding moisture to the stool as well as stimulating gut peristalsis and colonic mass movements.

The added bulk also reduces the incidence of spasmodic contractions of the bowel, which may contribute to the pain, and discomfort of irritable bowel syndrome, previously known as a spastic colon or spastic colitis. This is the type of fiber found in wheat bran and some vegetables. Dietary fiber is comprised of non-starch polysaccharides such as arabinoxylans, cellulose, resistant starch, resistant dextrins, inulin, lignin, waxes, chitins, pectins, beta-glucans, and oligosaccharides.

Lignin, a major dietary insoluble fiber source, may alter the rate and metabolism of soluble fibers. Lignin is found in high concentrations in tree bark and its difficulty in being digested and decomposed played a major role in the Carboniferous era when tree bark was a multiple of the thickness it is today. On the other hand, insoluble fibers like the resistant starches are fully fermented. The main disadvantage of a diet high in fiber is the increased intestinal gas production with bloating and being a social outcast as a possible consequence.

Soluble fiber can be found in foods such as oatbran, barley, nuts, seeds, beans, lentils, fruits (citrus, apples), strawberries and many vegetables

Insoluble fiber is found in foods such as whole wheat and whole grain products, vegetables, and wheat bran

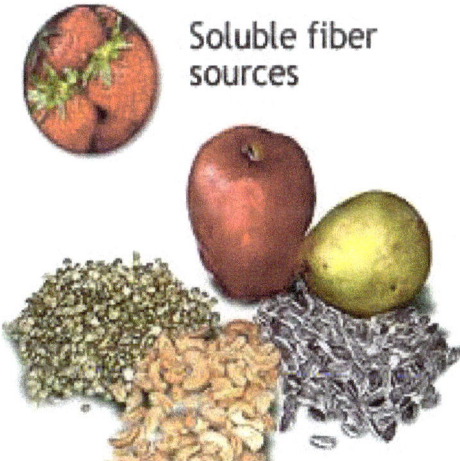

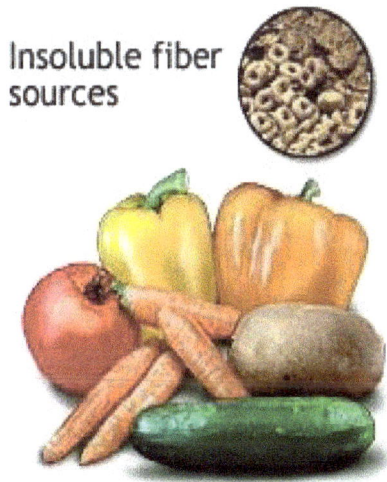

Soluble fiber sources

Insoluble fiber sources

The original definition of fiber was the components of plants that were not affected by digestive enzymes, a definition that includes lignin and polysaccharides. The definition was later expanded to include resistant starches, polysaccharides, lignin, and inulin with other oligosaccharides. While dietary fiber is present in nearly all fruits and vegetables, the type and quantity of fiber varies widely. Persimmons have safety issues and if eaten unripen the soluble tannin shiboul can lead to gastric phytobezoars a condition where a hardened wood like mass of fiber remains within the stomach for years or a lifetime.

Soluble fiber is present, in variable quantities, in plant food including legumes (peas, soybeans, lupins, beans), oats, rye, chia, and barley, some fruits and fruit juices (including prune juice, plums, berries, ripe bananas, apples, and pears), certain vegetables such as broccoli, carrots, Jerusalem artichokes, root tubers and root vegetables such as sweet potatoes and onions (skins of these are sources of insoluble fiber also), psyllium seed husk (a mucilage soluble fiber) and flax seeds, and nuts, with almonds being the highest in dietary fiber

Fiber Content Of Popular Foods			
Food Source	Soluble Fiber (g)	Insoluble Fiber (g)	Total Fiber (g)
Apple (1 med)	0.9g	2.0g	2.9g
Banana (1 med)	0.6g	1.4g	2.0g
Orange (1 med)	1.3g	0.7g	2.0g
Broccoli (1 stalk)	1.3g	1.4g	2.7g
Carrots (1 large)	1.3g	1.6g	2.9g
Tomato (1 small)	0.1g	0.7g	0.8g
Potato (1 medium)	1.0g	0.8g	1.8g
All Bran (1/2 cup)	1.4g	7.6g	9.0g
Oat Bran (1/2 cup)	2.2g	2.2g	4.4g
Corn Flakes (1 cup)	0g	0.5g	0.5g
Rolled Oats (3/4 cup)	1.3g	1.7g	3.0g
Wheat Bread (1 slice)	0.3g	1.1g	1.4g
White Bread (1 slice)	0.3g	0.1g	0.4g
Green Peas (2/3 cup)	0.6g	3.3g	3.9g
Kidney Beans (1/2 cup)	1.6g	4.9g	6.5g
Lentils (2/3 cup)	0.6g	3.9g	4.5g

source: USDA/ARS Nutrient Data Laboratory

Public Domain

Sources of insoluble fiber include, whole grain foods, wheat and corn bran, legumes such as beans and peas, nuts and seeds, potato skins, lignins, vegetables such as green beans, cauliflower, zucchini (courgette), celery, nopal, some fruits including avocado, and unripe bananas, the skins of some fruits, including kiwifruit, grapes and tomatoes. Vegetable gum fiber, such as guar gum and acacia Senegal gum, dissolve easily and have no aftertaste making them a popular fiber supplement additive.

To 'Air' is Human

Dietary fibers have three primary mechanisms: bulking, viscosity and fermentation. As they can change the nature and transit of the intestinal contents they may impact how other nutrients and materials are absorbed. Some soluble fibers bind to bile acids preventing their normal reabsorption in the small intestine this interruption in the normal enterohepatic circulation of the bile from the small intestine to the liver results in the loss of cholesterol in the form of bile acids via the stool. The cholesterol levels in the blood are subsequently lowered since the liver removes cholesterol from the circulation to synthesize replacement bile salts. Viscous soluble fibers may also inhibit the absorption of sugar thus reducing the sugar insulin response after meals.

Fatty foods and hypertonic solutions delay gastric emptying and gut transit time. The intestinal contents are called chyme once they leave the stomach. Chyme consists of food compounds, digestive enzymes, stomach acid and pancreatic and duodenal bicarbonate, bile acids, complex lipids in changing micellar, aqueous, hydrocolloid, hydrophobic, and hydrophilic phases all in a mixture of solid, liquid, colloidal and gas bubble phases. In other words, it is one chaotic churning, digesting, fermenting mass with selectively absorbs ion and secretion occurring throughout the process. Non-absorbed carbohydrates such as pectin, gum Arabic, oligosaccharides and resistant starch, are fermented by the gut flora to short-chain fatty acids (mainly acetic, propionic and n-butyric), carbon dioxide, hydrogen and methane. The colon will absorb nearly all of the short-chain fatty acids with the butyric acid being utilized as the main source of energy for colonic cells.

Soluble and insoluble fiber both increases food volume without additional caloric content. The increased volume can provide greater satiety, which may eat to decreased food intake and weight loss. Intestinal fermentation can increase the production of beneficial short chain fatty acids. Soluble fiber absorbs water and forms a viscous gel, known as a hydrophilic mucelloid that slows gastric emptying and intestinal transit. The increase bulk may shield carbohydrates from enzymes, delay the absorption of glucose, and reduce the fluctuations of blood sugar levels that result. On the other and the delayed transit allows more time for enzymatic activity as well as fermentation by the gut flora.

Insoluble fiber enhances gut motility and speeds transit time, as well as adding bulk and moisture to the stool promoting defecation and preventing constipation. Current recommendations for daily dietary fiber intake are 30 grams for the average adults. The average American consumes about half of that amount. Sugars and starches provide 4 Calories per gram as the digestive system has enzymes to break them down into the simple absorbable sugars of glucose, fructose, and galactose. Insoluble fiber cannot be digested so no calories are absorbed. Soluble fiber is partially fermented, and the caloric intake is determined by the degree that it is broken down into absorbable nutrients. As a result of the variability in calories generated there is controversy on their calorie count. 2 Calories per gram of soluble fiber is a reasonable compromise. Fibers with partial or low ferment ability include cellulose, hemicellulose, lignans, plant waxes, and resistant starches. Fibers with high ferment ability include beta-glucans, pectins, natural gums, inulins, oligosaccharides, and resistant dextrins.

Flatology

The scientific study of flatulence is termed flatology. Flatulence is defined as flatus (Latin blowing) expelled through the anus as well as the state of being affected with gases in the intestinal tract. The noises commonly associated with flatulence ("Blowing a raspberry") are caused by the vibration of the anal sphincter and occasionally by the buttocks. Both the noise and smell associated with flatus leaving the anus can be sources of embarrassment or comedy in many cultures. There are five general symptoms related to intestinal gas: pain, bloating and abdominal distension, excessive flatus volume, excessive flatus smell and gas incontinence.

Flatulence

Flatulence is defined as flatus (Latin blowing) expelled through the anus as well as the state of being affected with gases in the intestinal tract. The scientific study of flatulence is termed flatology .The noises commonly associated with flatulence are caused by the vibration of the anal sphincter and occasionally by the buttocks. Both the noise and smell associated with flatus leaving the anus can be sources of embarrassment or comedy in many cultures. Further characterizations of the nature of flatulence are found under the topics of fart, flatus, and intestinal gas, which are commonly used, interchangeably in the English language.

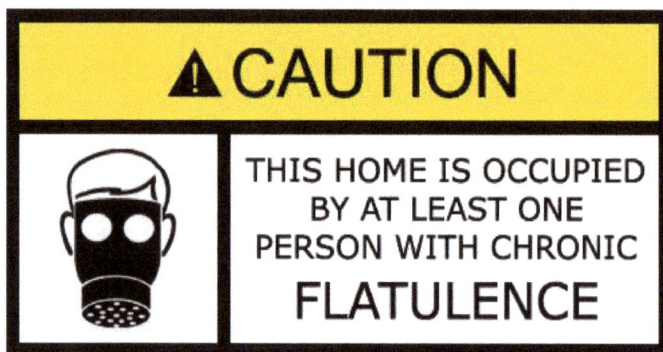

⚠ CAUTION

THIS HOME IS OCCUPIED BY AT LEAST ONE PERSON WITH CHRONIC FLATULENCE

unclestinky.files.wordpress.com Creative Commons License

FODMAP Diet

FODMAP is an acronym that stands for Fermentable Oligosaccharides, Disaccharides, Monosaccharides, And Polyols. These short chain carbohydrates and related sugar alcohols are poorly absorbed in the small intestine.. Many of the sugar alcohols including sorbitol, mannitol, xylitol, isomalt, and maltitol are added to commercial food products as non-nutritive bulk sweeteners. Originally developed at Monash University in Melbourne, Australia it has become popular worldwide as a means of reducing the symptoms of irritable bowel syndrome, functional gastrointestinal disorders, and excess intestinal gas

Foods suitable on a low-fodmap diet

fruit	vegetables	grain foods	milk products	other
fruit banana, blueberry, boysenberry, canteloupe, cranberry, durian, grape, grapefruit, honeydew melon, kiwifruit, lemon, lime, mandarin, orange, passionfruit, pawpaw, raspberry, rhubarb, rockmelon, star anise, strawberry, tangelo Note: if fruit is dried, eat in small quantities	**vegetables** alfalfa, artichoke, bamboo shoots, bean shoots, bok choy, carrot, celery, choko, choy sum, endive, ginger, green beans, lettuce, olives, parsnip, potato, pumpkin, red capsicum (bell pepper), silver beet, spinach, summer squash (yellow), swede, sweet potato, taro, tomato, turnip, yam, zucchini **herbs** basil, chili, coriander, ginger, lemongrass, marjoram, mint, oregano, parsley, rosemary, thyme	**cereals** gluten-free bread or cereal products **bread** 100% spelt bread **rice** **oats** **polenta** **other** arrowroot, millet, psyllium, quinoa, sorgum, tapioca	**milk** lactose-free milk, oat milk*, rice milk, soy milk* *check for additives **cheeses** hard cheeses, and brie and camembert **yoghurt** lactose-free varieties **ice-cream substitutes** gelati, sorbet **butter substitutes** olive oil	**sweeteners** sugar* (sucrose), glucose, artificial sweeteners not ending in '-ol' **honey substitutes** golden syrup*, maple syrup*, molasses, treacle *small quantities

3.bp.blogspot.com Creative Commons License

Eliminate foods containing fodmaps

excess fructose	lactose	fructans	galactans	polyols
fruit apple, mango, nashi, pear, tinned fruit in natural juice, watermelon **sweeteners** fructose, high fructose corn syrup **large total fructose dose** concentrated fruit sources, large serves of fruit, dried fruit, fruit juice **honey** corn syrup, fruisana	**milk** milk from cows, goats or sheep, custard, ice cream, yoghurt **cheeses** soft unripened cheeses eg. cottage, cream, mascarpone, ricotta	**vegetables** asparagus, beetroot, broccoli, brussels sprouts, cabbage, eggplant, fennel, garlic, leek, okra, onion (all), shallots, spring onion **cereals** wheat and rye, in large amounts eg. bread, crackers, cookies, couscous, pasta **fruit** custard apple, persimmon, watermelon **miscellaneous** chicory, dandelion, inulin	**legumes** baked beans, chickpeas, kidney beans, lentils	**fruit** apple, apricot, avocado, blackberry, cherry, lychee, nashi, nectarine, peach, pear, plum, prune, watermelon **vegetables** cauliflower, green capsicum (bell pepper), mushroom, sweet corn **sweeteners** sorbitol (420) mannitol (421) isomalt (953) maltitol (965) xylitol (967)

bp.blogspot.com Creative Commons License

Food Intolerance

Food intolerance is often very individualized and is not the same as food allergy. In food allergy the food that triggers the reaction is known as the antigen, and the allergic reaction is mediated by the body's immune and inflammatory response systems. The chart following identifies several of the other differences.

Allergy	Intolerance
Obvious symptoms	Subtle symptoms
Immediate reaction - within one hour	Delayed reaction - 12 to 72 hours
Rapid onset of symptoms and often reaction magnifies with each exposure	Slow onset and often slow magnification of symptoms, even after the often long delay
Often triggered by minute amount of food	Not predominantly affected by food quantity
Affects Immunoglobulin E (IgE)	Affects Immunoglobulin G (IgG) and/or other mechanisms (prostaglandins, leukotrienes, etc.)
Allergies are uncommon	Intolerances are very common
Generally non-reversible	Reversible
Well recognised by medicine	Just beginning to be recognised by medicine
Test : Prick or RAST (Radio-immunodiffusion Test)	Test : Electro-Dermal Screening (EDS) or Blood Immunoglobulin G (IgG)

lunar.thegamez.net Creative Commons License

In a number of cases of food intolerance the sensitivity is the result of lower levels of the necessary enzymes to digest specific foods. For example the milk sugar lactose requires the specific enzyme called lactase, to properly digest this complex sugar into absorbable simple sugars. If insufficient lactase is present the gut flora, which is comprised of various microorganisms, ferments the residual undigested sugar. This process leads to the release of various gases that may accumulate within the digestive tract and are eliminated as a fart. A portion of the gas is produced such as carbon dioxide are readily absorbed by the digestive tract and transported by the circulatory system to the lungs where they are eliminated through respiration.

The ability of the individual to produce the necessary lactase enzyme is often hereditary. Many populations have limited lactase production, which results in the common occurrence of lactose intolerance. If the intake of lactose is restricted the limited amount of lactase president may be sufficient to prevent the development of the symptoms of lactose intolerance. These symptoms such as excess intestinal gas diarrhea abdominal cramps are often dependent on the quantity of lactose ingested that exceeds the available lactase enzyme necessary for its digestion.

A number of the digestive enzymes, which are lacking in individual populations, can be supplemented either by purchased enzyme products, or by the production of the enzymes by the individuals gut flora. The flora may be supplemented with commensal organisms such as lactobacillus, which aid in the digestion of dairy products. Other commonly malabsorbed complex sugars include fructose, mannitol, sorbitol, and a variety of sugar substitutes.

Food Intolerance and Common Symptoms

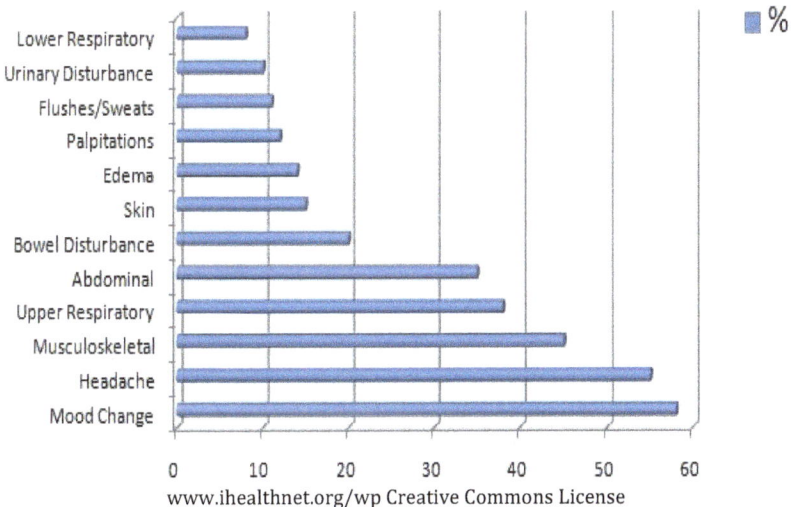

www.ihealthnet.org/wp Creative Commons License

Fructose in particular has limited enzyme available for its digestion and frequently leads to intolerance when ingested beyond the enzyme capacity. In some cases the necessary enzyme for digestion of the complex sugar or starch does not naturally occur in humans. One example is the enzyme cellulase, which is required for the digestion of cellulose a sugar commonly found in plants. This enzyme is found in herbivorous animals that consume grasses and cellulose containing food products.

To 'Air' is Human

The complex sugars found in legumes are in the raffinose class, which includes Stachyose and Verbascose. The enzyme required for their digestion is called Alpha galactosidase. This enzyme is not naturally occurring in humans and must be obtained from external sources. Without the availability of this enzyme the gut flora metabolism releases large quantities of gases, which are often released as a fart. The enzyme is found naturally in beans and legumes once the seed is germinated. The enzyme is also available commercially as over-the-counter products such as Beano, Say Yes to Beans, and other products.

Many individuals also have difficulty digesting the cereal grains, especially those that contain gluten. Gluten intolerance may range from mild excess gaseous us to true inflammation and damage of the intestinal lining. When the villi, which are the fingerlike projections of the bowel lining, are damaged malabsorption occurs. This condition known as gluten sensitive enteropathy (also known as celiac disease and celiac sprue) is a serious health concern. Adherence to a strict gluten-free diet is required to prevent further injury and complications from the malabsorption of nutrients and other features of the disorder.

A number of the food in tolerances may be addressed easily by avoiding the inciting foods in the diet. A number of food in tolerances are more challenging to control by diet alone as the commercial food products in the marketplace may contain small quantities. It is necessary to carefully read the ingredients of all commercial food products purchased or consumed if one has specific food intolerance. With further understanding of the gut microbiome, Pre-biotics and probiotics maybe used to have commensals microbes supplement the natural enzymes of the human host. There are a wide variety of food intolerances and enzyme deficiencies and that can be major contributors to gastrointestinal and other symptoms. Enzymes deficiencies are not uncommon and there are many possible enzymes to investigate including proteases such as pepsin, pepsinogen, trypsin, trypsinogen, chymotrypsin, and chymotrypsinogen. Other enzymes include amylase, lipase, invertase, sucrose, maltase, lactase, and about 1,600 others.

Taking a Sherlock Holmes approach and trying an elimination diet is certainly reasonable. Enzyme supplements are commercially available and are another approach for an empiric trial if the suspect foods are not well defined. It is important to take the appropriate enzyme with the appropriate food. The right enzyme for the wrong food, or the wrong enzyme for the right food, will not make a bit of difference in helping your digestion. The most common enzyme deficiency is lactase resulting in lactose intolerance. Medications can also interfere with enzyme activity and give rise to digestive symptoms

The most widely distributed naturally occurring non-enzyme food chemical capable of provoking reactions is salicylate, with tartrazine and benzoic acid sensitivity seen less often. Benzoates and salicylates occur naturally in many different foods, including fruits, juices, vegetables, tomatoes, spices, herbs, nuts, tea, wines, and coffee. Other natural chemicals, which commonly cause reactions and cross reactivity, include amines, nitrates, sulphites and some antioxidants. Reactions to chocolate, cheese, bananas, avocado, tomato or wine suggest that bioactive amines may be a likely candidate as a food chemical that triggers sensitivities.

Franklin, Benjamin

Benjamin Franklin (1706-1790) was a polymath scientist, author, statesman, philosopher, publisher, diplomat, inventor, and humorist. In 1781 he was serving as the United States ambassador to France and with his scientific background kept in close communication with the European community of scientists. As is typical for a scientific congress an announcement from the Royal Academy of Brussels was made calling for the presentation of scientific papers on a host of subjects.

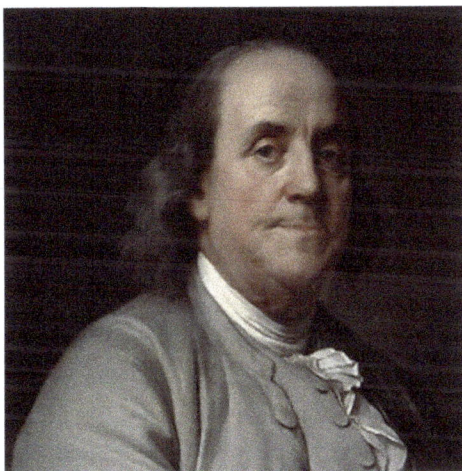

Portrait of Benjamin Franklin by Joseph Siffrein Duplessis c. 1785 National Portrait Gallery Washington D.C. Public Domain

Franklin found some of the proposals so pretentious that his "bawdy, scurrilous nature" was stirred to compose a satirical response in the form of a proposal for research. As an illustrious statesman and scientist his proposal would demand serious attention. His proposal to the Royal Academy of Brussels is reprinted in its entirety in the companion volume to this book *Artsy Fartsy, Cultural History of the Fart*.

"Let every fart count as a peal of thunder for liberty. Let every fart remind the nation of how much it has let pass out of its control. So fart, and if you must, fart often. But always fart without apology. Fart for freedom, fart for liberty… and fart proudly!"

"He that lives upon Hope, dies farting." is another of his famous quotes.

His proposal to the Royal Academy (reprinted in full below) called for scientific research to discover food additives that would provide a variety of attractive aromas to produce good smelling farts that would be socially welcomed.

Fructose

Fructose, fruit sugar, is a simple monosaccharide found in many fruits, berries, flowers, honey, artichokes, wheat, onions, and root vegetables. Fructose was discovered in 1847 by the French chemist Augustin-Pierre Dubrunfaut. It is prepared commercially from sugar cane, sugar beets, and corn. High-fructose corn syrup (HFCS) is made from the enzymatic conversion of cornstarch and is often added as a sweetener to soft drinks and other foods.

Apples and pears contain more than twice as much free fructose as glucose. High concentrations of free fructose in these fruits and their juices can cause diarrhea in children, as they are unable to absorb fructose as well as glucose and sucrose. The fructose creates higher osmolality in the small intestine drawing water into the gastrointestinal tract resulting in diarrhea. It is because of the fructose that apple juice; raisins, grape juice, and bananas will increase flatulence.

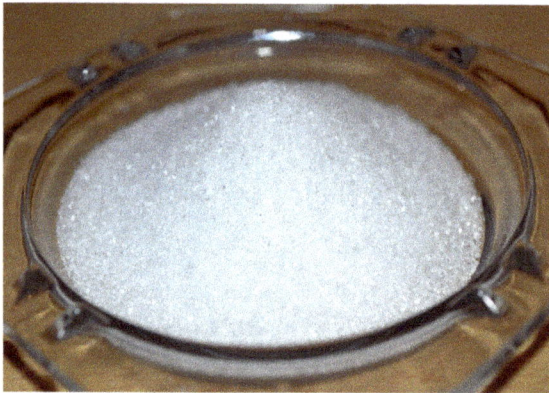

Crystalline fructose Creative Commons License

Fructose exists in foods either as a monosaccharide (free fructose) or as a unit of a disaccharide (sucrose). Fructose is seventy-three percent sweeter than sucrose. The enzyme sucrase catalyzes sucrose into glucose and fructose, both of which are absorbed by the small intestine, as is the other monosaccharide galactose. Fructose has a very low glycemic index of nineteen, compared with one hundred for glucose and sixty-eight for sucrose.

Fructose Intolerance, Hereditary

Dietary fructose intolerance is the decreased capacity to absorb fructose because of deficient fructose carriers in the small intestine's enterocytes. Hereditary fructose intolerance is a more serious liver enzyme deficiency that requires total abstinence from fructose. Hereditary fructose intolerance is a defect of fructose metabolism caused by an autosomal recessive gene mutation resulting in a deficiency of the enzyme aldolase B. Hereditary fructose intolerance individuals are asymptomatic until they ingest fructose, sucrose, or sorbitol. Symptoms can include vomiting, hypoglycemia, jaundice, hemorrhage, hepatomegaly, hyperuricemia and kidney failure.

The pathways of fructose in HFI & Fructose Malabsorption

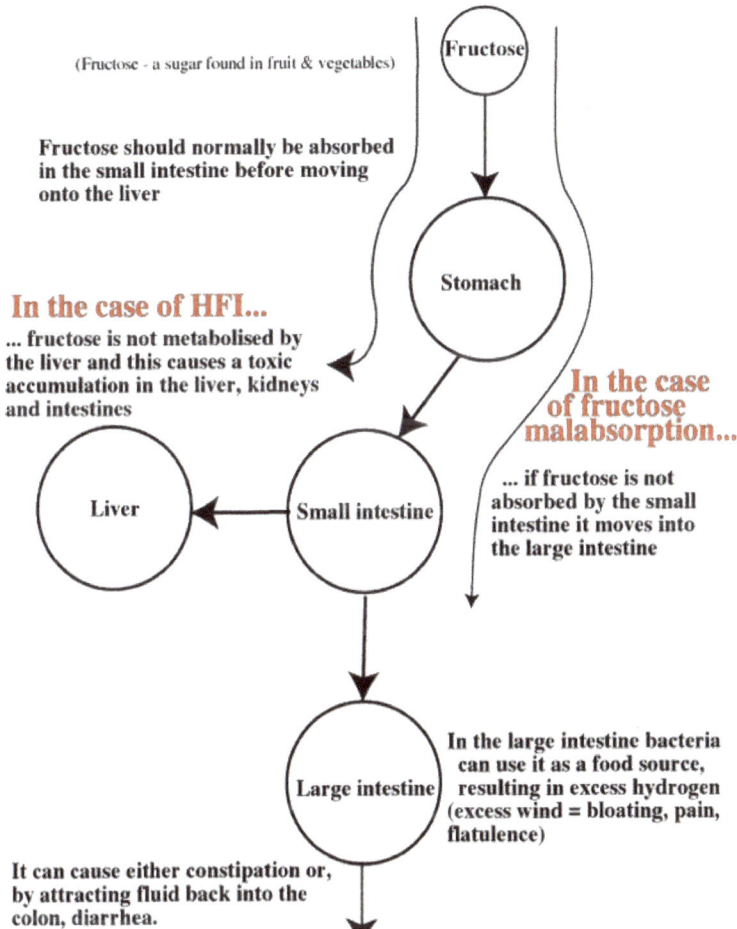

(Fructose - a sugar found in fruit & vegetables)

Fructose

Fructose should normally be absorbed in the small intestine before moving onto the liver

Stomach

In the case of HFI...
... fructose is not metabolised by the liver and this causes a toxic accumulation in the liver, kidneys and intestines

In the case of fructose malabsorption...

... if fructose is not absorbed by the small intestine it moves into the large intestine

Liver

Small intestine

Large intestine

In the large intestine bacteria can use it as a food source, resulting in excess hydrogen (excess wind = bloating, pain, flatulence)

It can cause either constipation or, by attracting fluid back into the colon, diarrhea.

Diagnosis of hereditary fructose intolerance is suspected in infants who become symptomatic when fructose-containing foods are introduced into their diet. Affected individuals are asymptomatic and healthy, provided they do not ingest foods containing fructose or its precursors sucrose and sorbitol.

To 'Air' is Human

Fructose is absorbed in the small intestine without the need for digestive enzymes. About 25–50 grams of fructose per intake can be properly absorbed in healthy people. People with fructose malabsorption cannot absorb more than 25 grams per intake. In the large intestine the fructose is metabolized into short chain fatty acids, producing hydrogen, carbon dioxide and methane. The increased osmotic load can cause diarrhea. The abnormal increase in hydrogen is detectable with the hydrogen breath test.

Foods that contain more glucose than fructose are usually well tolerated since glucose enhances absorption of fructose. Foods with a high fructose to glucose ratio like apples and pears can be difficult to process and sound are avoided. Additional foods to be avoided include those rich in fructans such as artichokes, asparagus, leeks, onions, wheat, sorbitol, xylitol, erythritol, inulin, fructo-oligosaccharide, and mannitol.

Fructose Malabsorption

Fructose malabsorption, formerly named hereditary fructose intolerance or dietary fructose intolerance, is the decreased capacity to absorb fructose because of deficient fructose carriers in the small intestine's enterocytes. This condition is common in patients with irritable bowel syndrome. It is not synonymous with the more serious hereditary fructose intolerance, a liver enzyme deficiency that requires total abstinence from fructose.

How Much Fructose Can I Eat Per Day?

We can only absorb 20 grams of Fructose per day. That's 4 ½ teaspoons or two apples.

Any more is harmful to the liver, causing fat deposits, obesity, and insulin resistance.

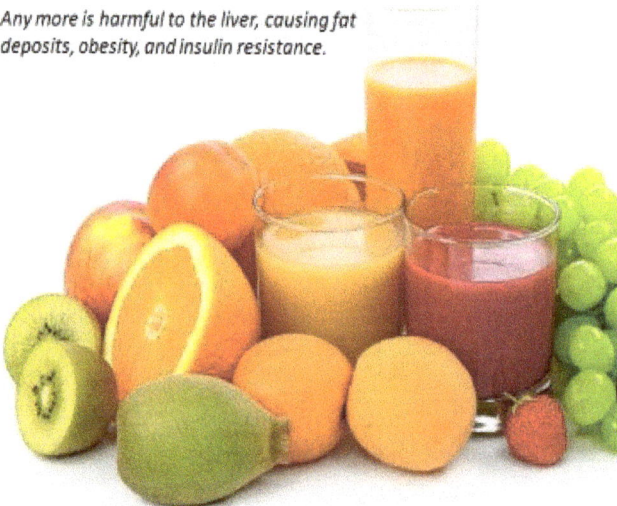

Fructose in fresh fruit

Fruit portion	Grams of Fructose
1 Lime	0.0
1 Lemon	0.6
1 cup cranberries	0.7
1 date	2.6
1/8 cantaloupe	2.8
1 cup raspberries	3.0
1 kiwi	3.4
1 slice pineapple	4.0
1 grapefruit	4.3
1 tangerine	4.8
1 peach/nectarine	5.8
1 orange	6.1
1/2 papaya	6.3
1 banana	7.1
1 cup blueberries	7.4
1 apple	9.5
1 pear	11.8
¾ cup raisins	12.3
1 cup grapes	12.4
1/2 mango	16.2
1 cup dry apricots	16.4
1 cup dry figs	23.0

Cells lining the small intestine

Cells lining the large intestine

Fructose

poor absorption
across the small
intestine

→ Fructose

fermented by bacteria
in the large intestine
into gases like
hydrogen which can
cause symptoms

gastronorth.com.au Creative Commons License

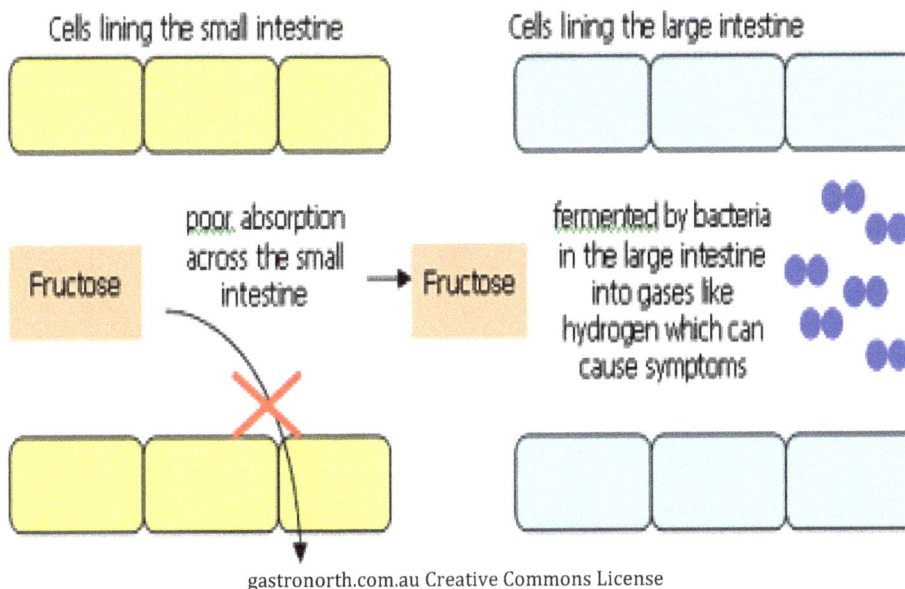

Gas, Therapy (see Intestinal Gas Therapy)

Gastroesophageal Reflux Disease (GERD)

Gastroesophageal reflux disease (GERD) is mucosal damage of the esophagus caused by the reflux of gastric acid, bile, and digestive enzymes. In Western populations GERD affects approximately ten to twenty percent of the population. The most common symptom is heartburn, formally known as pyrosis. In the United States twenty percent of people have symptoms in a given week, and seven percent every day.

GERD is usually caused by abnormal relaxation of the lower esophageal sphincter or hiatal hernia with contributing factors such as obesity, Zollinger-Ellison hypergastrinemia, hypercalcemia, scleroderma, and esophageal dysmotility. Carminatives, drugs, hormones, alcohol, tobacco, fried or fatty foods, and chocolate all of which can reduce the lower esophageal sphincter pressure can aggravate it.

Treatment is typically via lifestyle changes and medications such as proton pump inhibitors, H2 receptor blockers or antacids. Some Antacids can be absorbed leading to an alkalosis syndrome. Antacids also generate large volumes of carbon dioxide as they neutralize the gastric hydrochloric acid, Magnesium containing antacids can cause diarrhea, aluminum containing antacids can cause constipation, and often a combination of the two is used to minimize the impact on bowel movements, Calcium based antacids can lead to a rebound of acid secretion is calcium is a stimulant of gastric acid production.

177

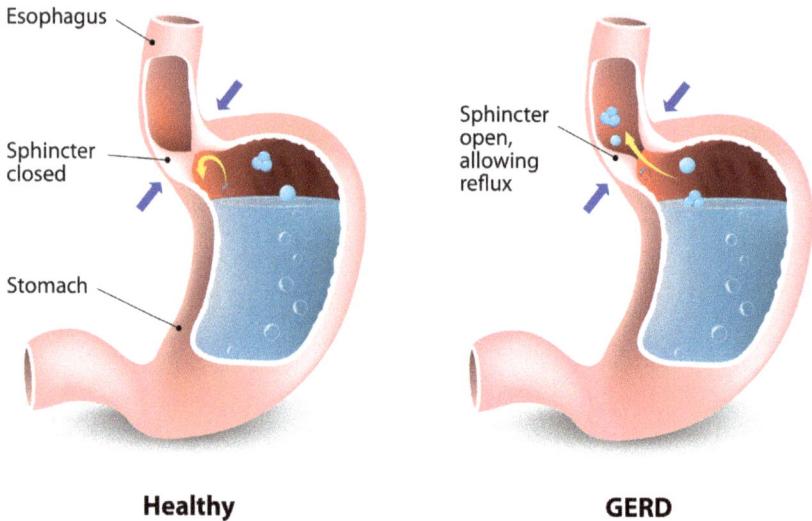

Healthy

GERD

Gastroesophageal Reflux Disease shutterstock/designua

Surgery treatment with tightening of the lower esophageal sphincter has a similar response rate as medications. If inadequately treated GERD may progress to Barrett's esophagus with intestinal metaplasia where the epithelial cells transition from the normal esophageal squamous epithelium to intestinal columnar epithelium. With the development of atypia and dysplasia this can progress to the development of adenocarcinoma of the esophagus. If Barrett's esophagus has developed a screening endoscopy with biopsies to evaluate for dysplasia is suggested.

The diagnosis of GERD is usually by history with typical symptoms of heartburn and reflux. Atypical manifestations of GERD include laryngitis, unexplained chest pain, chronic cough, sinusitis, pulmonary fibrosis, earache, recurrent ear infections, asthma, and obstructive sleep apnea. Another unusual symptom is called water brash, which is a rush of salivary secretions after an episode of regurgitation to dilute and clear the acid in the esophagus.

A possible cardiac cause of atypical chest should be excluded before ascribing the source to GERD. Approximately 40% of GERD patients have a Helicobacter pylori infection. The eradication of Helicobacter pylori can lead to a worsening of the GERD symptoms since the resolving gastritis leads to an increase in gastric acid secretion.

The current gold standard for diagnosis of GERD is esophageal pH monitoring. Endoscopy is advised if any alarm symptoms are present including dysphagia, anemia, and blood in the stool, wheezing, weight loss, respiratory or laryngeal symptoms. Long-standing or severe symptoms would also prompt endoscopic evaluation for Barrett's esophagus and dysplasia.

To 'Air' is Human

The treatments for GERD include lifestyle modifications, medications, and possibly surgery. Initial treatment is typically with a proton-pump inhibitor or histamine 2 blocker that usually provides prompt and significant relief. Weight loss, avoiding large heavy meals, not lying down, bending over, or doing headstands immediately after meals, decreasing or discontinuing tobacco, alcohol, and carminative can be helpful. Elevation of the head of the bed, not with pillows but with wood blocks under the legs at the head of bed as long as it is not a waterbed can be useful.

Antacids and mucosal protectants such as alginic acid or sucralfate can also be helpful but have a more frequent dosing schedule. Prokinetic agents to enhance esophageal motility and tighten the lower esophageal sphincter can also be used. The oldest generic prokinetic Metoclopramide has a high incidence of central nervous system side effects and is now rarely used. Newer prokinetics have a safer profile.

A variety of endoscopic therapies have been developed, including procedures designed to reduce the lumen diameter to reduce reflux. Laparoscopic procedures using magnets and other implantable devices have also been utilized to create a physical barrier to the reflux of gastric contents into the esophagus. The standard surgical treatment for severe GERD is the Nissen fundoplication, where the upper part of the stomach is wrapped around the lower esophageal sphincter. This corrects the hiatal hernia by keeping the stomach and LES below the diaphragm preventing reflux. Medical therapy and surgical therapies appear to be equally effective for this often-chronic condition.

Gastrointestinal Motility

Motilin

Motilin is a hormone secreted by endocrine M cells in the small intestine, especially in the duodenum and jejunum. It was named motilin because of its ability to stimulate gastric activity. Erythromycin and related antibiotics act as motilin agonists, and are sometimes used for their ability to stimulate gastrointestinal motility. Another hormone ghrelin can also induce motilin like effects.

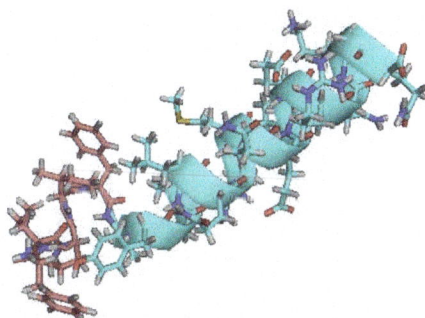

NMR solution structure of Motilin in phospholipid bicellar solution Author Adam Busch Pymol Structure Creative Commons License

To 'Air' is Human

Motilin triggers the migrating myoelectric complex component of gastrointestinal motility, which induces brief episodes of peristaltic activity several times an hour in between meals. Contractions of the gastric fundus and antrum triggered by motilin can cause stomach rumble or growls, borborygmi, and cramp like discomfort often described as hunger pains since they occur during a fasting period. The gastric emptying and peristaltic sweeping action clearing the stomach and small bowel of food residue or chyme has earned Motilin the moniker 'housekeeper of the gut'.

Gastrointestinal Pacemaker Cells

Interstitial cells of Cajal are pacemaker cells similar to the pacemaker cells of the heart, which cause the heart to beat regularly. They are present in the wall of the gut and communicate between the nervous system and the smooth muscle of the gut wall (Figure 1). When the signal arrives from the nervous system to the interstitial cells of Cajal that a person has eaten they begin their pacemaker function. This results in a coordinated and rhythmic set of contractions of the gut known as peristalsis, which propels food along the entire length of the digestive tract. The interstitial cells of Cajal were studied in relative obscurity for over one hundred years until the discovery that gastrointestinal stromal tumors (GIST) arise from interstitial cells of Cajal or an interstitial cell of Cajal-like precursor cell.

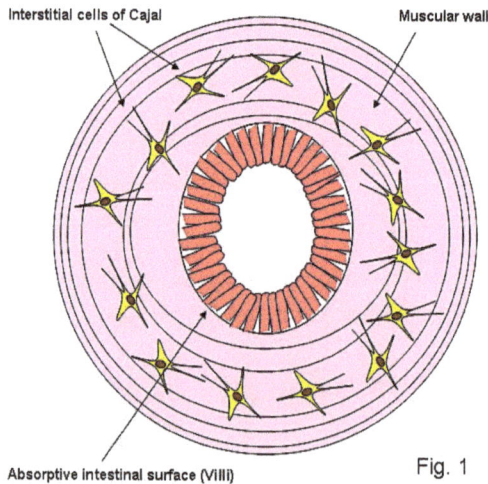

Fig. 1

Interstitial cell of Cajal are also thought to be the cells from which gastrointestinal stromal tumors (GISTs) arise. The interstitial cells of Cajal are derived from the mesoderm of the gastrointestinal tract and serves as a pacemaker for the peristaltic contractions of the smooth muscle. The interstitial cells of Cajal are named after Santiago Ramón y Cajal (1852 - 1934) a Spanish pathologist and Nobel laureate who was considered by many as the father of neuroscience.

To 'Air' is Human

The frequency of interstitial cell of Cajal pacemaker activity differs in different regions of the GI tract, 3 per minute in the stomach, twelve per minute in the duodenum, ten per minute in the ileum, and three per minute again in the colon. The loss of interstitial cells of Cajal may interrupt normal neural control of gastrointestinal contractions and lead to functional GI disorders, such as irritable bowel syndrome and chronic intestinal pseudo-obstruction. Diabetes mellitus often leads to gastrointestinal motility disorders.

Gastrointestinal motility disorders are a major source of morbidity and can have a profound influence on the quality of life. Irritable bowel syndrome is one of the most common of gastrointestinal disorders. Its prevalence in various countries around the world is between six and forty-six percent of the population. In the United States an estimated forty million people have the condition

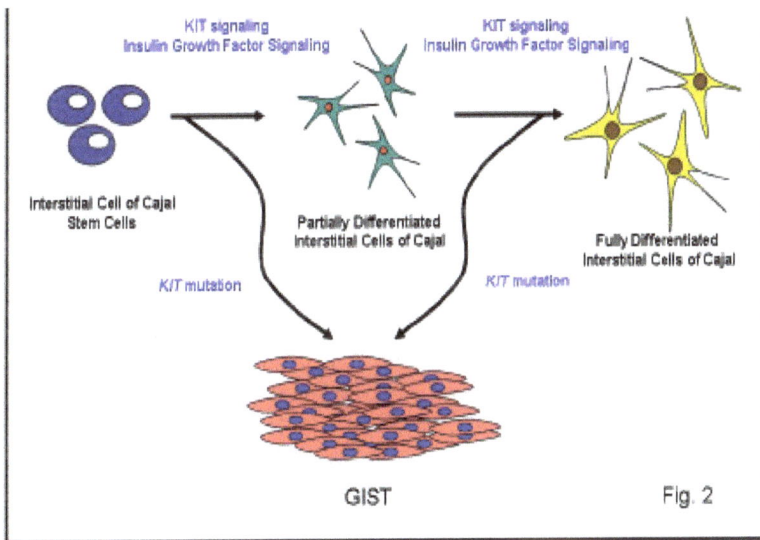

Pathway of interstitial cell of Cajal maturation and GIST formation. Interstitial cell of Cajal stem cells mature to partially differentiated and later fully differentiated interstitial cells of Cajal under the influence of KIT signaling and insulin growth factor signaling and likely many other growth and development factors. KIT or mutation in other genes such as platelet-derived growth factor receptor A leads to GIST formation.

Rapid Gastric Emptying

Rapid gastric emptying, also called dumping syndrome, occurs when undigested food empties too quickly into the small intestine. Early rapid gastric emptying begins during or right after a meal. Symptoms include nausea, vomiting, bloating, cramping, diarrhea, dizziness, and fatigue. Late rapid gastric emptying occurs 1 to 3 hours after eating. Symptoms include hypoglycemia (low blood sugar), weakness, sweating, and dizziness.

To 'Air' is Human

DUMPING SYNDROME

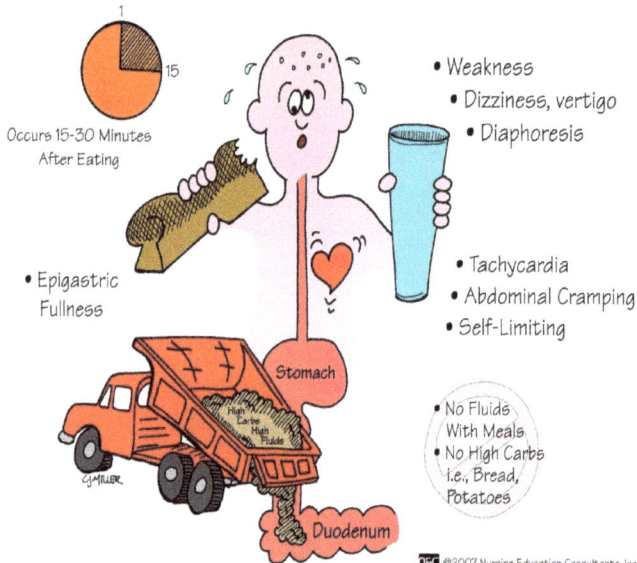

Occurs 15-30 Minutes After Eating

- Epigastric Fullness

Stomach

Duodenum

- Weakness
  - Dizziness, vertigo
  - Diaphoresis

- Tachycardia
- Abdominal Cramping
- Self-Limiting

- No Fluids With Meals
- No High Carbs i.e., Bread, Potatoes

©2007 Nursing Education Consultants, Inc.

Dumping syndrome arabnurses.com Creative Commons License

Rapid gastric emptying is usually the result of stomach surgery such as fundoplication or gastric bypass. The condition is also seen in people with Zollinger-Ellison syndrome, a rare disorder involving a gastrin hormone-secreting tumor in the pancreas. Treatment of rapid gastric emptying focuses on the underlying cause and may include changes in eating habits and medication. People who have the condition should eat several small meals a day that are low in carbohydrates. They should also drink liquids between meals and not with them. Prescription medications may also be utilized, with surgery as a last resort.

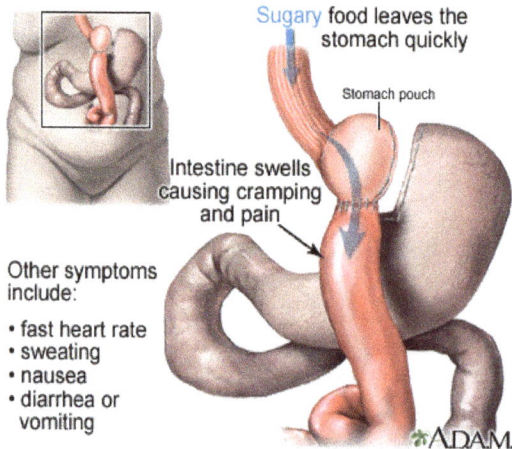

Sugary food leaves the stomach quickly

Stomach pouch

Intestine swells causing cramping and pain

Other symptoms include:

- fast heart rate
- sweating
- nausea
- diarrhea or vomiting

www.nlm.nih.gov Creative Commons License

Gastrointestinal Transit Time

Gastrointestinal transit time is the time period from ingestion of food or a biomarker until its elimination and exit from the digestive tract. The time period is highly variable and can be influenced by many factors including diet, physical activity, infection, inflammation, pharmaceuticals, etc. The gastrointestinal transit time can also be divided into the three subsets of gastric emptying, small intestinal transit and colonic transit.

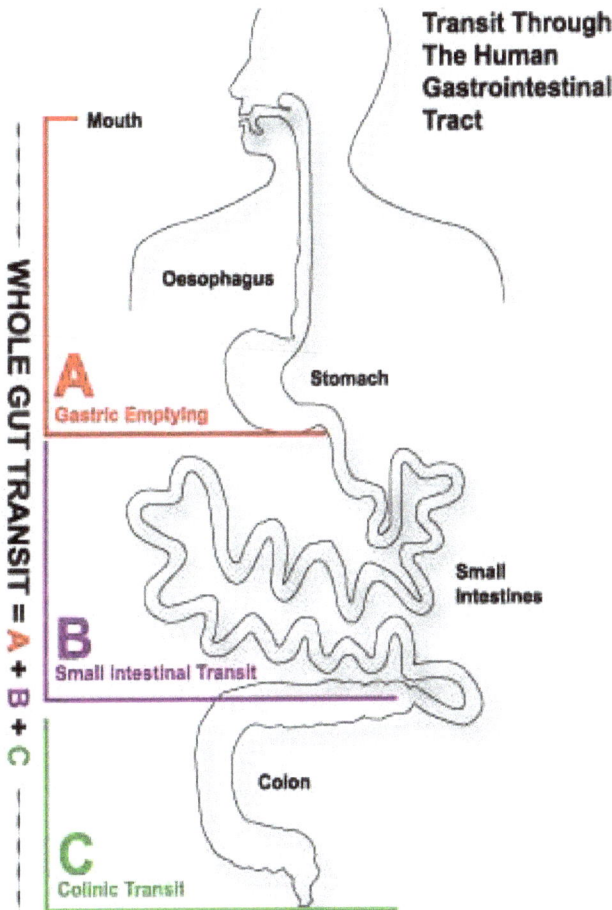

Transit Through The Human Gastrointestinal Tract

www.ibsresearchupdate.org Creative Commons License

The transit time is the general period of time it takes, from the swallow of ingestion to the elimination at defecation, for food to pass through the gastrointestinal track. Normal ranges are from half a day to two days but individuals vary. Certain conditions especially those with diarrhea may have a more rapid transit time, while those with neurologic conditions or diabetes may have a slow transit time.

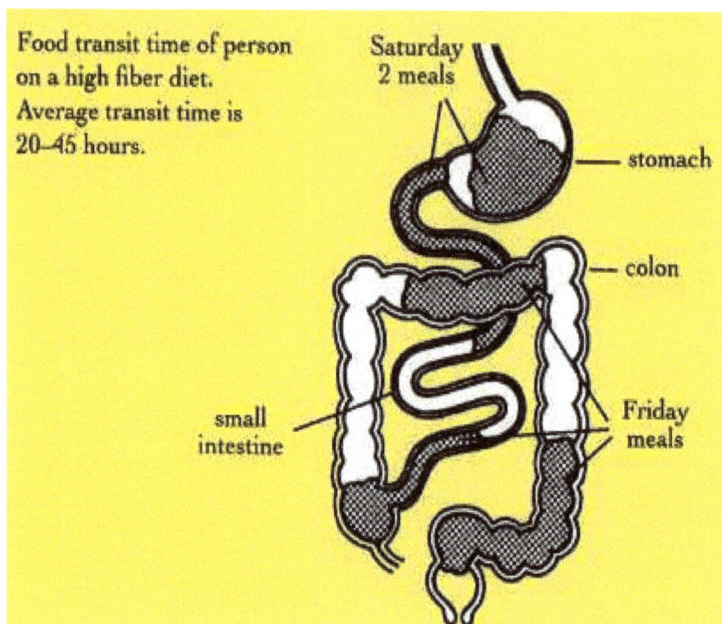

Food transit time of person on a high fiber diet. Average transit time is 20–45 hours.

Saturday 2 meals

stomach

colon

small intestine

Friday meals

www.elclorurodemagnesio.com Creative Commons License

In general it takes about one hour for half of the gastric contents to be processed and advanced into the duodenum and the stomach us usually empty two hours after ingestion. Approximately two to four hours is involved in digestion and absorption before the chyme is released into the colon for water absorption and packaging as feces. The material is eliminated approximately twelve to forty eight hours after ingestion.

Diabetics are particularly prone to a condition called gastroparesis, where the delay is primarily in gastric emptying. Although it is not uncommon to see certain undigested foods passed, like kernels of corn, more undigested foods may be seen with a rapid gut transit time.

Gastroparesis

Diabetes mellitus is one of the most common causes of delayed gastric emptying known as gastroparesis diabeticorum. It can also lead to generalized gastrointestinal motility disorder with delayed total gut transit times. Irritable bowel syndrome is also associated with gastrointestinal motility disorder.

This disorder of delayed gastric emptying is most often seen as a consequence of neuropathy secondary to diabetes mellitus. The delayed gastric emptying prevents both the nutritional intake as well as swallowed gasses from leaving the stomach. Meals that are high in fat cause the release of hormones that slows down gut motility and delays gastric emptying.

To 'Air' is Human

This can lead to increased burping and belching as well as distension. Side effects from medications, especially narcotic analgesics, and antidepressants are well-recognized causes of delayed gastrointestinal peristalsis and bloating. There are a number of pharmacological agents that have prokinetic actions that may be of value in treating delayed gastric emptying.

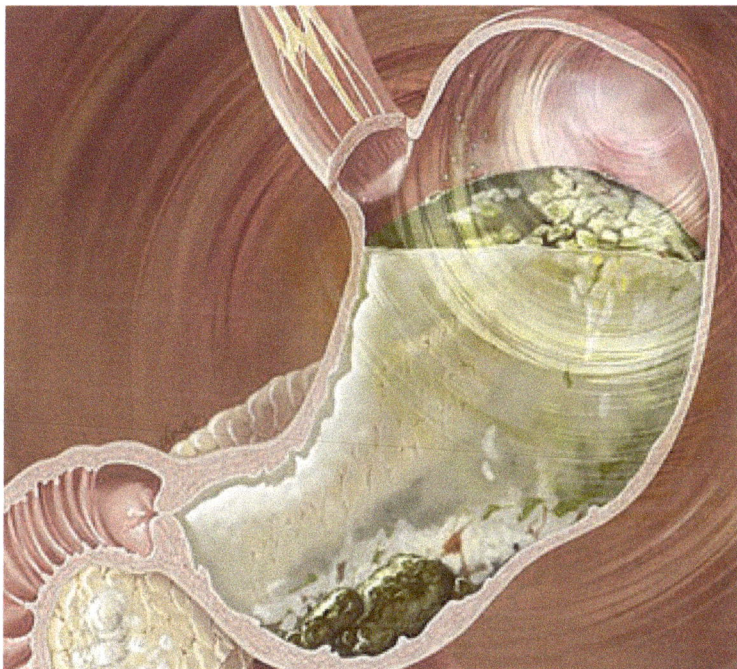

Gastroparesis is the delayed physiological emptying of the stomach with solids and liquids accumulating leading to discomfort, bloating, and distension and belching. Creative Commons License

Peristalsis & Segmental Contractions

Peristalsis (Greek peri-, "around" and stallein, "to place") is the propulsive wave of muscular contraction and relaxation, which advances digestive material through the intestinal tract. Earthworms use a similar mechanism in their movement. The process of peristalsis is controlled by the medulla oblongata of the brainstem. Segmental contractions are used to mix the chime with digestive juices and enzymes and to bring additional nutrient material in contact with the villi and microvilli of the small bowel mucosa.

Digestive material in the stomach is called chyme that in the esophagus and small intestine is called a bolus. The peristaltic wave in the esophagus advances the bolus in a wave lasting less than ten seconds. In the small intestine peristaltic waves lasts for a few seconds and the bolus is advanced a few centimeters. It serves to mix the chyme as digestion and absorption of nutrients occurs during the transit through the small intestine.

185

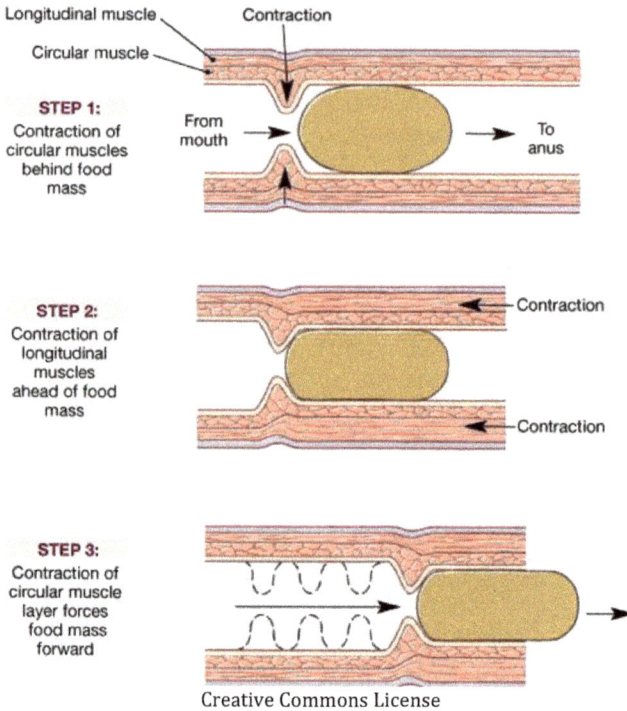

Longitudinal muscle

Circular muscle

Contraction

STEP 1:
Contraction of circular muscles behind food mass

From mouth

To anus

STEP 2:
Contraction of longitudinal muscles ahead of food mass

Contraction

Contraction

STEP 3:
Contraction of circular muscle layer forces food mass forward

Creative Commons License

Migrating motor complexes (MMC) are waves of gastric emptying followed by peristaltic activity that sweep through the stomach and small intestines in between meals. They each last for a moment or two and occur in a cyclic pattern several times an hour, advancing any remaining food residue or chyme through the small intestine into the colon. The maintenance of regular peristaltic activity during meals and intermittently during fasting is also thought to prevent the migration of colonic bacteria into the terminal Ileum.

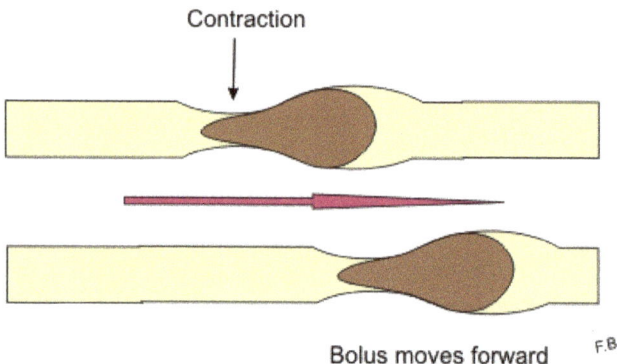

Contraction

Bolus moves forward   F.B

Peristaltic contractions in the gut. Author Boumphreyfr Creative Commons License

186

To 'Air' is Human

The hormone motilin triggers the MMC, as can motilin like agonists such as the antibiotic erythromycin. The at times audible borborygmi from the MMC are also referred to as stomach rumbles or growls and are also commonly thought of as hunger pains since the cramps occur during a fasting state.

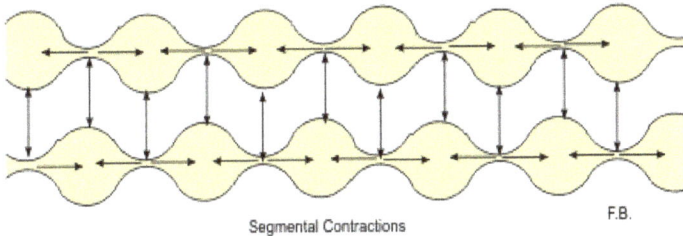

Segmental Contractions   F.B.

Segmental contractions in the gut. Author Boumphreyfr Creative Commons License

Gastrointestinal motility is also under the control of local enteric neurons that coordinate intestinal motility. Cholinergic neurons cause contraction and shortening of the circular muscle layer, shortening of longitudinal muscle, distension of the intestine. As chyme enters the duodenum, carbohydrates and proteins are only partially digested, no fat digestion has taken place. Digestion continues in the small intestine where hypertonic chyme has a low acidic pH and mixing is required for the enzymes and substrates to interact.

The most common motion of the small intestine is the motility action called segmentation. It is initiated by intrinsic pacemaker cells (Cajal cells) with the segmentation mixing the contents while peristaltic activity moves the bolus distally towards the ileocecal valve. After the bulk of the nutrients have been absorbed the gastroileal reflex and gastrin relax the ileocecal sphincter and allow chyme to pass into the large intestine. The colon absorbs the water and electrolytes from the still liquid chyme that is increasingly solidified by water absorption as it transits the large intestine.

Mass Movement

The large intestine (colon) does not have peristaltic activity like the small intestine illustrated above. Feces are propelled through the large intestine by mass movements, which occur one to three times per day. The stool stored in the rectum is expelled via the anus by defecation. Haustral contractions are slow segmenting movements that move the contents of the colon by peristaltic activity towards the rectum.. The haustra sequentially contract as they are stimulated by distension.

The defecation reflex is triggered by distension of rectal walls by feces. When stimulated the defecation reflex contracts the rectal walls and relaxes the internal anal sphincter. Voluntary signals stimulate relaxation of the external anal sphincter and defecation occurs.

To 'Air' is Human

Gastrointestinal Tract

The gastrointestinal tract is also known as the alimentary tract or alimentary canal. It consists of the esophagus, stomach, small intestine and large intestine. It may be considered to be the continuous passageway of the hollow viscous organs, from the mouth to the anus. It is also known as the digestive, intestinal, gastrointestinal, or GI tract. The gastrointestinal system is an expanded entity that includes structures other than the hollow viscus.

The gastrointestinal system includes the accessory organs necessary for digestion, such as the salivary glands, pancreas, liver, gallbladder, and their associated ducts. In an adult male human, the alimentary tract is twenty feet (five meters) long in a living subject. If the alimentary tract is measured at autopsy its length may be increased up to thirty feet (nine meters) because of the loss of the muscular tone and peristaltic contractions

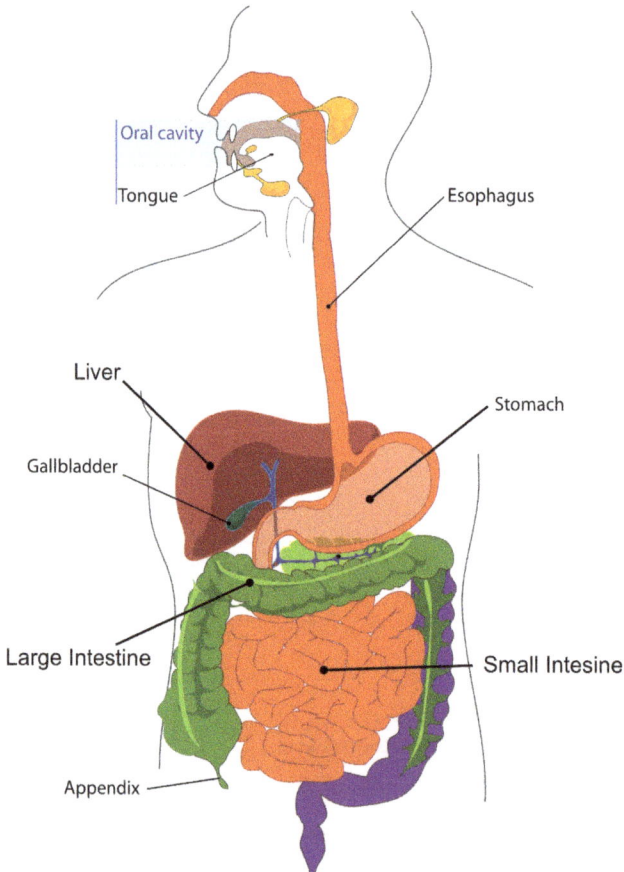

Digestive System. Creative Commons License

The alimentary tract may also be delineated as three distinct regions,

188

the foregut, midgut, and hindgut. This terminology reflects the embryological origin of each segment of the tract. The tissue of the gut actively secretes and releases hormones that help to regulate the digestive process. The long recognized gastrointestinal hormones, including gastrin, secretin, cholecystokinin, have now been joined by more recently discovered hormones. These include leptin, ghrelin, bombesin, neuropeptide Y and others that are mediated through either intracrine or autocrine mechanisms. The multiple hormones may have individual effects, as well as acting with their counterparts in both positive and negative feedback loops. They have powerful effects not only on the digestive tract, but also on the brain and enteric nervous system. They have a profound influence on the satiety center, the area of the brain that plays a vital function in the control of appetite and weight.

The upper alimentary tract consists of the esophagus, stomach, and duodenum. The ligament of Treitz is considered the anatomical landmark that serves as the dividing line between the upper and lower alimentary tracts. The lower alimentary tract includes most of the small intestine, including the jejunum and ileum. The lower alimentary tract also includes all of the large intestine, consisting of the appendix, cecum, ascending colon, transverse colon, descending colon, sigmoid colon, rectum, and anus. The intestines may also commonly be referred to as the alimentary tract, alimentary canal, digestive tract, gastrointestinal (GI) tract, bowels, small bowel, large bowel, hollow viscus, gut, entrails, viscera, or innards. The lumen is the hollow distensible cavity where digestion and absorption take place.

The swallowed food is described as a bolus as it leaves the mouth. When the bolus leaves the stomach and exits through the pyloric sphincter and enters into the duodenum it is now known as chime. The chime has already been partially digested by salivary and gastric enzymes and acids, as well as having gone through a churning and mixing process in the stomach. When the chime leaves the last portion of the small intestine, known as the ileum, it passes through the ileocecal valve. Once it has passed through the ileocecal valve it has entered the cecum, the first portion of the colon, also known as the large intestine or large bowel. The material, which was known as chime on the small intestine side of the ileocecal valve, is now described as feces as it has entered into the colon. The major function of the colon is the absorption of water from the liquid feces that enters the cecum.

As the water is absorbed through the colonic epithelium the feces is solidified and finally stored in the rectum until defecation and elimination take place. The absorption of water is important to conserve the body's fluid balance and maintain adequate hydration. If too little water is absorbed from the feces it may remain liquid or loose and contribute to diarrhea. If excess water removal takes place the feces can become firm and difficult to eliminate resulting in constipation.

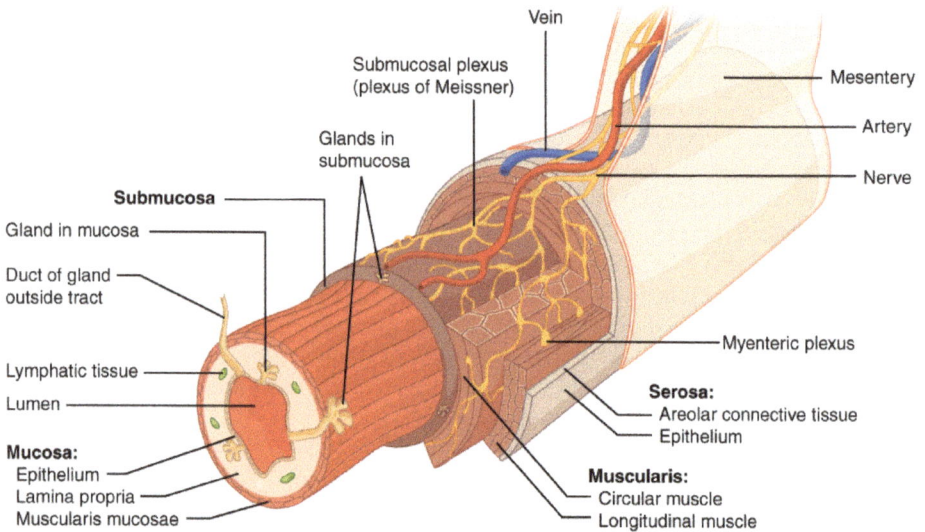

Connexions, OpenStax College, Rice University, Anatomy & Physiology, Overview of the Digestive System Creative Commons License

Going from the inside of the lumen towards the outer wall, there are several layers of tissue found in the anatomy of the gastrointestinal organs. The layers of the intestine, starting from the lumen, includes the mucosa (glandular epithelium and muscularis mucosa), sub mucosa, muscularis externa (made up of inner circular and outer longitudinal muscles), and the covering serosa. The sensory nerve fibers of the small intestine and colon can sense distension and spasm, but not other pain sensations such as those that would normally be felt by the skin if cut or burned.

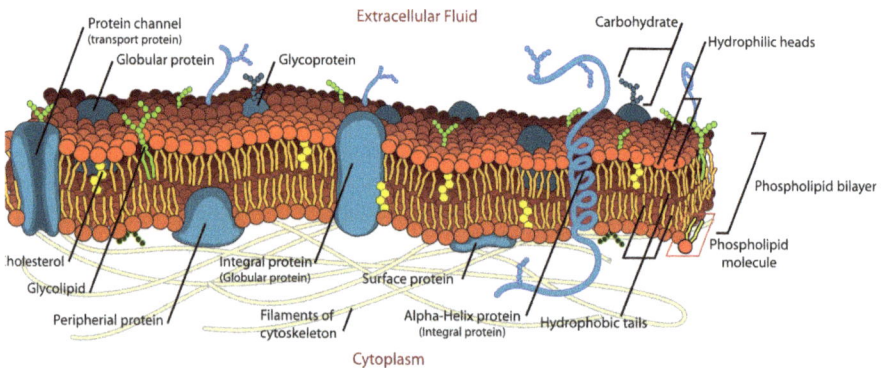

Cell wall anatomy. Creative Commons License

The small intestine is divided into three anatomical segments. The short first portion is immediately distal to the pyloric sphincter, the valve that empties the stomach. This first portion of the duodenum following the stomach is called the duodenum. The term duodenum comes from the middle Latin phrase, duodenum digitorium "space of twelve digits,". A translation of the Greek dodekadaktylon, literally "twelve fingers long," was described by the Greek physician Herophilus (c. 353-280).

The first portion of the duodenum has the critical function of receiving the highly acidic gastric contents. It secretes sodium bicarbonate to neutralize the potent stomach acid. Without its natural ability to neutralize gastric acid, the duodenal mucosa may become injured or inflamed, possibly resulting in an ulcer and internal bleeding.

Brunner glands (Duodenal glands) are secretory compound tubular submucosal glands. They are commonly found in the proximal duodenum. The main function of Brunner glands is to produce mucus and an alkaline solution containing sodium bicarbonate. It protects the duodenal mucosa from the potent gastric acid and neutralizes the chyme leaving the stomach and entering the duodenum Brunner's glands also secrete the polypeptide hormone urogastrone, Urogastrone inhibits the gastric parietal and chief cells from secreting hydrochloric acid and as well as their digestive enzymes. The hormone was given the name urogastrone because it can be identified and isolated from the urine as a fluorescent pigment. The hormonal structure is derived from epidermal growth factor.

Additional quantities of sodium bicarbonate enter into the second portion of the duodenum after being secreted by the pancreas. The pancreatic duct, as well as the bile duct, typically enter the second portion of the duodenum together. They enter the duodenum via an anatomical structure called the Ampulla of Vater. Within the Ampulla of Vater is a muscular valve known as the Sphincter of Oddi. The Sphincter of Oddi controls the flow of bile and pancreatic juice into the duodenum. The bile is produced in the liver and may be stored in the gallbladder for later release as needed. The pancreas also produces and secretes digestive enzymes, in addition to the sodium bicarbonate it secretes to neutralize gastric acid.

The neutralized chime is mixed with the potent digestive enzymes and bile furthering the digestive process and preparing nutrients for absorption.. The jejunum, the middle portion of the small intestine between the duodenum and the ileum, was given its name after the Latin word jējūnus, which means empty or poor, so called because it was always thought to be empty after death.

The ileum, from the Latin Ilium meaning flank or groin, is the final segment of the small intestine and enters the cecum of the colon close to the appendix at the ileocecal valve. The small intestine is described as small because the lumen is narrower than the lumen of the large intestine. The average length of the small intestine is twenty-three feet (seven meters) and is approximately one inch (two and one half centimeters) in diameter. It is substantially longer than the approximately five-foot length of the large intestine, also called the colon.

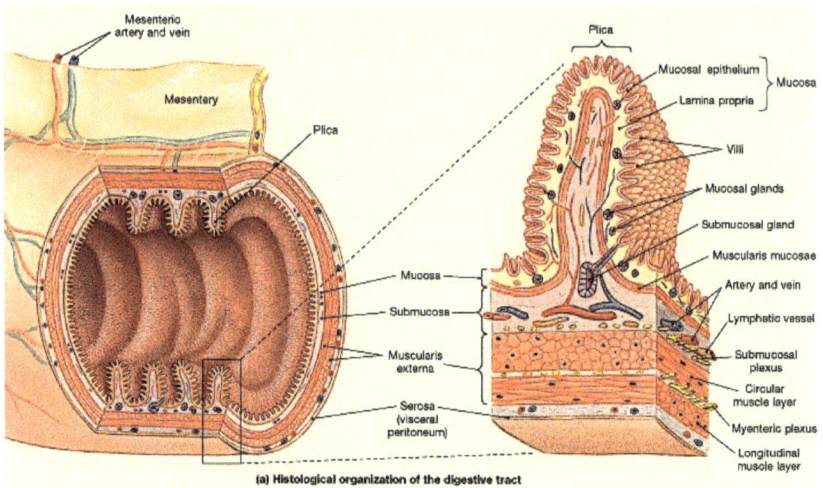

(a) Histological organization of the digestive tract
Creative Commons License

In spite of the relatively long length of the small intestine, its absorptive capacity would not be sufficient to maintain nutrition for an organism the size of humans, if it were a simple hollow tube. Without modifications to increase its surface area, the nutritional needs of a large mammal such as humans would exceed its absorptive ability. The small intestine has several remarkable features that dramatically increase its absorptive capacity. These consist of deep circular folds of the mucosa and sub mucosa known as plica circulares or plica. These folds work in conjunction with millions of fingerlike extensions of the mucosa called villi.

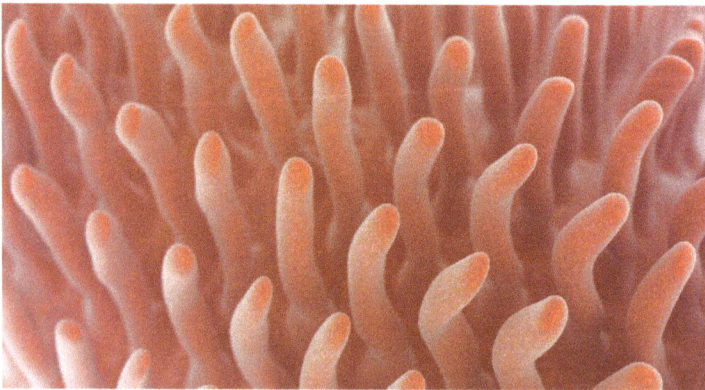

Villi increase the surface area for absorption. Creative Commons License

These villi are provided with additional microscopic projections of the mucosal cell plasma membranes called microvilli. Each of these modifications dramatically increases the surface area available to meet the nutritional needs of larger animals such as humans.. The surface area available to the average human adult for digestive processes, enzymatic activity, and absorption exceeds that of a championship tennis court.

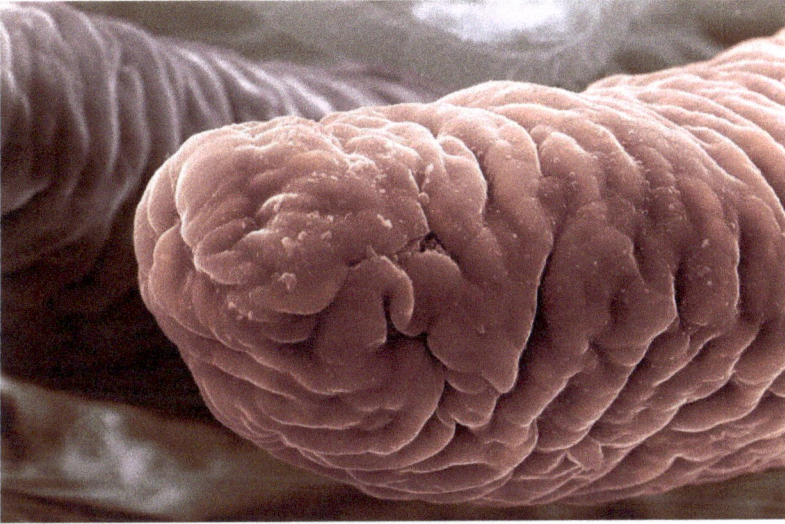

wellcomeimages.org Close up of intestinal villi Creative Commons License

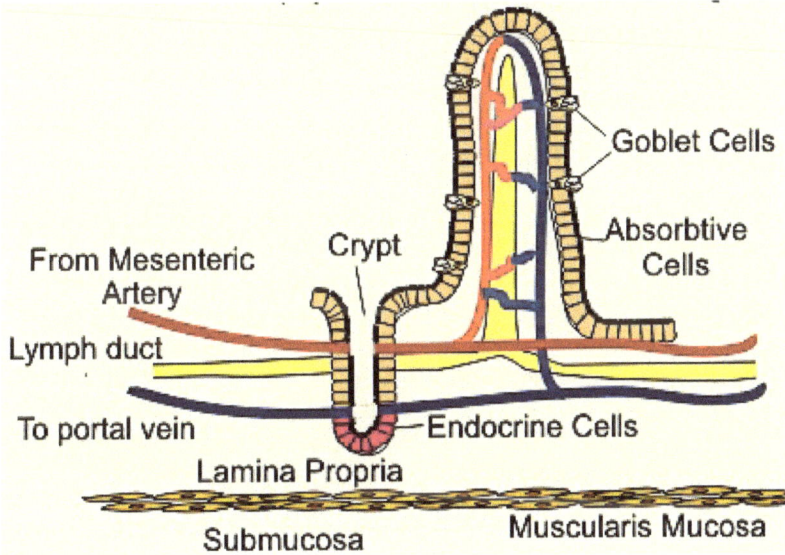

Diagrammatic anatomy of a villous. Wikibooks Gastrointestinal Physiology Frank Boumphrey, MD Creative Commons License

The small intestinal mucosal epithelial cells consist of absorptive cells, mucus secreting goblet cells, entero-endocrine cells that secrete gastrointestinal hormones, and interspersed intraepithelial lymphocytes and T cells. The lymphocytes and T cells are important in the immune response, as the gut is exposed to the vast majority of foreign pathogens introduced into the body.

To 'Air' is Human

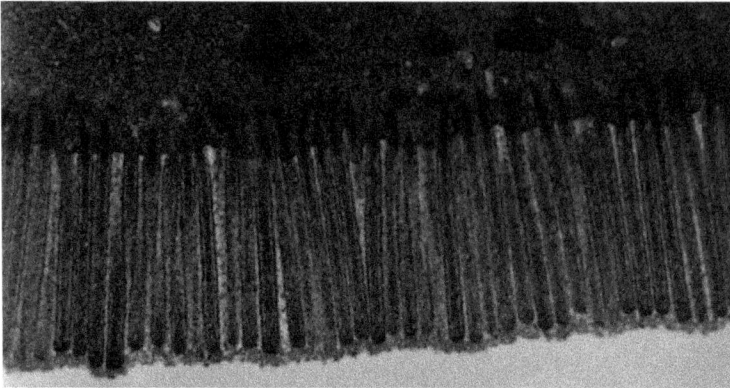

Each villous has thousands of microvilli, as demonstrated on this scanning Transmission electron microscope image of a human jejunal epithelial cell. Image shows absorptive cell with the densely packed microvilli that make up the absorptive border. Eac Louisa Howard, Katherine Connolly Creative Commons License

There is growing evidence that exposure to microorganisms during a normal childbirth leads to a healthy gut flora. Those who were delivered via a Caesarian section are more prone to a number of gastrointestinal disturbances as well as other systemic conditions. The microbiome are the microorganisms that live within our digestive tracts, on our skin, and in several regions on and in our body. The vast majority of these organisms are beneficial. They may provide active benefits, including supplying nutritional metabolic products that humans cannot manufacture. In addition these beneficial organisms, known as commensals, prevent pathogens from establishing colonies, which could lead to illness.

The cells of the intestinal crypts also secrete an intestinal juice in response to irritation of the mucosal lining. This solution is slightly alkaline and isotonic with blood plasma. It is predominantly water, with some mucus, and with very little enzymatic activity. A number of intestinal infections, toxins, or inflammatory processes may stimulate the release of intestinal juice, which may lead to diarrhea. The liquid chyme has over ninety percent of its nutritional value digested and absorbed by the small intestine. The chyme exits the small intestine via the ileocecal valve, entering into the cecum of the large intestine, also called the colon. The lumen of the gastrointestinal tract, although commonly thought of as being deep within the body, is actually contiguous with and exposed to the external environment. It is a potential pathway for pathogenic microorganisms. Peyer patches are lymphoid nodules located in the laminae propria layer of the mucosa and submucosa of the ileum. They are located only in the ileum and are not present in the duodenum or jejunum of the small intestine

There are approximately thirty Peyer patches, each a few centimeters long. They are involved in the immune surveillance of the gastrointestinal tract and have a response and defense mechanism Peyer patches are covered by specialized epithelial cells called microfold cells (M cells). They contain B and T lymphocytes and are an important feature of the gastrointestinal immune response. The cells of Peyer patches allow the sampling of antigens in the gut lumen. The antigen may stimulate a response from the Peyer patches T cells, B cell lymphocytes, and memory cells. Activated lymphocytes may stimulate and magnify the immune response. They can pass into the mesenteric lymph nodes and travel via the lymphatic thoracic duct into the blood stream. From there, they may circulate throughout the gastrointestinal tract as a defense.

Pathogenic microorganisms and other antigens that enter the intestinal tract may encounter several layers of the body's immune defense. Besides the B-lymphocytes, and T-lymphocytes from Peyer patches, the antigen may also encounter macrophages, and dendritic cells. The Mucosa Associated Lymphoid Tissue (MALT) also provides immunological defenses. If injured, the ability of the small bowel to digest and absorb nutrients may be compromised. A condition that temporarily damages the small intestine, like diarrhea from a viral or bacterial gastroenteritis, often called a stomach flu, can cause a blunting or shortening of the villi. This decreases the absorptive capacity of the small intestine and may lead to diarrhea.

The damage to the villi will also lead to the loss of digestive enzymes that reside on the villi. This is one of the reasons people are often advised to avoid dairy products for a week or so after stomach flu. The villi need time to recover and return enzyme levels to normal. If you eat or drink lactose without waiting until the recovery is complete, you may end up with symptoms of lactose intolerance such as gas and diarrhea.

When the liquid chyme leaves the jejunum and ileum of the small intestine, it goes through the ileocecal valve and becomes feces. In the cecum of the colon lies the infamous appendix, which for thousands of years was a mystery as to its purpose. Its function has only very recently been identified. It stores as a reservoir of intestinal bacteria, representing the healthy gut microbiome, from which the gut flora can be replenished after a bout of intestinal dysentery. The gut microbiome is much more important than most people, including physicians and research scientists, have given it credit for. The microbes of the body far outnumber the number of human cells. The vast majority are commensals, and are engaged with us in a symbiotic relationship from which we both benefit.

The colon, unlike the small intestine, is less involved in the digestion of foods and nutrients. It is primarily involved in the absorption of water and sodium, as well as the absorption of some fat-soluble vitamins such as vitamin K. The colon removes the excess moisture from the watery chyme, and the stool solidifies as it transits the gut. It is stored in the rectum and sigmoid colon, awaiting the right opportunity to be eliminated through defecation. A process or illness that impairs the colon's absorption of water will lead to more fluid stool and diarrhea. If the elimination is delayed moisture continues to be absorbed and the stools can become harder resulting in constipation. The colon is not a vital organ, and people can live a normal life span without it, in spite of the challenges of avoiding dehydration.

To 'Air' is Human

Global Warming

Global warming due to greenhouse gas production from human activity is mainly due to deforestation, the combustion of fossil fuels, livestock enteric fermentation and manure management, and landfill emissions. In terms of biomass bacteria would be the main contributors to global warming by their methane production. Other contenders nominated have been termites, which have over 2000 species and are prolific methane producers (initial reports suggested that they produce 40% of global methane), livestock such as cows, sheep, and pigs, and lastly dinosaurs, which are no longer around to defend their reputations.

A ruminant (Latin *ruminare* - to chew over again) is a mammal that digests plants in a multi compartment stomach through bacterial fermentation. It regurgitates the semi-digested mass, called cud, and chews it again and repeats the swallow. The process of re-chewing the cud is called "ruminating". There are about 150 species of ruminants, which include both domestic and wild species. Ruminating mammals include cattle, goats, sheep, giraffes, yaks, deer, camels, llamas, and antelope. Ruminant bacterial fermentation is a significant contributor to global methane production, which is over twenty times as potent a greenhouse gas as carbon dioxide. To incentivize efforts to reduce livestock methane production a number of countries have proposed taxes on the release of greenhouse gasses.

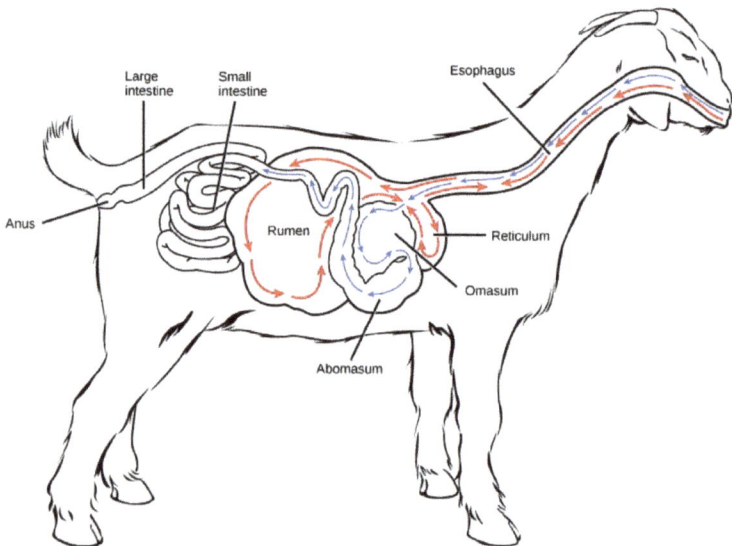

www.rice.edu Creative Commons License

It took extensive scientific experimentation to collect the intestinal gasses of herds of cattle before it was discovered that the methane production was coming from the other end of the cows and other ruminants. It is the burps and belches from the multi compartment ruminant stomach that is the primary source of methane. The Great Chicago Fire, which destroyed the city in 1871, has traditionally been blamed on Mrs. O'Leary's cow kicking over a kerosene lamp. With the large volume of methane produced it is just as likely to have been caused by her cow farting and belching,. But that would not have been an acceptable cause in Victorian times.

Kangaroos are herbivores and as marsupial their burps and farts contain little or no methane, a potent greenhouse gas. It appears that the reduced methane emissions are due to the microbes in the kangaroos' gut flora. Australian researchers hope that introducing a similar gut flora to other methane producing herbivores such as cattle and sheep will contribute to a reduction in greenhouse gasses and the resultant global warming. Methane can cause about 20 times as much atmospheric warming as an equivalent volume of carbon dioxide.

Kangaroos, like cattle and sheep, are ruminants that re-chew their cud with the assistance of the gut flora to digest the and metabolize their cellulose based grazing diet. In the foregut the meal is broken down by fermentation with carbon dioxide and hydrogen released. In cows and other ruminants, microbes called methanogens transform these gases into methane. But in the kangaroos' guts the same hydrogen and carbon dioxide may be utilized by bacteria called acetogens to produce acetate, a volatile fatty acid.

These microbes compete with methanogens to use the carbon dioxide and hydrogen, so the more acetogens the less methane production. The odds are in generally in favor of methanogens, since the process of methane production is generally more energy efficient than producing acetate. One of the acetogen microbes, *Blautia coccoides*, live in cows as well as in kangaroos. Further research is being undertaken to understand why the organism is more successful in competing with the methanogens in kangaroos than in other herbivores.

Carbon dioxide, methane, nitrous oxide, and three groups of fluorinated gases (sulfur hexafluoride, hydro fluorocarbons , and per fluorocarbons) are the major greenhouse gases impacted by human activity. These are regulated under the Kyoto Protocol an international treaty that was adopted in 2005. Nitrogen dioxide (NO_2) warms the atmosphere three hundred and ten times more than carbon dioxide, and methane twenty-one times more than carbon dioxide. Although CFCs are greenhouse gases, regulations were initiated because CFCs' cause ozone depletion, not because of their contribution to global warming. Ozone depletion itself has a relatively minor effect on greenhouse warming.

Dinosaurs are no longer around to defend themselves and have been accused of contributing to global warming. We do not know if they were ruminants and contributed by belching up gasses as well, but there should be no doubt that they were big time farters. Their nickname "thunder lizards" may have more to do with their farts than their footsteps.

Gluten

Gluten (Latin gluten, "glue") is a protein composite of gliadin and glutenin found conjoined with starch in the endosperm of various grass grains related to wheat, and some forms of oats. In barley the gluten component is known as hordein, in rye it is known as secalin. Corn, maize, and rice do not contain gluten. Gluten gives elasticity to dough and gives the final product a chewy texture. Bread flours are high in gluten (hard wheat); pastry flours have a lower gluten content. Kneading promotes the chewiness of a product by the formation of gluten strands and cross-links. In wheat, alpha-gliadins are not only seed storage proteins, but also act as inhibitors of alpha-amylase activity. About 1 in 133 people in developed nations have sensitivity reactions to gluten, which can damage the villi and microvilli of the small intestine. This can lead to malabsorption, gas, diarrhea, and a variety of metabolic disorders and physical ailments. The treatment is a strict gluten free diet.

Buddhist monks discovered gluten in the 7th century. The monks, who were vegetarians, were trying to find a substitute for meat. They discovered that when they submerged dough in water, the starch washed off and all that was left was a meat-like, textured, gummy mass, the gluten. Gluten sensitivity as the cause of Celiac Disease was discovered during the World War Two occupation of the Netherlands where celiac patients actually improved when all of the wheat was confiscated by Nazi Germany for their military.

Gluten, a substance in wheat and other grains, may be found in a variety of foods including breads, cakes, cereals, pasta, commercial dairy products and alcoholic beverages

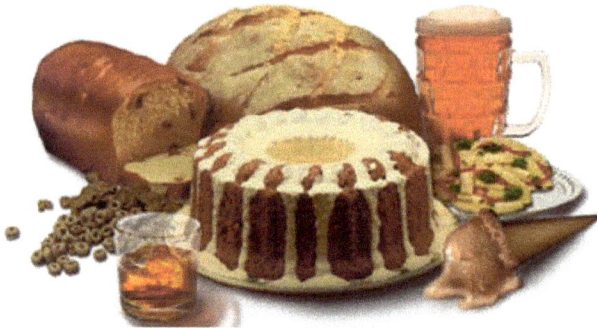

digestivedisease.uthscsa.edu Creative Commons License

Gluten Sensitive Enteropathy

Gluten Sensitive Enteropathy is also known by a number of other names, including, Celiac Sprue, Celiac Disease, Sprue, and Non-Tropical Sprue. It is not synonymous with gluten intolerance although it may be considered a more severe form of intolerance leading to physical and physiological changes in the gut and other areas of the body.

Celiac (Greek κοιλιακός (koiliakós, "abdominal") disease is an autoimmune disorder of the small intestine that occurs in genetically predisposed people and is thought to occur in up to 1% of United States population. It may also be called celiac sprue, nontropical sprue, endemic sprue, sprue, gluten enteropathy, gluten-sensitive enteropathy, and gluten intolerance. It is caused by a reaction to gliadin, a prolamin protein of gluten, found in wheat, rye, barley, and sometimes oats.

Humans first started to cultivate grains in the Fertile Crescent of Western Asia about 9500 BCE) it is probable that coeliac disease did not occur before this time. Aretaeus of Cappadocia, living in the second century described a malabsorptive syndrome presumed to be celiac disease with pain, flatulence, and a malodorous intractable diarrhea. While a role for carbohydrates had been suspected, the link with wheat was not made until the 1940's by the Dutch pediatrician Dr. Willem Karel Dicke. He noticed that during the Dutch famine of 1944 the scarcity of wheat and bread led the rate among children affected by CD to drop essentially zero, but returned to over 35% once wheat was again available after the war.

On exposure to gliadin the enzyme tissue transglutaminase modifies the protein triggering an immune response causes an inflammatory reaction in the small bowel. This leads to damage and atrophy of the villous lining of the small intestine that is critical for digestion and absorption of nutrients. Treatment requires a gluten free diet to avoid the offending protein. is a lifelong gluten-free diet.

Typical and Atypical Symptoms of Celiac Disease

Typical Symptoms

Abdominal distention	Failure to thrive
Chronic diarrhea	

Atypical Symptoms

Independent of malabsorption

Alopecia	Myasthenia gravis
Ataxia	Polyneuropathy
Dental enamel hypoplasia	Primary biliary cirrhosis
Dermatitis herpetiformis	Psoriasis
Dilative cardiomyopathy	Recurrent aphthous
Epilepsy	stomatitis
Hyperthyroidism	Recurrent pericarditis
Hypothyroidism	Vasculitis
Isolated hypertransaminasemia	

Secondary to malabsorption

Flatulence	Recurrent spontaneous
Hepatic stenosis	abortion
Osteopenia	Short stature
Recurrent abdominal pain	Sideropenic anemia

Celiac disease can present with malabsorption, steatorrhea weight loss, anemia, fatigue, and other symptoms related to the nutritional deficiencies. Milder or subclinical cases may present without symptoms, often discovered by abnormal results on a routine blood test. When chronic diarrhea is present in celiac disease it is often pale, voluminous, malodorous because of fat absorption leading to steatorrhea. Abdominal pain, cramping, bloating, distension, and gaseousness with mouth ulcers may be present. It is my unusual for lead patients to be seen and treated for irritable bowel or other conditions for several years before the correct diagnosis becomes apparent.

Untreated celiac disease has an increased risk of adenocarcinoma and lymphoma of the small bowel. Malabsorption may lead to nutritional deficiencies such as minerals and the fat-soluble vitamins A, D, E, and K. Anemia may develop from iron insufficiency as well as from deficiencies of folic acid and vitamin B_{12} which may give rise to megaloblastic anemia and neuropathy. Calcium and vitamin D malabsorption (and secondary hyperparathyroidism) may cause osteopenia (decreased mineral content of the bone) or osteoporosis. Vitamin K deficiency interferes with to the bloods ability to clot and can present as abnormal bleeding. Bacterial overgrowth of the small intestine can occur aggravating malabsorption or preventing the resolution of malabsorption with a gluten free diet.

A variety of other conditions, especially autoimmune disorders are more common in those with celiac disease. These include those IgA deficiency, dermatitis herpetiformis, diabetes mellitus, autoimmune thyroiditis, primary biliary cirrhosis, hyposplenism, and microscopic colitis, abnormal liver function tests, delayed growth and development., Addison disease (adrenal insufficiency), alopecia areata, Down syndrome (trisomy 21), osteoporosis, Sjögren syndrome, systemic lupus erythematosis, and Turner syndrome.

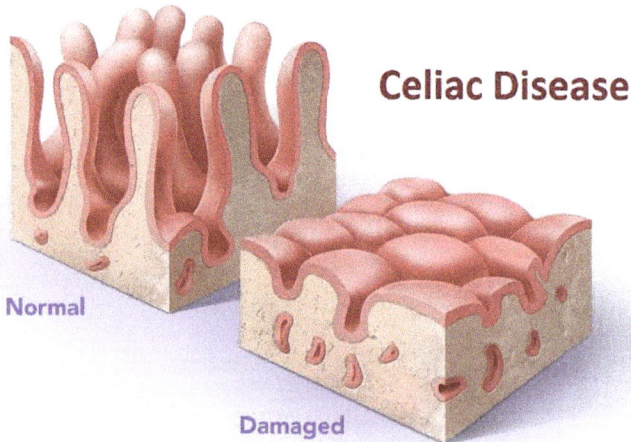

Celiac Disease

Normal

Damaged

Intestinal villi in celiac disease are atrophic ih.constantcontact.com Creative Commons License

There are several tests that can be used to assist in diagnosis. The level of symptoms may determine the order of the tests, but all tests lose their usefulness if the person is already eating a gluten-free diet. Intestinal damage begins to heal within weeks of gluten being removed from the diet, and antibody levels decline over months. For those who have already started on a gluten-free diet, it may be necessary to perform a challenge with some gluten-containing food in one meal a day over 6 weeks before repeating the investigations.

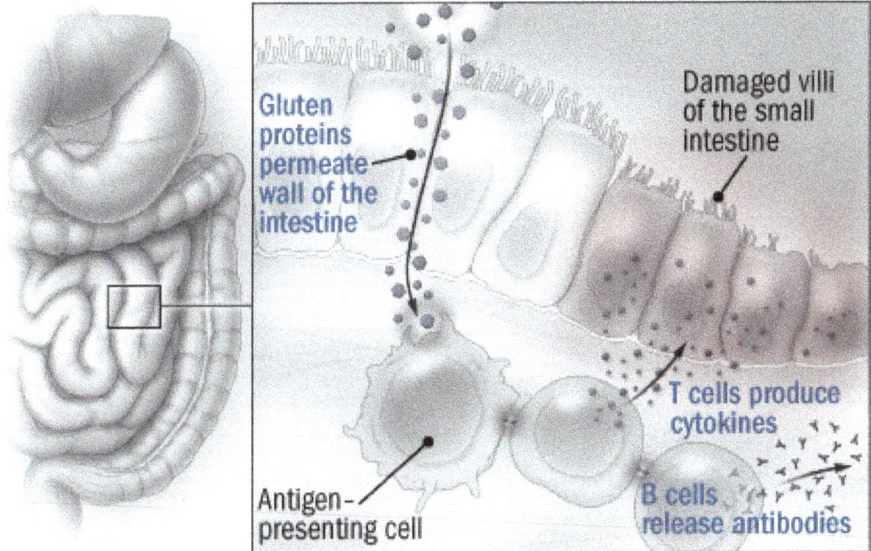

www.health.harvard.edu Creative Commons License

Diagnostic tests are very accurate unless a gluten free diet was instituted before testing. The tests accuracy is diminished with longer time periods from gluten exposure. Serological blood tests have high sensitivity and specificity for celiac disease but endoscopy and small bowel biopsy is usually necessary for a definitive diagnosis of celiac disease. Anti-endomysial immunoglobulin A (IgA) antibodies and IgA tissue anti-transglutaminase (tTG) have over 90% sensitivity and nearly 99% specificity.

Gut-Brain-Microbiome-Food Axis

A relatively recent discovery has been that the gut brain axis has a very important third component, the microbiome. The gut microbiome is also known as the gut flora and consists of the multitude of other life forms residing within the gut. These include bacteria, viruses, protozoans, Archaea, parasites, prions, fungi, and probably other undiscovered or unidentified organisms. By number of cells, the human cells of our body are outnumbered ten to one by the over one hundred trillion microbes living on and within the average human. If instead of cell population the comparison were based on genes that can be expressed and control biological functions, the human genes are outnumber one hundred to one. In addition to the gut microbiome, there are unique microbiomes on all aspects of the human body exposed to the external environment. Research activities are studying all areas of the human microbiome including, skin, oral, nasal, genitourinary, etcetera. The research findings to date are so dramatic that many scientists describe the microbiome as if a new major organ system of the body has just been discovered.

The organisms that make up the gut flora are a major source of the intestinal gasses produced during digestion and fermentation. The interaction between these organisms, food, and the human gut and brain are just beginning to be uncovered. More important than their major contribution to intestinal gas is their even more important contribution to human health and vitality.

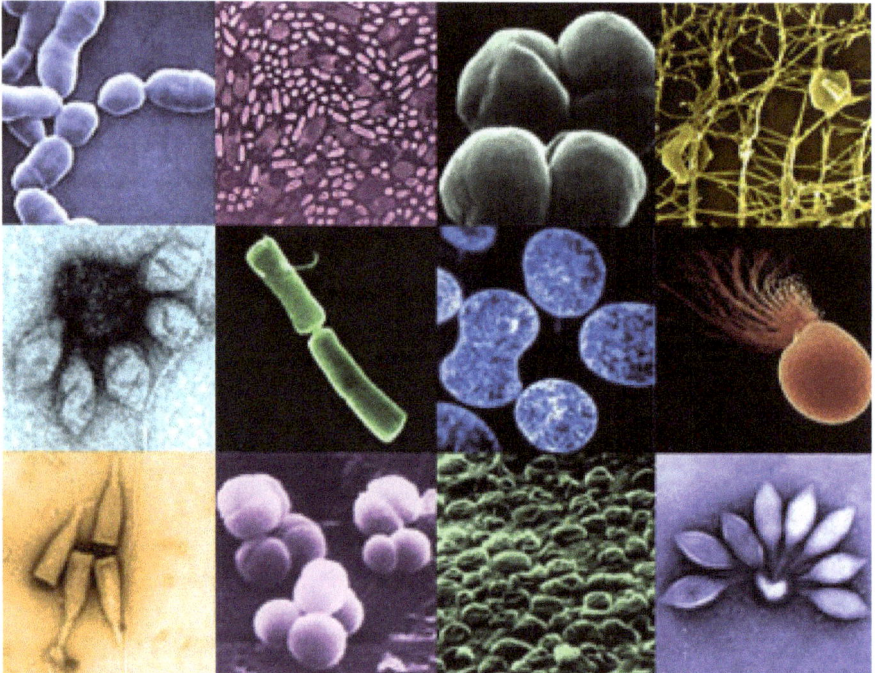

The human gut microbiome is made up of hundreds of trillions of organisms including Archaea, bacteria, parasites, prions, protists and viruses. They produce gasses such as hydrogen and methane that are constituents of intestinal gas.

The brain gut axis has been recognized for over a century. It has also been well recognized that information and influence travels in both directions. The brain can trigger digestive system symptoms and disorders including the common functional conditions such as irritable bowel syndrome. Digestive disorders frequently send signals to the brain and may lead to systemic anxiety, fear, depression, and distress. The brain central and autonomic nervous systems are intimately connected with the enteric nervous system of the gastrointestinal tract.

Gut intuition, know it in your gut, gut wrenching experience, gut wrong, gut check, butterflies in the stomach, gut instinct, gut reaction, listen to your gut, go with your gut, are all common expressions to describe the common experiences of intuition most commonly known as gut feelings. The gastrointestinal tract is sensitive to stress and emotion. Anger, anxiety, sadness, fear, elation are all among the many feelings that can trigger symptoms in the gut ranging from mild spasm to intense nausea, vomiting, cramps, diarrhea, and fecal incontinence.

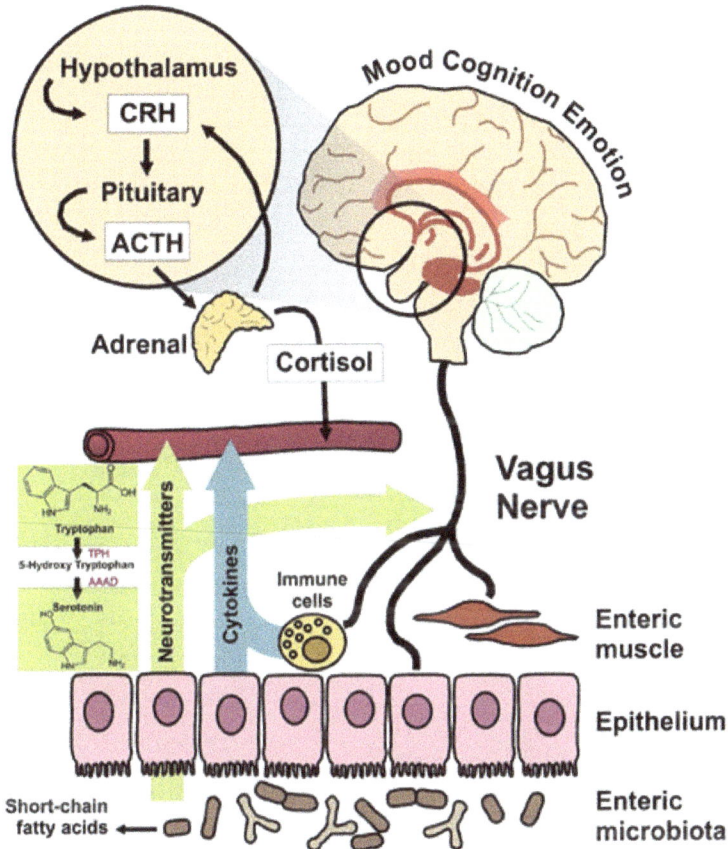

The brain has a direct effect on the digestive tract. As demonstrated by Ivan Pavlov, dogs accustomed to hearing a bell before being fed begin to salivate with just the sound of the bell even if no food is offered. The release of saliva, digestive enzymes, hormones, and gut motility can all be stimulated by thoughts generated by the brain alone.

Ninety-five percent of the body's supply of the well-recognized and critically important neurotransmitter serotonin is found in the gut. The brain and its serotonin receptors, representing only five percent of the body's serotonin, is a frequent target of prescription medications such as Prozac (fluoxetine). These pharmaceuticals are known as a selective serotonin re-uptake inhibitor (SSRI). The gut and the brain each have fifty percent of another important neurotransmitter, dopamine.

Gut Fermentation Syndrome

Gut fermentation syndrome is also known as the auto-brewery syndrome and is a rare medical condition in which not only gas but alcohol is produced within the gastrointestinal tract through endogenous fermentation. The alcohol produced is absorbed and can lead to intoxication if sufficient substrate is ingested into the digestive system. Numerous cases have been documented in the medical literature with isolation of the fermenting organism *Saccharomyces cerevisiae*. Interestingly enough many people use *Saccharomyces* and Brewer's yeast as a probiotic supplement. It has also been investigated, but eliminated, as a possible cause of sudden infant death syndrome.

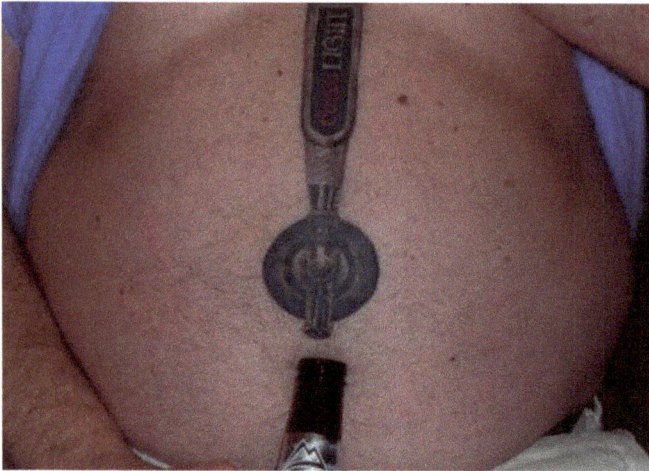

www.egotastic.com Creative Commons License

Claims of endogenous fermentation of this type have also been used as a defense against drunk driving charges. Often the defendant is required to submit to medical isolation and documentation that their blood alcohol level will rise spontaneously if given a fermentable carbohydrate rich meal. If the blood levels do not confirm the existence of the extremely rare disorder they are convicted of the driving while intoxicated charge and have additional medical expenses added to their penalty.

Alcoholic beverages, typically containing <1% to 40% ethanol by volume, have been produced and consumed by humans since pre-historic times. Ethanol is obtained fermentation using glucose that is produced from the hydrolysis of starch in the presence of yeast. Several of the benign bacteria in the intestine use fermentation as a form of anaerobic metabolism, which produces ethanol as a waste product. Human bodies contain some quantity of alcohol produced by these bacteria. In rare cases, this can be sufficient to cause "auto-brewery syndrome" in which intoxicating quantities of alcohol are produced by the bacterial flora of the gastrointestinal tract. Ethanol is further metabolized by the liver.

To 'Air' is Human

High Altitude Living (see Atmospheric Pressure, Ideal Gas Laws)

The majority of the world's population lives close to the seashore and have the standard atmospheric pressure of one atmosphere found at sea level. A significant percentage of the world's population lives at higher altitudes with atmospheric pressures less than one atmosphere. One hundred and forty million people live at altitudes above 2,500 meters (8,200 ft.). M The higher above sea level you are, the lower is the atmospheric pressure you are subjected to. As a consequence, although the number of molecules of gas produced is identical, it will require a larger volume of space to contain it.

Those who travel to higher altitudes, whether by climbing a mountain, driving up a mountain road, or traveling by air, experience an increase in flatulence. The underlying principle is the same, according to the gas laws of physics a reduction in atmospheric pressure results in an increase in the volume of intestinal gas. Those who reside in high altitude communities become used to this degree of flatulence as normal for their elevation.

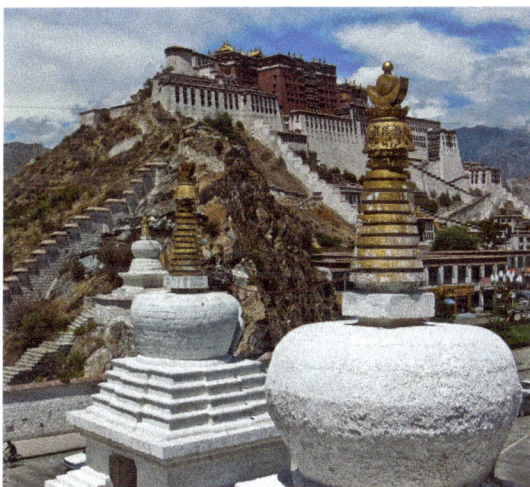

The Potala Palace, Lhasa, Tibet is higher yet at 11,450 feet altitude. Photo by Antoine Taveneaux
Creative Commons License

If you live in Denver Colorado, the mile high city with an elevation of five thousand one hundred and eighty three feet (one thousand six hundred and nine meters) feet above sea level, the volume will be larger than residing in Los Angeles or New York City. It is all relative as residing in Mexico City, which is at seven thousand three hundred and fifty feet (two thousand two hundred and forty meters), will produce a much larger volume than Denver. Working or living in high-rise buildings may also give rise to changes in atmospheric pressure. This is most readily demonstrated by taking a high-speed elevator in a high-rise building. The rapid decrease in atmospheric pressure traveling from the lower to the higher floors often results in pressure changes on the eardrum (tympanic membrane). The equalization of pressure on both sides of the tympanic membrane may give rise to an ear popping sensation.

Another important consideration for those engaged in high altitude activities is the recognition that the oxygen content of air decreases with an increase in altitude. The percentage saturation of hemoglobin with oxygen determines the oxygen content of the blood. Atmospheric pressure decreases exponentially with altitude, so while the O_2 fraction remains relatively constant the absolute amount of oxygen in a given volume of air decreases exponentially as well. At an altitude around 2,100 m (7,000 feet) above sea level, the oxygen saturation of hemoglobin begins to decrease dramatically.

Many air travelers are under the false impression that pressurization of the aircraft means the oxygen content of the air is the same as that on the ground at sea level. The aircraft is typically pressurized to maintain a cabin pressure equivalent to an altitude of approximately eight thousand feet. This leads to a reduction in the oxygen content of the air on the aircraft. Some normal individuals find this reduction in oxygen uncomfortable and develop headaches and other symptoms. Others are more sensitive, or recognize that their underlying medical condition requires that they have access to supplemental oxygen for their safe travel.

At an altitude of 5,000 m (16,000 ft.), the altitude of the Mount Everest base camp, hemoglobin oxygen saturation is reduced by fifty per cent. At the and only a third at the summit of Mount Everest at an altitude of 8,848 m (29,029 ft.) above sea level the oxygen saturation is reduced by two thirds. Travel to high altitude regions can lead to medical problems, from the mild symptoms of acute mountain sickness to life threatening high altitude pulmonary edema and cerebral edema. The higher the altitude, the greater the risk. For those with underlying circulatory or lung conditions the additional stress of even mildly lower oxygen content of the air can be potentially life threatening. Altitude sickness can develop rapidly and is a life-threatening condition requiring an immediate descent in altitude.

Hydrogen

Hydrogen and methane are two explosive gasses produced by the gut microbes. Their presence in farts make the fart ignitable and flammable, used to the amusement of some and the chagrin and painful burns of others. These same microorganisms continue their gas production in the feces after it exits the host digestive tract. Both hydrogen and methane are odorless. Hydrogen sulfide and other aromatic and volatile substances are also produced by the microorganisms in feces that produces its characteristic odor.

Hydrogen is lighter than air and lighter than helium. Unfortunately it is also explosively flammable. Hydrogen fires are less destructive to immediate surroundings because of the buoyancy of H_2, which causes heat of combustion to be released upwards as it ascends in the atmosphere. On May 6, 1937, the hydrogen filled German airship Hindenburg burst into flames while attempting to land at Lakehurst, New Jersey. In little more than 30 seconds, the largest object ever to soar through the air was incinerated.

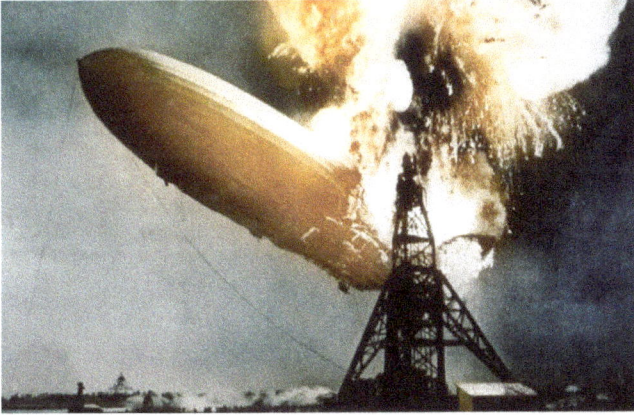
Public Domain

Hydrogen is a chemical element the symbol H and atomic number 1. It is the lightest element and in its single atom form it is by far the most abundant element in the universe, comprising approximately 75% of its total mass. In the earth's atmosphere as the diatomic H2 molecule it is a colorless, odorless, tasteless, non-toxic, highly explosive gas. Most of the hydrogen on Earth is in molecules such as water and organic compounds because hydrogen readily forms covalent bonds. In 1766 Henry Cavendish was the first to identify hydrogen gas. In 1783 Antoine Lavoisier gave the element the name hydrogen (Greek ὕδρω hydro water and γενῆς genes creator) when he and Laplace confirmed Cavendish's finding that water is produced when hydrogen is burned.

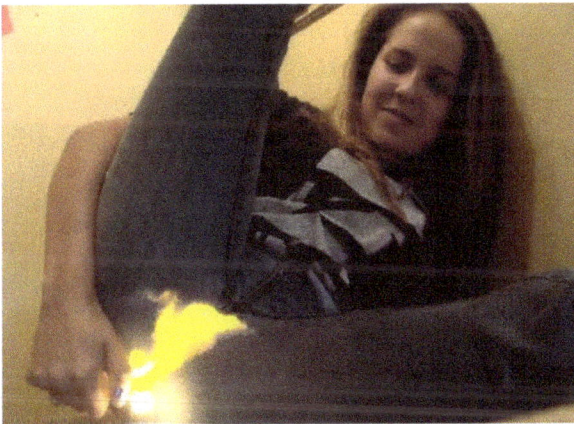
Moment of ignition of a fart, video is at youtu.be/Zt9rvaijpPY

Hydrogen and methane are the two flammable gasses that may be found in a fart making them flammable. Lighting a fart to see if one produces these gasses is actually a dangerous activity. Significant burns to the anogenital area have occurred as a result, especially when ignited without a clothing barrier. The popular television show *Mythbusters* filmed an episode confirming that many farts are indeed flammable. It appears that the network found the episode too provocative, and perhaps for liability concerns that children watching might attempt their own demonstrations decided to not 'air' the episode.

Hydrogen, The Big Bang

For those entertained by the lighting of the hydrogen or methane of farts, there is another 'big bang' associated with hydrogen gas. According to the Big Bang theory of the origin of the universe, atoms were created as the super-heated and compressed dense mass of the universe expanded and cooled. It is virtually beyond our ability to comprehend the astronomical numbers of atoms in the universe. All the more remarkable is that after billions of years the cooling and expansion continues yet 90% plus of the energy and matter in the universe remains invisible to our scientific instruments and exploration to date.

Through the process of nuclear fusion within stars two atoms of hydrogen combined into one atom of helium. The process of fusion continued to create the heavier elements through stars and supernova. In spite of the billions of years that have passed since the Big Bang the development of the heavier elements is still in its infancy. 98% of all known matter in the universe is the simplest element hydrogen. Another 1% is the next earliest element helium. All of the other elements that populate our universe and that were created from stardust are less than 1% of the known elements.

The known universe is 99% hydrogen and helium, the two lightest elements and nearly always found as gases. Planets are the extreme oddity of being comprised of heaver elements of liquids and solids as well as gasses. Our planet Earth is a remarkable find with heavier elements as well as the primary element hydrogen. Most of the planets hydrogen has been oxidized in a ratio of two hydrogen atoms to one oxygen atom into H_2O, liquid water, frozen ice, or water vapor depending on its local environment. The primary elements are gasses but as compounds they form other states of matter as liquids or solids. If you think of the human body we are primarily and predominantly hydrogen and oxygen gasses that have formed a liquid compound water.

When we observe an object with our vision what we are seeing are the photons of light energy being reflected back to us. The object is absorbing all of the wavelengths of light except those that are reflected back. So we are not actually seeing the object, what we are seeing is a reflection of what it did not absorb. Even though our reality may be an illusion, for the sake of our sanity I think it best to accept the illusion as reality and leave the details to the quantum physicists and scientists!

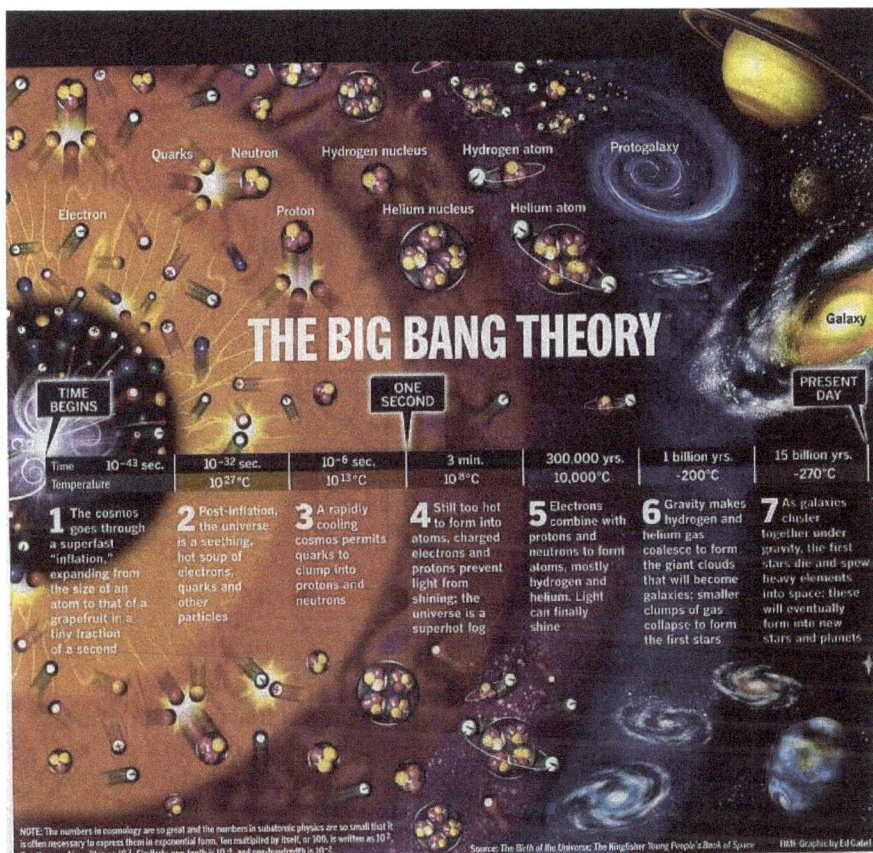

Big Bang Theory illustrated Time Magazine graphic

Hydrogen Sulfide

Hydrogen sulfide with the formula H_2S is a colorless gas with the characteristic foul odor of rotten eggs. It is heavier than air, poisonous, corrosive, flammable, and explosive and often results from the bacterial fermentation of organic material in anaerobic environments such as in swamps and sewers. H_2S also occurs in volcanic gases, natural gas, and well water.

Hydrogen sulfide (HS) is also produced by some cells and has biologically active signaling functions. Nitric oxide (NO) and carbon monoxide (CO) are the only other gases known to have this property. It acts as a relaxant of smooth muscle and as a vasodilator. It is also active in the brain where it may play a role in memory as well as Alzheimer's Disease, where the brains hydrogen sulfide concentration is markedly decreased. Hydrogen sulfide's ability to act as a vasodilator may be protective against cardiovascular disease. The sulfur group in allicin, garlic's bioactive component, is catabolized to hydrogen sulfide and may explain garlics reported cardio protective properties. Like nitric oxide, hydrogen sulfide is involved in the relaxation of the smooth muscle that causes vasodilation and erection of the penis. Nitric oxide and hydrogen sulfide appear to work via different mechanisms suggesting that new therapeutic options for erectile dysfunction and a variety of medical conditions may be possible.

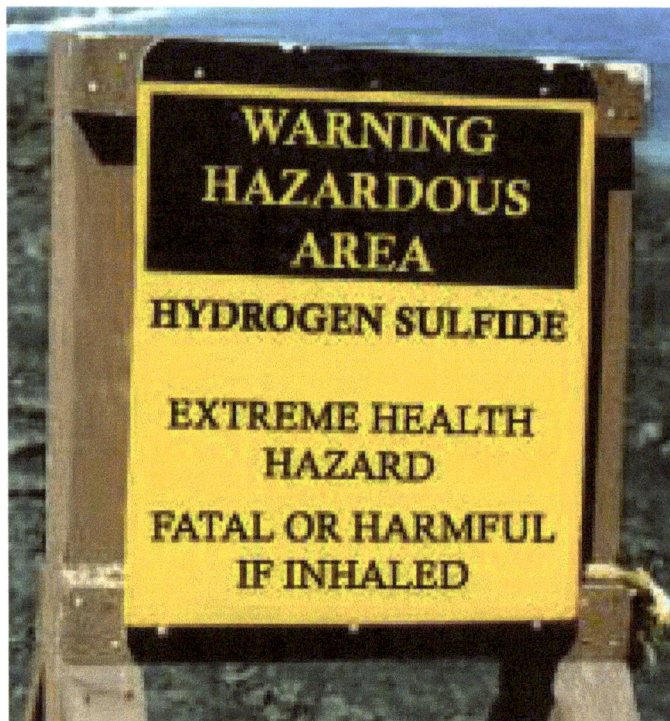

Public Domain

An excess of hydrogen sulfide can also be detrimental. The overproduction of HS is involved in the pathogenesis of type 1 diabetes and leads to the injury and death of the insulin producing beta cells. The injurious effects of Hydrogen sulfide have been implicated in mass extinctions that have occurred in the Earth's past. Buildup of hydrogen sulfide in the atmosphere, perhaps from major volcanic eruptions, may have caused the Permian-Triassic extinction event 252 million years ago.

Hydrogen Sulfide is found in high concentrations in the calderas of volcanoes, which is also where significant mining activity for sulfur takes place. In spite of the harsh conditions and dangerous gasses active mining for sulfur takes place in the crater of Kawah Ijen volcano in Java, Indonesia. Next to a sulfuric acid lake with a measured pH as low as 0.5 a number of vents in the caldera emit volcanic gasses like sulfur dioxide (SO_2) and hydrogen sulfide (H_2S). These gasses are channeled through ceramic pipes where the gasses are condensed into liquid sulfur as the gas cools. Deep red molten sulfur pours out of the pipes, further cools to the yellow mineral, which forms solid yellow cakes of sulfur, and are ten carried out of the area by miners in baskets. The miners work without protective equipment and have to hike up and down out of the high altitude volcanoes caldera twice a day. Typical miners earn the equivalent of $13 U.S. per day.

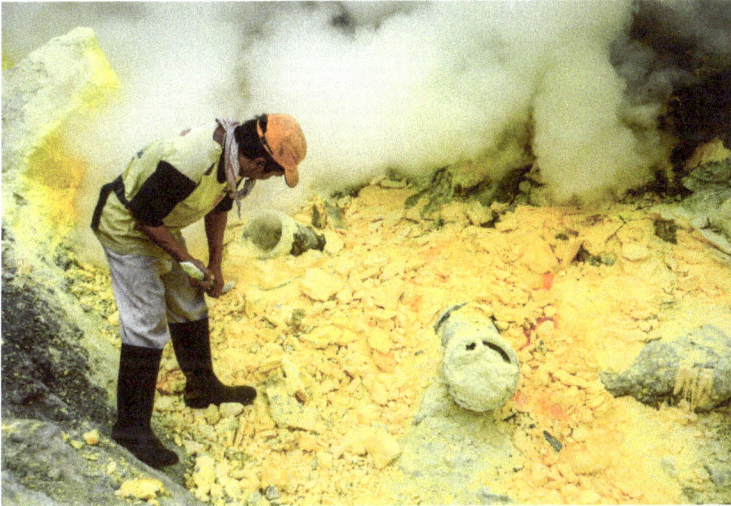

Sulfur mine. shutterstock/Zephyr_p

A number of Archaea organisms utilize hydrogen sulfide, and even elemental sulfur as an energy source. The relatively recent discovery of Archaea, and the organisms that are considered extremophiles, has revolutionized our understanding of life itself. These organisms can exist, and thrive in environments previously considered incompatible with life.

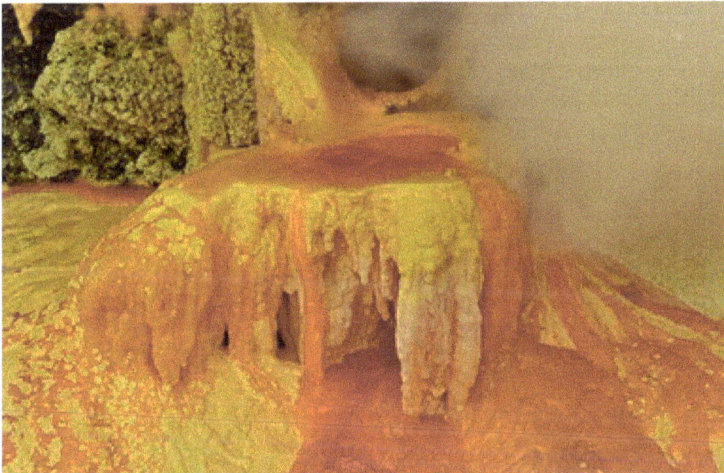

Olivier Grunewald.

Stanley Miller and Harold Urey became famous for their pioneering studies of what the early earth's atmosphere was like and what might have been brewing there millions of years ago. Using discharges of electricity as a substitute for lightning they used a few basic chemicals, water, methane, hydrogen and ammonia, to simulate the atmospheric conditions on Earth before life began. They demonstrated that some of the early building blocks of life were spontaneously created in this environment. Early experiments showed five to ten different amino acids, the building blocks for plants, animals, and fungi were generated.

Creative Commons License

In 1958 they added hydrogen sulfide to the mix and the long forgotten vials from their primordial-soup-in-a-bottle experiments were rediscovered just a few years ago. Using much more sophisticated analysis than was available over fifty years ago shows that the volcanic activity seeping hydrogen sulfide helped create the rich environment from which early life evolved. The recent analysis showed that by adding hydrogen sulfide the number of amino acids generated increased up to 23, with additional compounds and amines generated as well. Included in the new amino acids was methionine, which is a required building block for many life forms

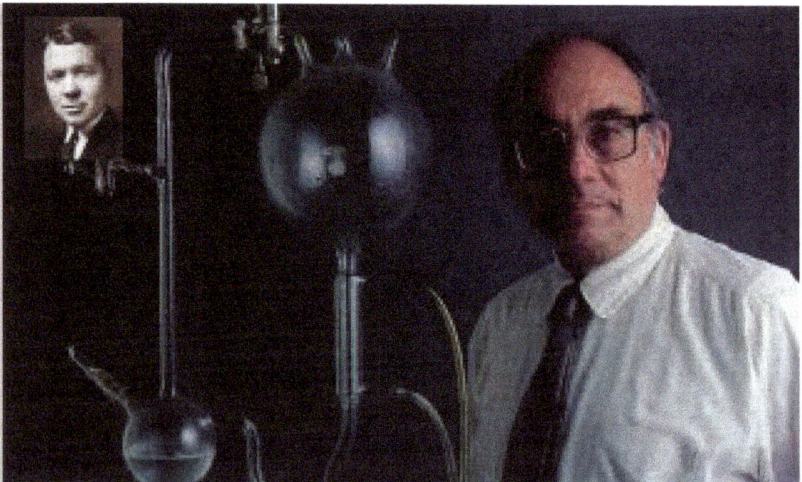

Harold Urey (inset) and Stanley Miller devised an experiment that revealed the earliest building blocks of life may have been generated in early planetary atmosphere of the Earth. Creative Commons License

Ideal Gas Law

Many aspects of the human body that deal with gasses, in particular the respiratory system and the gastrointestinal systems both deal with large volumes of gas. Unlike solids and liquids the gasses in nature are dramatically impacted by changes in temperature, pressure and volume. For example when the temperature of a gas increases its volume increases or if its volume cannot increase because it is contained than its pressure increases. The individual laws of physics discovered and named after Avogadro, Boyle, Charles & Gay-Lussac dealing with gas at different temperature, volume, and pressure have been combined into the ideal gas law: PV = nRT. The symbols represent the properties of the gas, P is pressure, V is volume, n is the amount in moles, R is the ideal gas law constant and T is temperature.

Ideal Gas Law

| Boyle's Law | Charles' Law | Avogradro's Law |

Ideal Gas Law

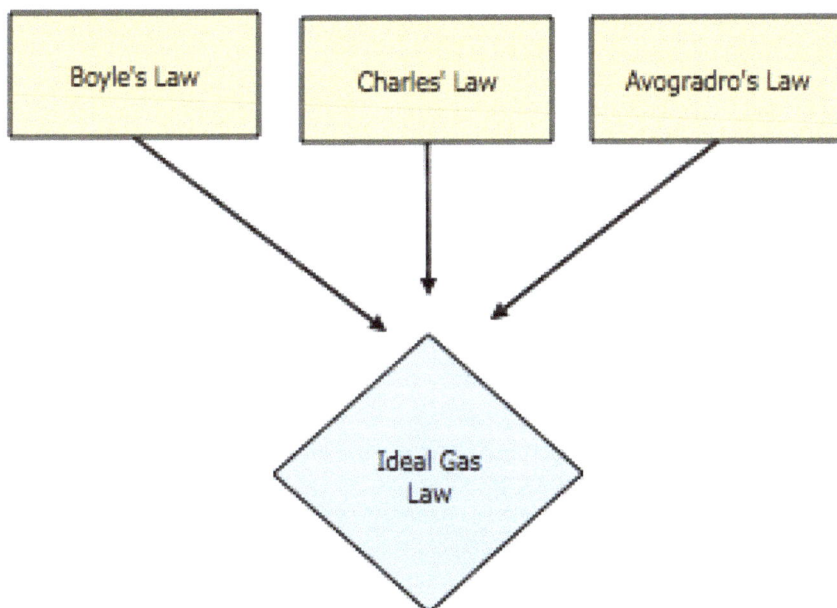

http://chemwiki.ucdavis.edu Creative Commons License

Farts are no exception and obey the ideal gas laws. The volume of a fart is related to its temperature and pressure. As an example, if you happen to have a fever and your body temperature is elevated the pocket of gas in your intestines will expand or the pressure will increase, or you will release a fart with more power volume and sound than usual. The laws of physics are the basis for the changing behavior of intestinal gas in scuba diving, mountain climbing, airplanes, and a wide variety of situations you may or may not have thought about.

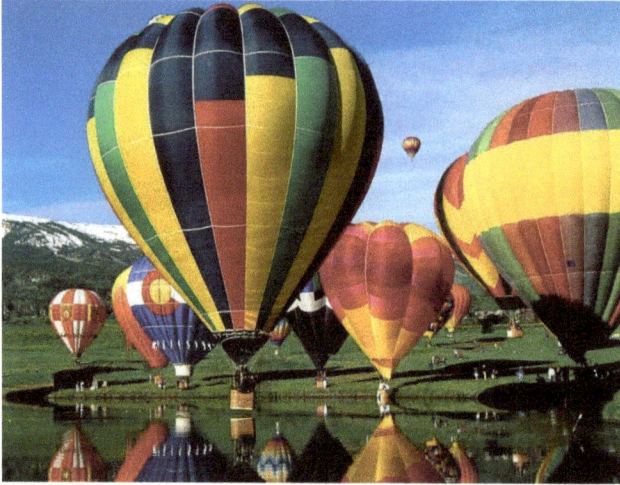

Hot air balloons are an example of hotter temperature leading to volume expansion. Creative Commons License.

Intestinal Gas, Therapy

When it comes to therapy for intestinal gas the first attempt is to identify foods or products that exacerbated, and avoid them. One can try an elimination diet, where one food or food group at a time our abstained from. If there is no improvement in the degree or symptoms related to intestinal gas a different food or food group is substituted for an elimination period.

One of the most common foods to which people are sensitive, which results in excess of gaseousness, is lactose intolerance. Lactose is the complex sugar found in milk and requires the enzyme lactase for its conversion to the two simple sugars, glucose and galactose, to allow its absorption. Most individuals have some degree of lactose intolerance, and can adequately digest small amounts of dairy product without symptoms. The symptoms of lactose intolerance become manifest when the amount of lactose consumed exceeds the individual's ability to produce lactase. The ability of the digestive track cells of the villi to produce lactase diminishes with age especially after infancy and childhood.

The avoidance of dairy products particularly in excess of the individual's lactase production results in symptom resolution. The most common symptoms are those of excessive gaseousness including distension and flatulence, and diarrhea. There are many dairy substitute products in the marketplace including those manufactured from rice, soy, various nuts such as almonds and cashews, coconuts, and others. Another approach is the commercial availability of the enzyme lactase itself. It may have already been added to the dairy product and is commonly found in the marketplace. Lactase supplements, which are taken orally with dairy products, are also available and effective.

To 'Air' is Human

Another common source of excessive gaseous and this is a diet high in legumes and cruciferous vegetables. A number of vegetables have a high content of complex sugars known as raffinose, verbascose, and stachyose. The enzyme required to metabolize and digest these complex sugars is known as alpha-galactosidase. Humans as well as other animals do not have this enzyme, which is found only in plants. When the undigested complex sugar reaches the gut flora we microbes ferment and metabolize it releasing gases in the process. One approach is to reduce the quantity of these food products in the diet. In the case of beans soaking them for several hours, and in particular and allowing them to sprout, starts the process of alpha-galactosidase production within the bean itself. A simpler approach is taking an alpha-galactosidase supplement such as beano just prior to the meal. Alpha-Galactosidase is destroyed by heating, and that should not be added to foods prior to cooking or preparation.

Other food sensitivities such as to gluten are controversial. There is a known condition of gluten sensitive enteropathy also known as celiac disease, sprue, and nontropical sprue. In this condition a portion of the gluten known as gliadin damages the villi of the intestinal tract. As the damage continues the villi are blunted and shortened, eventually resulting in malabsorption. The inability to digest and process foods provides material for they gut microbiome to metabolize and release gases as well as causing diarrhea. A much larger portion of the population has reported sensitivity to gluten, and indeed a significant number do have difficulty digesting wheat and the other cereal grains that do contain gluten including rye, barley, and oats.

The sugar fructose most commonly found in fruits is a frequent source of intestinal gas and diarrhea if consumed in excess. All humans have a limited capacity to process the fruit sugar fructose. Nonnutritive sugars such as mannitol sorbitol and other food additives such as polysorbate-80 may cause excessive gaseousness as well. The most common foods related to belching and burping, known as eructation, are those, which contain gases in dilution such as carbonated beverages, beer, and champagne. Many foods also have very high air content. This includes whipped foods, baked goods including bread, fruit, ice cream, and others.

Some individuals are also prone to aerophagia. Everyone swallows air but those prone to aerophagia gulp down more than the average amount of air. The activities that can result in excess of aerophagia include rapid eating, drinking with the strong or from a bottle, tilting the head and neck back while swallowing, poorly fitting dentures, chewing gum or tobacco products, sucking or chewing on hard candies, as well as smoking. Talking while eating will also result in excessive swallowing. Individuals with sinus condition or postnasal drip tend to swallow their secretions frequently, every swallow also including about one teaspoonful of air.

Most of the individuals who have excessive burping and belching also have a hiatal hernia and gastroesophageal reflux disease GERD. In this condition the most common problem is inappropriate relaxation of the lower esophageal sphincter, when it should be closed tight after each swallow to prevent regurgitation. The gastric contents are usually very acidic from the addition of hydrochloric acid produced by the gastric glands. When this acidic material is refluxed into the esophagus irritation and damage of the esophageal lining may occur. If it occurs on a chronic basis the development of a change in the mucosal lining, known as a Barrett esophagus, may arise with an increased risk of the development of esophageal cancer.

The usual treatment for gastroesophageal reflux disease includes conservative measures such as reducing excess weight above normal, avoidance of foods and social habits that relax the lower esophageal sphincter. This includes fried foods, fatty foods, alcohol, tobacco, chocolate, and peppermint. Other measures may include elevating the head of the bed and avoiding any recumbent position until at least one hour after mealtime. Over-the-counter antacids and gastric acid suppressants are frequently used. If symptoms persist stronger prescription medication may be required to suppress the stomachs hydrochloric acid production. Fortunately, conservative treatment or acid suppressants are very effective. In some individuals the symptoms of heartburn is not present or minimal.

The gas symptomatology of bloating and distension is most frequently seen in irritable bowel syndrome. It is considered a functional gastrointestinal disorder most probably related to altered motility and heightened sensitivity to intraluminal pressure. Recent evidence suggests that alterations in the gut microbiome maybe playing a very important role in this condition. Some individuals benefit from introduction of the FODMAP dietary modification. Other conditions may also cause such symptoms including inflammatory bowel disease, bacterial infections, parasites, and others. One condition in particular that causes great concern in women is a possibility of ovarian cancer. This is typically a silent disease and bloating may be one of its first manifestations because of fluid buildup within the abdomen known as ascites.

Chronic pancreatitis and pancreatic insufficiency can result in enzyme deficiencies leading to malabsorption of fats, proteins, and carbohydrates. Fat malabsorption often leads to a form of diarrhea known as steatorrhea. In this condition the gas as well as the oily floating stool have the particularly characteristic offensive odor. Fortunately and pancreatic enzyme replacement supplements are commercially available and effective.

The approach to the intestinal gas problem of flatulence is addressed in the same manner as those above, as any unresolved burping, belching, and distension will nearly always eventually result in the gas passing down below. Because flatulence is of great social concern various treatment approaches have been attempted. One of the most important issues is to exclude significant underlying disease such as inflammatory bowel disease, bacterial overgrowth, parasites, and others.

To 'Air' is Human

Dietary modification or the usage of enzyme supplements can be very helpful. If this approach does not provide symptomatic improvement there are several over-the-counter safe products designed to be internal deodorants. The use of bismuth subgallate as well as chlorophyll products have been particularly successful. The use of pre-biotics, probiotics, and changes in the gut microbiome may be attempted. The use of antibiotics is usually limited to proven small intestinal bacterial overgrowth. Individuals who have undergone bariatric surgery, particularly with a gastric bypass, are especially prone to gas issues.

The use of activated charcoal has a long history of adsorbing toxins and gases. It has been used in chair cushions and other external modalities with some degree of effectiveness. Oral ingestion of activated charcoal has been less successful, presumably because the absorptive capacity of activated charcoal is markedly diminished by the time it reaches the colon. The addition of activated charcoal pads, as well as impregnating fabric with activated charcoal, the potential to provide a significant benefit. To be effective all of the gas released has to pass through activated charcoal. Formfitting underwear made with activated charcoal impregnated fabric has been very successful, albeit more expensive. The successful use of activated charcoal pads is dependent on the consumer placement of the pad in not allowing gas to escape. New product development including the use of other adsorbent material and metal ions hold promise for the availability of additional approaches.

As with all issues of health and wellness each person needs to be assessed individually. With the advances in the human genome project it is now recognized that it is not just the genetic blueprint in the DNA that makes up the individuals uniqueness. Although humans have approximately 23,000 genes these genes are also controlled by external factors in a process described as epigenetics. It is also now recognized that the human body is in essence more than just human cells. The human system includes the microbiome, the microorganisms that live on and within us. The gut-brain-microbiome-food axis demonstrates the intimate interconnectivity of these four elements. If one were to analyze the human system by the number of cells a human is comprised of approximately 10% human cells and 90% microbial cells. If one were to analyze the system on the basis of the number of genes, humans are approximately 1% human genes and 99% microbial jeans.

The era of personalized medicine will advance the understanding of both health and disease. The previous approach of using population-based medicine will be abandoned as technology and bioinformatics allows treatments to be specifically tailored to the individual's genome, microbiome, and metabolome. The effectiveness of therapy should increase dramatically along with a significant reduction in adverse reactions to medications. This approach will also avoid the time and monetary expense of medications that did not provide a benefit, even if fortunately they did not cause an adverse reaction. In the interval as these advances are being brought into clinical practice it remains the best approach to tailor the treatment plan to the individual. What works for one may not work for another. Until the science and technology sufficiently evolve it often takes a trial and error approach to find the best treatment approach for the individual. And it is the individual who can be the only judge if the treatment is successful or the search for a solution must continue.

Irritable Bowel Syndrome

Irritable bowel syndrome (IBS) also known as spastic colon is a functional disorder with the diagnosis based on symptoms of abdominal discomfort, bloating, and alteration of bowel habits. It may be predominated by diarrhea or constipation or alternation between the two. It is more common in women and symptoms can vary with the menstrual cycle. In the US there is an incidence of about 15% of the entire population. A diagnosis of irritable bowel syndrome is made on the basis of symptoms if celiac disease, lactose intolerance, parasites, and bacterial overgrowth have been excluded and there are no signs of weight loss, gastrointestinal blood loss, infections or family history of inflammatory bowel disease.

Irritable bowel syndrome occurs more commonly after an intestinal infection, or a stressful life event. A history of sexual abuse is found in thirty percent of women with irritable bowel syndrome. A serum test for anti-vinculin antibodies, which are elevated after intestinal infections is being investigated as a possible tool to identify irritable bowel syndrome. The cause of irritable bowel syndrome is unknown and there may be several different cause and conditions all pooled together under this diagnosis until further advances are made. The most popular theory is that IBS is a disorder of the complex neuroendocrine pathway between the brain and the gastrointestinal tract. Alternative approaches to the mind-body interactions have been proposed for irritable bowel syndrome and yoga, exercise, tai chi, meditation, and other modalities may offer benefits.

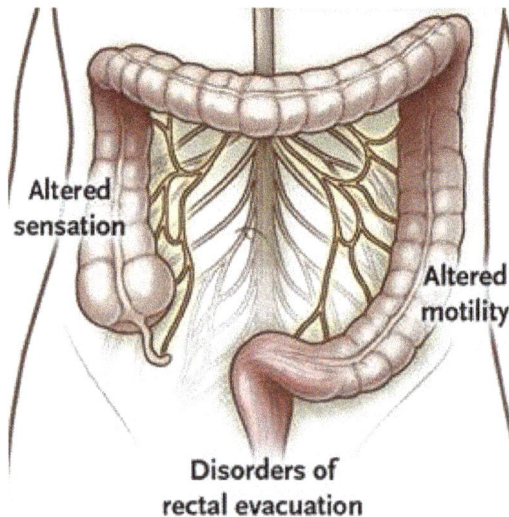

Altered sensation

Altered motility

Disorders of rectal evacuation

Treatments have included dietary adjustments, medication and psychological interventions. FODMAP is an acronym that stands for Fermentable Oligosaccharides, Disaccharides, Monosaccharides, And Polyols. Restricting these short chain carbohydrates and related sugar alcohols, which are poorly absorbed in the small intestine. May be of benefit in irritable bowel syndrome. Many of these sugar alcohols including sorbitol, mannitol, xylitol, isomalt, and maltitol are added to commercial food products as non-nutritive bulk sweeteners. See entry on FODMAP diet for more details.

Newer prescription agents involving the neuroendocrine pathways, particularly serotonin agonist and antagonist are being studied. Other approaches using non-absorbable antibiotics such as rifaximin have provided relief for some patients, as has the use of probiotic agents to modulate the gut flora. Some believe the condition is triggered by changes in the gut flora and associated changes to the immune system. Fortunately irritable bowel syndrome is not associated with a higher risk if cancer or other conditions that would reduce life expectancy. It has a significant impact on quality of life and the economy. In the United States irritable bowel syndrome has been estimated to cost $10 billion a year in direct medical costs and an additional $20 billion in indirect costs.

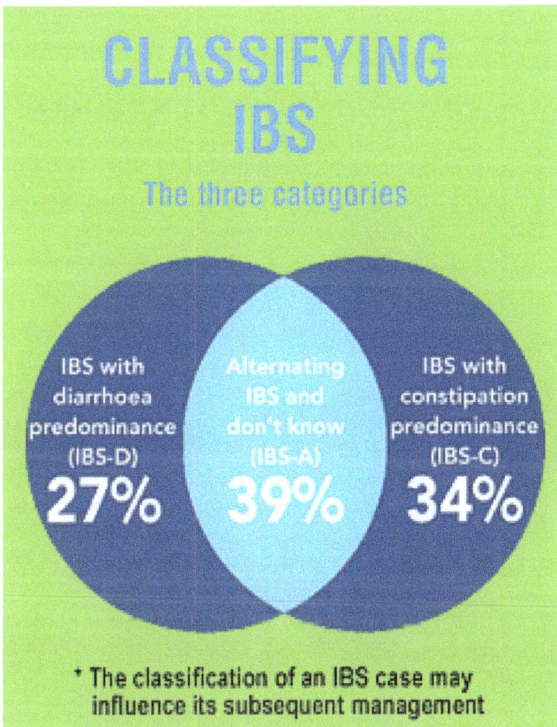

CLASSIFYING IBS

The three categories

IBS with diarrhoea predominance (IBS-D) 27%

Alternating IBS and don't know (IBS-A) 39%

IBS with constipation predominance (IBS-C) 34%

* The classification of an IBS case may influence its subsequent management

media2.onsugar.com Creative Commons License

To 'Air' is Human

Lactase

Lactase is an enzymes involved in the hydrolysis of the disaccharide lactose into galactose and glucose. Lactase is located on the tips of microvilli along the lining of the small intestine. Levels of lactase decrease with weaning in a significant proportion of the human population. Other populations benefit from a mutation that is thought to have occurred over 5,000 years ago with the rise of the domestication of herd animals that allowed the continued ingestion of dairy products into adulthood. If the intake of lactose exceeds the availability of lactase to digest it the gut flora ferments the disaccharide. This gives rise to the symptoms of lactose intolerance, gas, cramps, and possibly diarrhea.

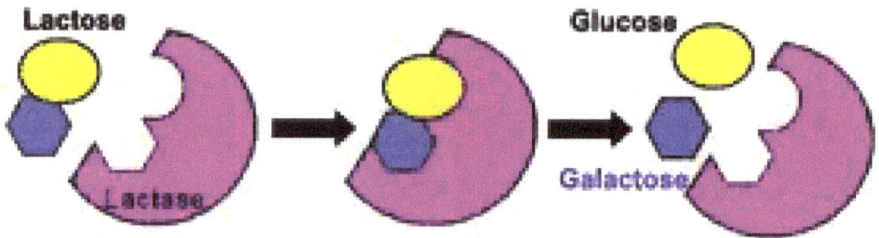

www.pharmaceutiucal-materials.com Creative Commons License

Lactose free foods are available where the lactase enzyme has already been added to the product to break down the lactose. The enzyme itself is also commercially available and should be taken with dairy products that contain lactose. Some dairy products, such as most hard cheeses, are lactose free on the basis of the production process. Acidophilus and Lactobacillus in yogurt and other foods also provides some lactase activity. Most people with lactose intolerance still have a nominal amount of the lactase enzyme and can digest lactose in very small quantities such as milk used as a creamer for coffee. Other dairy substitutes such as almond, rice, and soy 'milk' are lactose free.

Lactobacillus

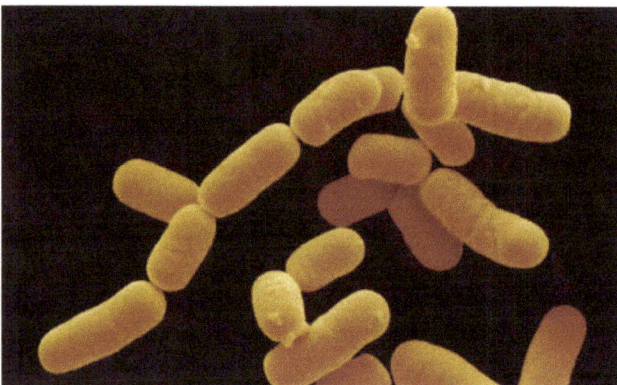

Lactobacillus rhamnosus, a probiotic bacterium www.theguardian.com Creative Commons License

To 'Air' is Human

Lactobacillus is a Gram-positive anaerobic rod-shaped bacterium that converts lactose and other sugars to lactic acid. The production of lactic acid makes its environment acidic which inhibits the growth of some harmful bacteria. In humans they are present in the vagina and the gastrointestinal tract where they make up a small portion of the gut flora. The genus Lactobacillus currently consists of over 180 species and encompasses a wide variety of organisms. Bifidobacterium was previously called *Lactobacillus bifidus* and has a separate entry under bifidobacterium.

Lactose

Lactose is a disaccharide of galactose and glucose that is found in milk from the Latin word lactis (milk). Lactose was discovered in milk in 1619 AD by Fabriccio Bartoletti. Varying between mammalian (the term derives from the distinctive characteristic of mammary glands). Lactose comprises between 2~8% of milk by weight. It is commercially extracted from whey, several million tons of which are produced annually as a by-product of the dairy industry. Whey is the liquid remaining after milk is curdled and strained, often for the production of cheese.

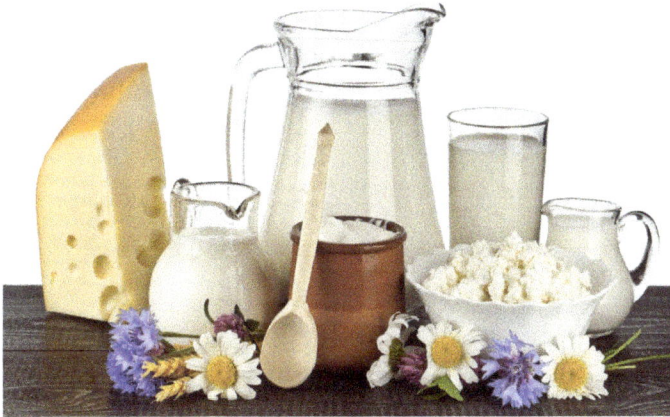

Dairy products. Creative Commons License

As a natural sugar found in milk and milk products it is found in cheese, ice cream, and processed foods, such as bread, cereal, and salad dressing. Hard cheeses typically have markedly reduced lactose content. Acidophilus milk and products that contain live Lactobacillus cultures such as in yogurts have reduced lactose content. Lactose free dairy products are also commercially available, as is the enzyme supplement lactase, which can be taken with the ingestion of lactose to help with its digestion, and processing.

Mammals nurse their infants on milk, which is rich in lactose. The villi of the small intestine secrete the enzyme lactase (β-D-galactosidase), which hydrolyses the lactose molecule into the simple sugars glucose, and galactose, which are easily absorbed. In most mammals the production of lactase decreases with the decreased consumption of reaching maturity.

Humans have continued to supplement their diet with milk from other mammals, especially those who developed herding practices of livestock, such as cattle, sheep, goats, camels, etc. The descendants of these populations appear to have induced the genetic tendency to maintain lactase production into adulthood. Other people have lost the ability to maintain significant lactase production and when the ingestion of lactose exceeds their enzymes capacity, the symptoms of lactose intolerance become apparent. When lactose is not digested by lactase the gut flora ferment it with the production of bloating, flatulence and occasional diarrhea from the osmotic properties if the sugar molecules drawing water into the digestive tract.

Any illness that damages the villi will result in a decrease if all of the enzymes and can aggravate underlying food intolerance. A viral or bacterial gastroenteritis, commonly referred to as a 'stomach flu or bug', will damage the villi and reduce the enzymes that would normally aid in digestion. The cell lining and villi of the small intestine tend to recover rapidly and thus for the few days following an infection dairy products are best avoided until the enzyme levels have recovered.

A major use of lactose is in the pharmaceutical industry where it is commonly used as inexpensive filler for pills because of its compressibility. It is also commonly used as inexpensive filler in a wide variety of food products. It is not unusual for individuals with known lactose intolerance to be unaware that they are ingesting sizable amounts of lactose in foods or pharmaceuticals. Reading the ingredient labels is important but the consumer has to be aware that lactose may be present if whey, whey protein, nonfat dry milk, milk sugar, powdered dairy product, etc. are included on the ingredient list. Unfortunately, lactose filler in pharmaceutical and nutraceutical products as well as nutritional and dietary supplements are rarely identified.

Lactose Intolerance

Lactose intolerance, also known as hypolactasia or lactase deficiency is the condition that arises when there is an insufficient quantity of the enzyme lactase, which is needed to metabolize the lactose commonly found in milk and dairy products. Hippocrates (460-370 BCE) was one of the first to recognize that many individuals had a difficult time digesting cow's milk. Lactase is an enzyme involved in the hydrolysis of the disaccharide lactose into galactose and glucose. Lactose intolerance is not an allergy and is not due to an immune response, it is due to the lack of a key digestive enzyme.

Lactase is located on the tips of microvilli along the lining of the small intestine. Levels of lactase decrease with weaning in a significant proportion of the human population. Other populations benefit from a mutation that is thought to have occurred over 5,000 years ago with the rise of the domestication of herd animals that allowed the continued ingestion of dairy products into adulthood. If the intake of lactose exceeds the availability of lactase to digest it the gut flora ferments the disaccharide. This gives rise to the symptoms of lactose intolerance, gas, cramps, and possibly diarrhea.

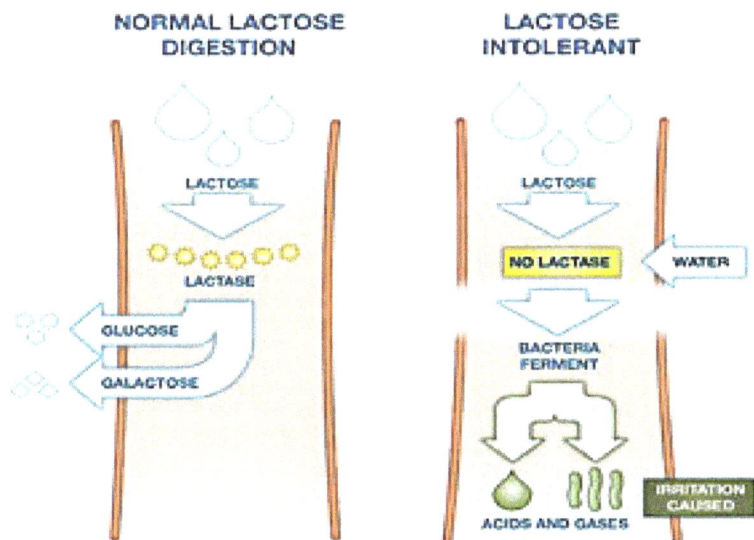

NORMAL LACTOSE DIGESTION	LACTOSE INTOLERANT
LACTOSE	LACTOSE
LACTASE	NO LACTASE ← WATER
GLUCOSE	BACTERIA FERMENT
GALACTOSE	
	ACIDS AND GASES — IRRITATION CAUSED

www.avonmorelactosefree.ie Creative Commons License

Lactose is a disaccharide of galactose and glucose that is found in milk from the Latin word lactis (milk). Lactose was discovered in milk in 1619 AD by Fabriccio Bartoletti. Varying between mammalian (the term derives from the distinctive characteristic of mammary glands). Lactose comprises between 2~8% of milk by weight. It is commercially extracted from whey, several million tons of which are produced annually as a by-product of the dairy industry. Whey is the liquid remaining after milk is curdled and strained, often for the production of cheese.

Mammals nurse their infants on milk, which is rich in lactose. The villi of the small intestine secrete the enzyme lactase (β-D-galactosidase), which hydrolyses the lactose molecule into the simple sugars glucose, and galactose, which are easily absorbed. In most mammals the production of lactase decreases with the decreased consumption of milk upon reaching maturity, a condition known as primary lactase deficiency. Secondary lactase deficiency arises when the intestinal villi are damaged, such as by gastroenteritis, celiac disease, parasites, etcetera. Congenital lactase deficiency is a very rare autosomal dominant inherited condition most often seen in the Finnish population. Certain populations, which developed dairy herds and persisted in milk consumption favored those who had a genetic variation now known as the lactase persistence allele. DNA evaluation of ancient skeletons revealed that this beneficial mutation developed in Europe and Russia over four thousand years ago. Seventy-five percent of African-American, Jewish, Native American, and Mexican American populations are lactose intolerant.

As a natural sugar found in milk and milk products it is found in cheese, ice cream, and processed foods, such as bread, cereal, and salad dressing. Hard cheeses typically have markedly reduced lactose content. Acidophilus milk and products that contain live Lactobacillus cultures such as in yogurts have reduced lactose content. Lactose free dairy products are also commercially available, as is the enzyme supplement lactase, which can be taken with the ingestion of lactose to help with its digestion, and processing.

Worldwide prevalence of lactose intolerance in recent populations (schematic)

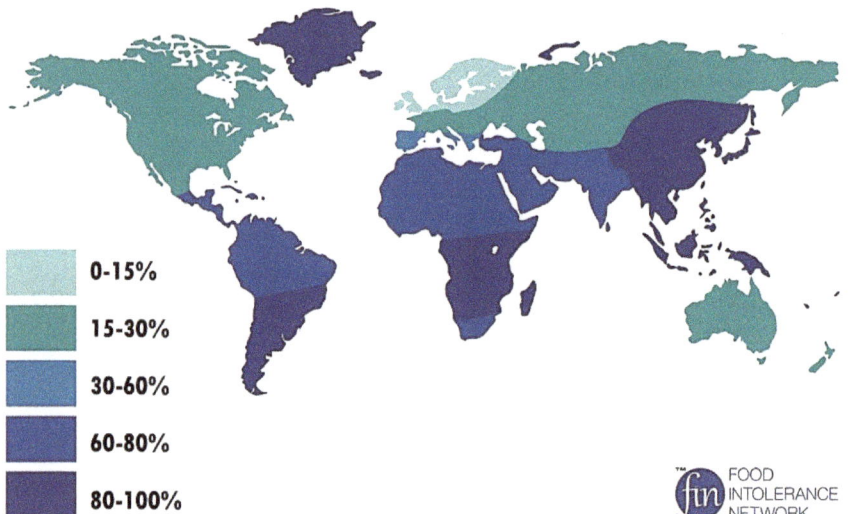

0-15%

15-30%

30-60%

60-80%

80-100%

FOOD INTOLERANCE NETWORK

upload.wikimedia.org/wikipedia/commons Author: NmiPortal Creative Commons License

Humans have continued to supplement their diet with milk from other mammals, especially those who developed herding practices of livestock, such as cattle, sheep, goats, camels, etc. The descendants of these populations appear to have induced the genetic tendency to maintain lactase production into adulthood. Other people have lost the ability to maintain significant lactase production and when the ingestion of lactose exceeds their enzymes capacity, the symptoms of lactose intolerance become apparent. When lactose is not digested by lactase the gut flora ferment it with the production of bloating, flatulence and occasional diarrhea from the osmotic properties if the sugar molecules drawing water into the digestive tract.

Any illness that damages the villi will result in a decrease if all of the enzymes and can aggravate underlying food intolerance. A viral or bacterial gastroenteritis, commonly referred to as a 'stomach flu or bug', will damage the villi and reduce the enzymes that would normally aid in digestion. The cell lining and villi of the small intestine tend to recover rapidly and thus for the few days following an infection dairy products are best avoided until the enzyme levels have recovered.

A major use of lactose is in the pharmaceutical industry where it is commonly used as inexpensive filler for pills because of its compressibility. It is also commonly used as inexpensive filler in a wide variety of food products. It is not unusual for individuals with known lactose intolerance to be unaware that they are ingesting sizable amounts of lactose in foods or pharmaceuticals. Reading the ingredient labels is important but the consumer has to be aware that lactose may be present if whey, whey protein, nonfat dry milk, milk sugar, powdered dairy product, etc. are included on the ingredient list. Unfortunately, lactose filler in pharmaceutical and nutraceutical products as well as nutritional and dietary supplements are rarely identified.

Dairy Product	Lactose (grams)	Dairy Product	Lactose (grams)
American Cheese, processed (1 slice, 1 oz)	1.17	Butter (1 tbsp)	0.01
Blue Cheese, crumbled (1/2 cup)	0.34	Sour Cream, cultured (1 tbsp)	0.02
Brie Cheese (1 oz)	0.13	Half and Half Creamer (1/2 cup)	0.19
Cheddar Cheese (1 oz)	0.15	Heavy Whipping Cream (1/2 cup)	0.07
Cottage Cheese, creamed, large curd (1/2 cup)	2.80	Milk: Fluid Whole, 2%, 1% (1 cup)	12.32
Cottage Cheese, creamed, small curd (1/2 cup)	3.00	Milk: Dry (1/4 cup)	12.29
Cream Cheese (1 tbsp)	0.32	Milk: Evaporated (1/2 cup)	12.65
Feta Cheese (1/2 cup)	3.07	Milk: Goat (1 cup)	10.85
Mozzarella Cheese, shredded (1/2 cup)	0.58	Milk: Human (1 cup)	16.95
Parmesan Cheese, hard (1 oz)	0.23	Milk: Lactaid (1 cup)	0.00
Provolone Cheese (1 oz)	0.16	Yogurt, Greek, plain (6 oz container)	5.51
Ricotta Cheese (1/2 cup)	0.33	Yogurt, plain, 8 grams protein (8 oz container)	10.58
Swiss Cheese (1 oz)	0.37	Yogurt, plain, 12 grams protein (8 oz container)	15.98

Source: USDA, ARS National Agricultural Library; Nutrient Data Laboratory
Amount of lactose may vary by brand. Read labels carefully.

Creative Commons License

Lactose free foods are available where the lactase enzyme has already been added to the product to break down the lactose. The enzyme itself is also commercially available and should be taken with dairy products that contain lactose. Some dairy products, such as most hard cheeses, are lactose free on the basis of the production process. Acidophilus and Lactobacillus in yogurt and other foods also provides some lactase activity. Most people with lactose intolerance still have a nominal amount of the lactase enzyme and can digest lactose in very small quantities such as milk used as a creamer for coffee. Other dairy substitutes such as almond, rice, and soy 'milk' are lactose free.

Le Pétomane

Joseph Pujol (1857 – 1945) was a stage performer from 1887 to 1914, and first performed on the Moulin Rouge stage in Paris in 1892. He had the unusual ability to inhale air into his colon through his anus and expel it at will. With the stage name Le Pétomane, French for the fart maniac, he was also affectionately known as 'the fartiste'.

With sufficient colonic inhalations and exhalations he was able to minimize the odor and control the sounds emanating from his anus to such a degree that he could play musical tunes. To assure that there was no odor he also underwent regular colonic irrigations before performances. Appearing on stage in red cape, white cravat, and black trousers, with a pair of white gloves held in the hands, he displayed the incongruous touch of elegance that added to his charm. A program of fart impressions followed, including contrasting the hearty fart of the miller with the timid fart of the young girl.

To 'Air' is Human

He proceeded to demonstrate the diffidence of the fart of the bride on her wedding night (almost inaudible) compared to the fart of the bride a week later (a lusty raspberry). His musical impersonations included an imitation of a tuba player on his instrument. He stunned the audience with a majestic ten-second fart, which he likened to a couturier cutting six feet of calico cloth. He would play *Le Marseilles* on his personal human wind instrument, his colon, even though he could only produce four notes do, mi, so, and the octave do. To add to his musical repertoire he would insert a tube offstage into his rectum and attach it to the musical instrument the ocarina. Then playing *O' Sole Mio* he would invite the audience to sing along.

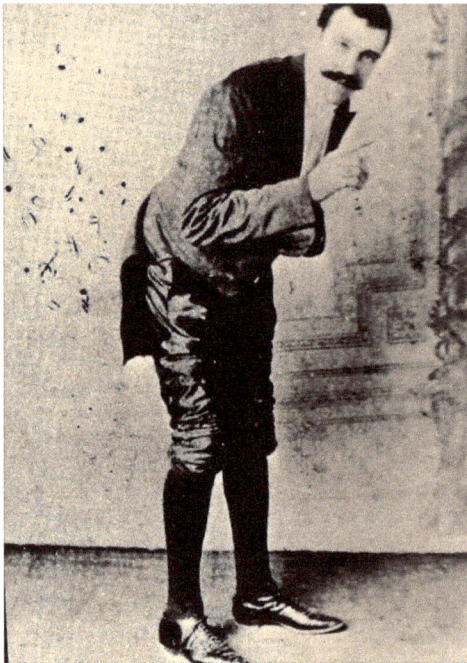

Joseph Pujol (Le Pétomane) 1857, Public Domain

Replacing the musical instrument at the end of the tube with a cigarette he used his colon to inhale. After withdrawal of the tube he would exhale the cigarette smoke out of his behind. For the grand finale he would imitate a twenty-one-gun salute, and the Great 1906 San Francisco earthquake with a thunderous roar that went on for over five continuous minutes. He would end his performance by blowing out a candle at a distance of three feet. Other than Harry Houdini, he was the highest paid stage performer in Europe and was earning a salary of twenty thousand francs per week. This was substantially more than the eight thousand francs per week salary of his contemporary Sarah Bernhardt who was considered the leading lady of the stage at that time. King Leopold II of Belgium and Edwards Prince of Wales came incognito to see Le Pétomane perform. Sigmund Freud attended a performance, and perhaps inspired, went on to describe his theory of anal fixation.

At one point he was embroiled in a disagreement with his stage manager and was going to perform in a different venue. The manager went to the courts and got a judicial injunction preventing Le Pétomane from performing elsewhere. During the court hearing Le Pétomane demonstrated his unique abilities in front of the court (he judge did not rule him out of order, or in contempt of court). Le Pétomane decided to offer his farting services and performance for free in a public display, but the manager and the court decision forbade him to fart in public.

When he died, the physicians of the day wanted to do a postmortem examination to find out how he had such remarkable anal control. The family held onto his body until enough decomposition set in that they no longer had to fear grave robbers retrieving the body for science. Joseph Pujol's memorable life lives on in the cinematic and stage arts. In Mel Brooks' 1974 movie Blazing Saddles, with many memorable fart scenes, there is an inside joke. It is an artistic acknowledgement to Joseph Pujol with Mel Brooks himself playing Governor William LePetomane.

Methane

Methane is produced in the human intestinal tract by microbial organisms. Methanogens are microorganisms of the Kingdom Archaea, not bacteria as previously thought. They produce methane as a metabolic byproduct in anaerobic conditions when oxygen is not present. Methanogens have been found in a variety of extreme environments and an thrive and reproduce in boiling water as well as in ice cores taken miles down in arctic glaciers. They are common in wetlands, where they produce marsh gas, and in the digestive tracts of animals and humans where they generate the methane content of flatulence as well as the ruminant belch. Higher methane concentrations in intestinal gas have been associated with decreased gastrointestinal tract motility and constipation.

Hydrogen and Methane are combustible gasses. In the presence of oxygen and an ignition source you have a potent flammable commodity. When methane burns it has a characteristic blue flame that you may see in a pilot light if you have a gas stove or furnace. Adolescent males and those who remain as adolescents intellectually have a fondness for demonstrating their dragon like ability to be human flamethrowers by igniting their farts. This is not a recommended activity and severe injury has resulted from successful attempts to ignite farts.

Hydrogen and methane are the two flammable gasses that may be found in a fart making them flammable. Lighting a fart to see if one produces these gasses is actually a dangerous activity. Significant burns to the anogenital area have occurred as a result, especially when ignited without a clothing barrier. The popular television show *Mythbusters* filmed an episode confirming that many farts are indeed flammable. It appears that the network found the episode too provocative, and perhaps for liability concerns that children watching might attempt their own demonstrations decided to not 'air' the episode.

On occasion dung and excrement can be more than just flammable, it can be explosive. The microorganism that produce hydrogen and methane that lead to ignitable farts continue their activity while sitting in a pile. For those foolish enough to light a match in a pile of cow dung to see what happens up close and personal the link to the video above should be convincing.

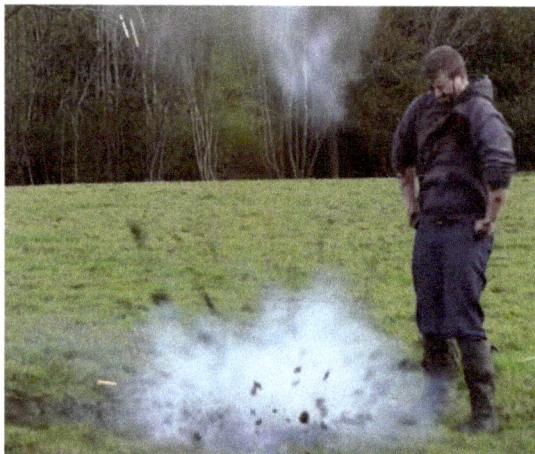

Lighting a match to a pile of cow dung is not a sign of higher intelligence. The methane and hydrogen generated by the microbes active in the dung pile may accumulate to explosive levels.
youtu.be/bZI1eeV88lQ

One of the more unusual injuries from a lit fart was second and third degree burns on the buttocks and a broken arm. The heavy gentlemen was sitting on the toilet defecating and farting extensively for a period of time. Being overweight his buttocks formed a firm seal around the toilet seat retaining all of the gasses in the enclosed space of the toilet bowl. He was smoking at the time and made a little space under his cheeks to innocently toss the lit cigarette into the toilet bowl. It promptly ignited blowing him off the seat, shattering the toilet bowl and causing extensive burn injuries to his buttocks. His wife called the paramedics and as he was being carried down the stairwell to the waiting ambulance he told them what caused the explosion. They laughed so hard they dropped the gurney thus breaking his arm.

Methane, Greenhouse Gases & Global Warming

'The primary greenhouse gases in the Earth's atmosphere are water vapor, carbon dioxide, methane, nitrous oxide, and ozone. Venus is a prime example of the planetary temperature consequences of the greenhouse effect. Nitrogen (N 2), oxygen (O 2), and argon (Ar), major components of the atmosphere are not greenhouse gases because they are minimally affected by infrared radiation. Clouds, composed of water droplets or ice crystals, do contribute to the greenhouse effect since they absorb and emit infrared radiation.

Water vapor accounts for about 50% of the Earth's greenhouse effect, with clouds contributing 25%, carbon dioxide 20%, and the minor greenhouse gases and aerosols accounting for the remaining 5%. Methane has a twenty fold greater impact on the greenhouse affect then carbon dioxide, when measured by weight. As a percentage however methane has a much smaller effect since it is found in relatively small amounts. The most important constituents of the greenhouse gasses are water vapor, clouds, carbon dioxide, methane, and ozone. Less important contributors include sulfur hexafluoride, hydro fluorocarbons, and per fluorocarbons.

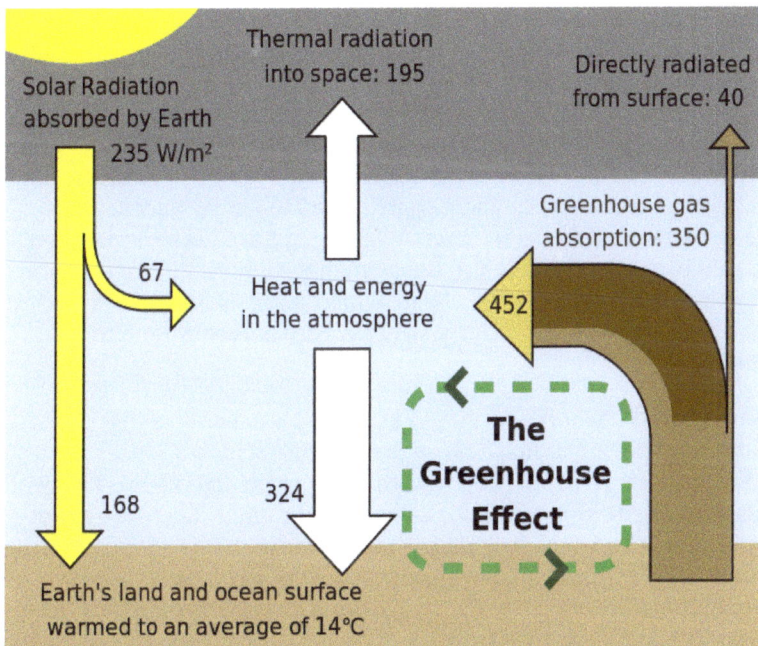

The figure shows the flows of energy between space, the atmosphere, and the Earth's surface, and how these flows trap heat near the surface and create the greenhouse effect. Energy exchanges are expressed in watts per square meter (W/m²). The sun is responsible for virtually all energy that reaches the Earth's surface. Of the surface heat captured by the atmosphere, more than 75% can be attributed to the action of greenhouse gases that absorb thermal radiation emitted by the Earth's surface. The atmosphere in turn transfers the energy it receives both into space (38%) and back to the Earth's surface (62%). The process by which energy is recycled in the atmosphere to warm the Earth's surface is known as the greenhouse effect. Creative Commons License

The atmospheric lifetime measures the time required to restore equilibrium in its concentration in the atmosphere. Water vapor has an atmospheric lifetime of approximately nine days in striking contrast to carbon dioxide of 30 years and N2O 114 years. The Earth's surface temperature is partly dependent on the balance between the absorption of radiant energy from the sun, and its reflection and re-radiation of energy back to space.

To 'Air' is Human

An earlier period of widespread glaciation (Snowball Earth) came to abrupt end about 550 MYA when a colossal volcanic outgassing raised the atmospheric CO2 concentration to 12%, about 350 present day levels. The extreme greenhouse conditions resulted in the deposition of calcium carbonate as limestone at the rate of over a foot each year. This brought a close to the Precambrian eon, and was succeeded by the warner Phanerozoic times with the appearance of multicellular animal and plant life. There has not been a recurrence of such a dramatic greenhouse effect since. No volcanic carbon dioxide emissions today are less than 1% of human production.

Based on measurements from Antarctic ice cores, the concentrations of carbon dioxide in the atmosphere are now 30% higher than levels before the industrial revolution. The levels had not changed appreciably in over 10,000 years. Although human activity only accounts for 5% of the greenhouse gasses, the naturally occurring amount was closely balanced by the Earths capacity to utilize the carbon sink of photosynthesis. Greenhouse gas production from human activity is mainly due to deforestation, the combustion of fossil fuels, livestock enteric fermentation and manure management, and landfill emissions. In terms of biomass bacteria would be the main contributors to global warming by their methane production. Other contenders nominated have been termites, which have over 2000 species and are prolific methane producers (initial reports suggested that they produce 40% of global methane), livestock such as cows, sheep, and pigs, and lastly dinosaurs, which are no longer around to defend their reputations.

A ruminant (Latin *ruminare* - to chew over again) is a mammal that digests plants in a multi compartment stomach through bacterial fermentation. It regurgitates the semi-digested mass, called cud, and chews it again and repeats the swallow. The process of re-chewing the cud is called "ruminating". There are about 150 species of ruminants, which include both domestic and wild species. Ruminating mammals include cattle, goats, sheep, giraffes, yaks, deer, camels, llamas, and antelope. Ruminant fermentation is a significant contributor to global methane production, which is over twenty times as potent greenhouse gas. Actually it is not the ruminant itself but the protist within its microbiome that generates hydrogen from the breakdown of cellulose. Within the protist is another organism Archaea, acting as a mutualist that converts the hydrogen to methane. To incentivize efforts to reduce livestock methane production a number of countries have proposed taxes on the release of greenhouse gasses. In spite of it being labeled as a flatulence tax, the predominant source of global warming from ruminants comes from fermentation in their multi compartment stomachs. It should really be called a burping and belching tax, but that is not as newsworthy.

Carbon dioxide, methane, nitrous oxide (N_2O) and three groups of fluorinated gases (sulfur hexafluoride (SF_6), hydro fluorocarbons (HFCs), and per fluorocarbons (PFCs)) are the major greenhouse gases impacted by human activity. These are regulated under the Kyoto Protocol an international treaty that was adopted in 2005. Nitrogen dioxide (NO_2) warms the atmosphere 310 times more than carbon dioxide and methane 21 times more than carbon dioxide. Although CFCs are greenhouse gases, regulations were initiated because CFCs' cause ozone depletion, not because of their contribution to global warming. Ozone depletion itself has a relatively minor effect on greenhouse warming.

Methane, Natural Gas

Natural gas is a naturally occurring mixture of hydrocarbon gases that consists primarily of methane. Smaller quantities of the higher alkanes such as ethane, propane, butanes, and pentanes are also often present. Other components that are commonly removed before marketing as a fuel can include hydrogen sulfide, carbon dioxide, water vapor, nitrogen, oxygen, and helium.

Natural gas is often used as an energy source for heating, cooking, and electricity generation. It is also used as fuel for vehicles and as a chemical feedstock in the manufacture of plastics and other commercially important organic chemicals. It contributes to less global warming as it produces 30 per cent less carbon dioxide than using petroleum and forty-five percent less than using coal as a fuel source.

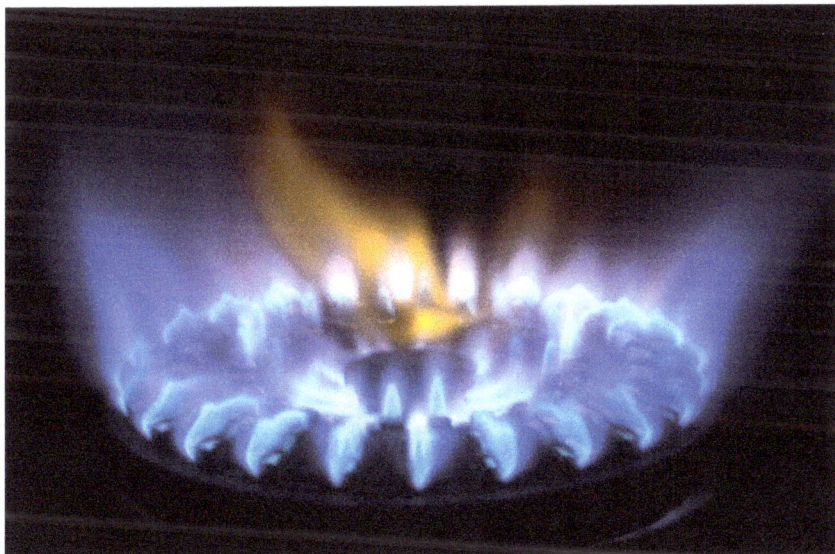

Creative Commons License

Natural gas is found in deep underground natural rock formations or associated with other hydrocarbon reservoirs in coal beds and as methane clathrates. Petroleum is also another resource found in proximity to and with natural gas. Most natural gas was created over time by two mechanisms: biogenic and thermogenic. Biogenic gas is created by methanogen organisms in marshes, bogs, landfills, and shallow sediments. Deeper in the earth, at greater temperature and pressure, thermogenic gas is created from buried organic material.

The location of shale gas compared to other types of gas deposits.

To 'Air' is Human

Shale gas in the United States is rapidly increasing as a source of natural gas. Led by new applications of hydraulic fracturing technology and horizontal drilling, development of new sources of shale gas has offset declines in production from conventional gas reservoirs, and has led to major increases in reserves of US natural gas. Large quantities of methane exist in the form of hydrates on offshore continental shelves and in the permafrost of the arctic regions. Hydrates are formed in the presence of a combination of high pressure and low temperature. Technology has yet to be developed yet to make the extraction economically viable.

Methane, Biogas

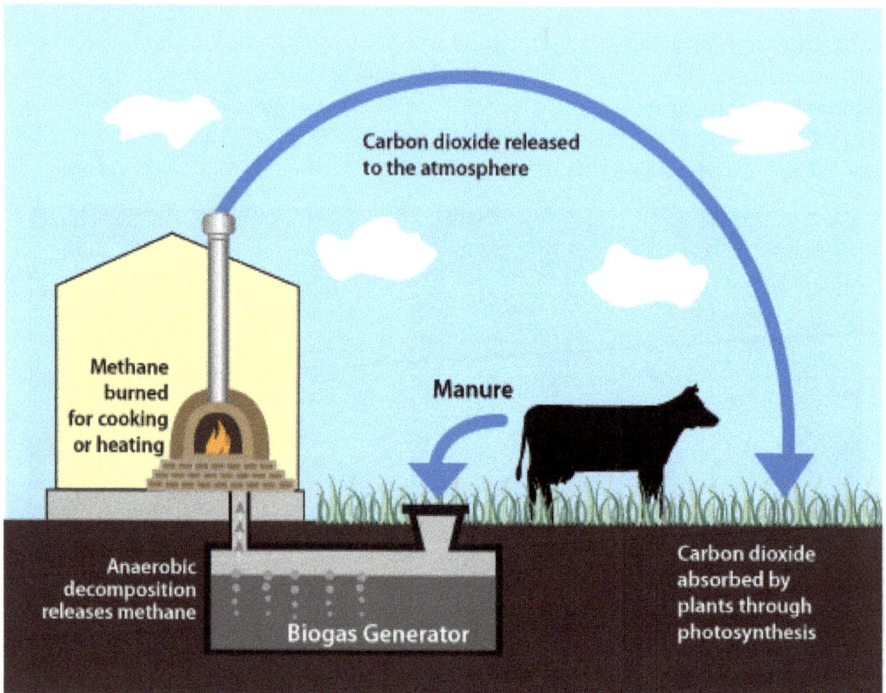

Creative Commons License

Biogas is produced by the anaerobic breakdown of organic biomass. The breakdown may require several different organisms acting in concert. For example the ruminant animal cannot digest cellulose without assistance from protist that reside in its gut microbiome. The protist generate hydrogen in the process of cellulose breakdown, which would be detrimental to the protist without the assistance of Archaea. The methanogenic Archaea actually reside within the protist and convert the hydrogen to methane. The sources of methane actually live in symbiotic relationships with other life, including termites, ruminants, and cultivated crops. When methane is produced with the decay of biomass it is referred to as biogas. Sources of biogas include swamps, marshes, landfills, manure, sewage sludge, and enteric fermentation.

To 'Air' is Human

Landfill gas has methane concentrations of approximately fifty percent. Waste treatment technologies can produce biogas of up to seventy-five percent methane. Biogas can be cleaned and upgraded to natural gas standards and is referred to as bio methane. One cow produces the manure in one day to generate three-kilowatt hours of electricity, enough to power a one hundred watt light bulb for twenty-four hours. If you imagine every cow having a one hundred watt light bulb illuminated from its digestive tract end product, you would have a new definition of a taillight.

Methane, Dinosaurs

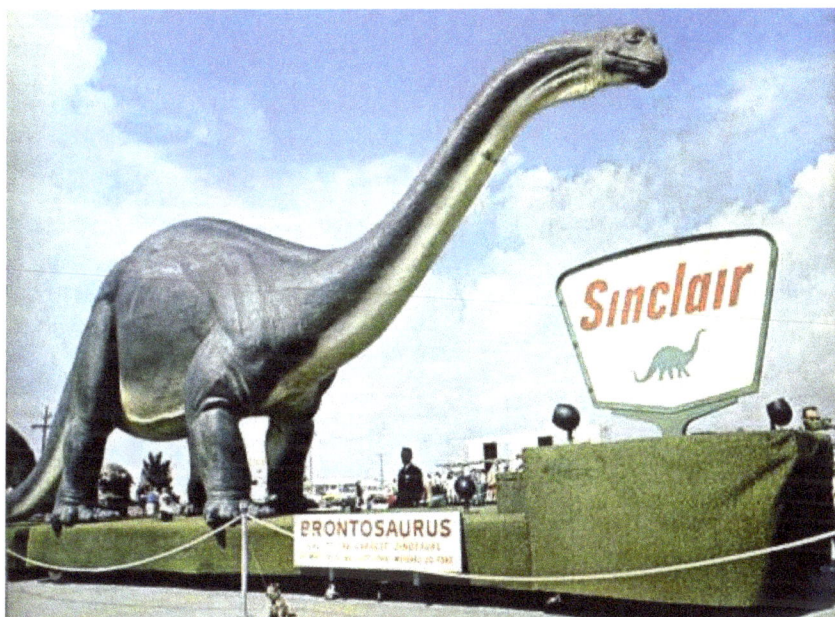

American Oil & Gas Historical Society

In 1933, the Sinclair Oil Corporation had an exhibit at the World's Fair in Chicago, suggesting that the world's oil reserves were created from material from the dinosaurs of the Mesozoic Era. Sinclair Oil featured advertisements in one hundred and four newspapers and five national magazines displaying a dozen different dinosaurs, from the menacing tyrannosaurus red and three-horned triceratops to the peace loving passive yet massive forty ton vegetarian Apatosaurus (brontosaurus) with a tail thirty feet long. Sinclair used 'Dino' a big green Apatosaurus (Brontosaurus) as its official mascot and corporate symbol, trademarking the dinosaur in 1932.

P. G. Allen, developer of life-like papier-mâché animals for the motion picture industry, was working on an exhibit for the 1933 Century of Progress Exposition in Chicago, the equivalent of a World Fair. Sinclair Oil sponsored the dinosaur exhibition and to enhance the academic stature of its promotions financed the

233

dinosaur-fossil search expeditions of Dr. Barnum Brown, curator at the American Museum of Natural History. After Doctor Brown's death in January 1963, Sinclair retained Dr. John H. Ostrom of Yale University's Peabody Museum of Natural History as consultant on the Sinclair sponsored Paleontology exhibit at New York World's Fair in 1964.

Sinclair's marketing was a masterstroke, but led to the common public misperception that petroleum is predominantly derived from the organic remains of the great dinosaurs. Rather than the enormous dinosaurs, it was microscopic bacteria that produced the petroleum reserves if our time period. Single-celled bacteria evolved in the earth's oceans about three billion years ago, and were the dominant life form on the planet until about 600 million years ago. In fact, if dominant is qualified as largest by biomass, bacteria retain that distinction today.

As microscopic as the individual bacteria may be, the bacterial colonies known as "mats" were of enormous proportions. They had masses of millions of tons compared to the hundred tons for the largest dinosaur, the sauropods. As these massive colonies died off and decayed they subsided to the bottom of the sea and were covered by layers of accumulating sediments. Over millions of years these layers of sediment thousands of feet underground were compressed under tremendous pressure and temperature, and developed into the liquid hydrocarbons we recognize as petroleum.

The vast majority of the world's coal deposits date back to the Carboniferous period, about three hundred million years ago. The first dinosaurs would not make their grand entrance in the evolutionary timetable until seventy-five million years later. During the Carboniferous period the earth was heavily forested. With the death and decomposition of these trees and plant life buried under great pressure and temperature under heavy layers of sediment, they were transformed into solid coal rather than liquid petroleum. As the search for petroleum and coal preserves often entails drilling and excavation of deep layers of sediment, it is not uncommon for fossils of dinosaurs and other prehistoric forms of life to be uncovered. The discovery of a theropod dinosaur during fossil fuel exploration in China has been given the appropriate name Gasosaurus. It looks as though Dino's story may have come full circle.

Microbiology

The microbes of the gastrointestinal flora are major contributors to intestinal gas. Although unseen, an invisible world had been theorized for centuries. The ancient Greeks thought about it and wrote comprehensively about a world of atoms, molecules, and microscopic life forms far beyond the technology of their day. The glass lens makers from the thirteenth through sixteenth centuries provably developed ever improving prototypes of the microscope after first developing the telescope. It was only in the late 1674 that Antoine Van Leeuwenhoek, a glass lens maker, used an improved optical microscope of his own design to identify red blood cells, spermatozoa, and microorganisms. His advance began the field of microbiology, brining a previously invisible world into view. The field continues to bring new discoveries and understanding of life on earth and the interdependence of various life forms.

Microorganisms gave been found to survive and thrive in extreme locations from many miles underground in rocks, under the ice of Antarctica, in volcanic vents under seas, and the vacuum of outer space. The world of microorganisms has expanded from knowledge of bacteria, to discovery of other microorganisms such as the virus, prion, and Archaea. The future will probably yield further discoveries as continuing research and advancing technology allow.

From the time of Van Leeuwenhoek to the present dramatic advances have taken place in the understanding of the role of microorganisms in human health and disease, as well as life in general. Louis Pasteur was a pioneering influence and identified the role of microorganisms in the fermentation process leading to enhanced production of wine, cheese, and vinegar. He developed an immunization program to protect cattle from anthrax, as well as to treat people exposed to the previously uniformly fatal rabies. He was able to disprove the prevailing theory of spontaneous generation of life and developed the process of disabling most pathogenic organisms by boiling in a process that was named after him, pasteurization.

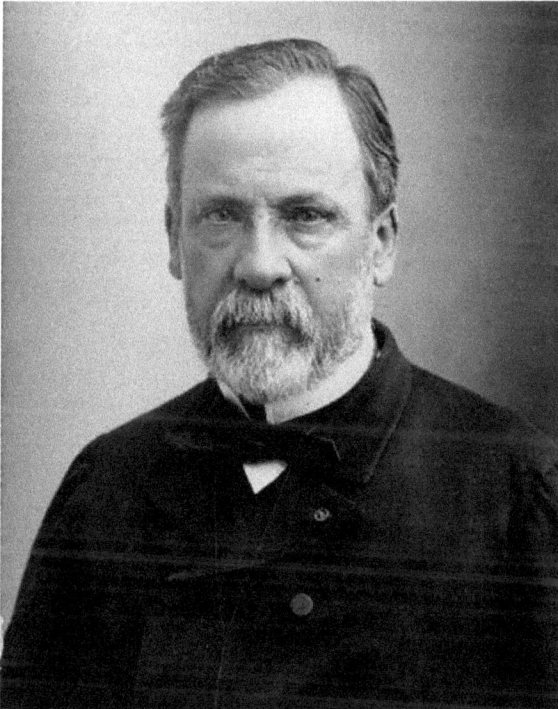

Louis Pasteur, Public Domain

To 'Air' is Human

It took many more years for the concept of pathogenic organisms to bring hygiene to a new level of awareness. Even in medical circles there was great reluctance to embrace hand washing and the use of disinfectants. Joseph Lister was preceded by Ignatz Semmelweis who fought an ignorant medical establishment that used to operate on trusting patients with their bare hands. Semmelweis was able to prove that infections were transmitted from the autopsy room to the operating room because hands were not washed. In spite of this proof he was ignored and ridiculed, which led to his mental collapse and death in a psychiatric hospital because he could not save thousands of innocent people who were condemned to death because of arrogance and ignorance.

Similar stories can be found in many areas of science and medicine where lifesaving advances were delayed for decades or centuries. The story of anesthesia is a prime example where excruciatingly painful and gruesome surgeries were performed on awake subjects who were forcibly restrained, while the anesthetic of nitrous oxide was being used as laughing gas purely for entertainment purposes. The discoverer of nitrous oxide, Sir Humphrey Davies, an esteemed scientist suggested that it be studied as an anesthetic but the physicians and surgeons of his day simply ignored him. The rediscovery of it and other products as anesthetics is a remarkable story that has been told by several books on the subject.

Another interesting aspect of the story of microbiology is how it took hundreds of years for scientists and physicians to recognize that pathogenic organisms were responsible for many diseases. It has also taken a similar period of time for the recognition that ,most organisms are not pathogenic but are commensals ort actually improve health. One of the pioneers in this investigation was a scientist working at the Pasteur Institute in Paris, Dr. Élie Metchnikoff (1845-1916). He investigated the extreme longevity of centenarians in Bulgaria and believed their long lives were due to the yogurt and sour milk consumed as a regular part of their diet.

He received the Nobel Prize in Medicine for his work on immunity, and identified the *Lactobacillus delbrueckii subspecies bulgaricus* organism in yogurt that is considered an ideal probiotic. His theory of aging being due to toxic bacteria, and that lactic acid producing organisms could prolong life, were very influential. His advocacy of probiotics was embraced by the Japanese scientist Minoru Shirota who developed a stronger strain of the probiotic organism *Lactobacillus casei* found in Yakult and kefir. Dr. John Harvey Kellogg, the medical director of the Battle Creek Sanitarium, also embraced Dr. Metchnikoff's theory. Dr. Kellogg administered series of colonics to cleanse the bowels then had his patients eat half a bowl of yogurt, with the other half administered as an enema. Dr. Kellogg also advocated a high fiber high roughage diet and developed a corn flake cereal, founding the very successful Kellogg Cereal Company

To 'Air' is Human

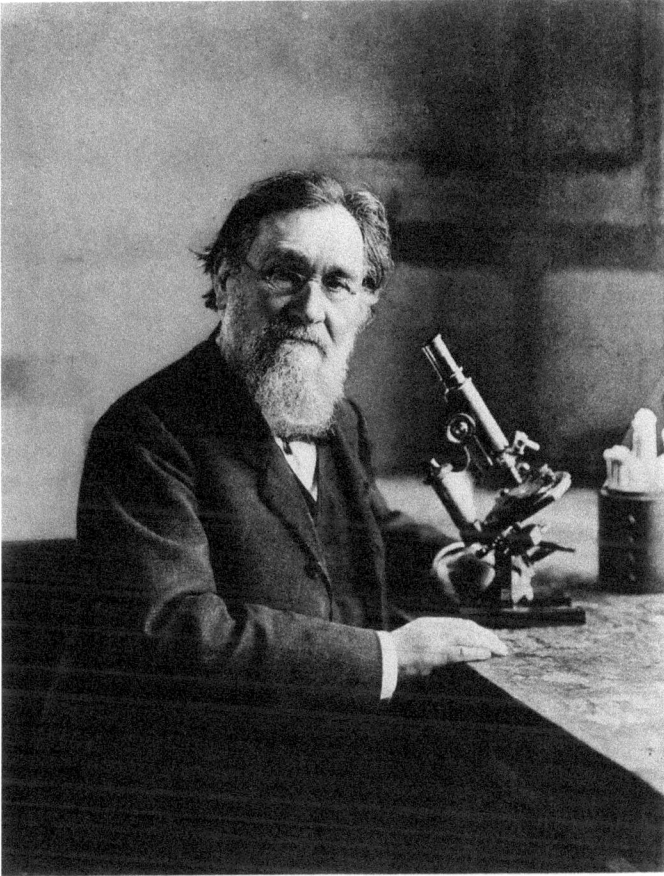

Élie Metchnikoff, Nobel Prize winning scientist at the Pasteur Institute in Paris

Unfortunately science and medicine are replete with many instances where personality flaws, greed, arrogance, jealousy, stupidity, ignorance, and a hundred and one other human failings led to missed opportunities to prevent or cure disease, and improve human health. Even more unfortunately these failings show no sign of abating, with conflicts of interest, desire for personal financial gain, overreaching for recognition, and the securing of patents, too often leading to fraud and deception. Of course dedicated and compassionate professionals are the majority, but progress is hindered nonetheless leading to the illness and death of innocents.

Microbiome

The micro biome includes microbes, their genomes, and their environmental interactions. Gut flora consists of the microorganisms that live in the digestive tract and are the largest component of the human flora. The gut flora contains approximately one hundred trillion microorganisms in its intestines, a number much greater than the ten trillion cells of the human body. The gut flora has approximately one hundred times as many genes as the human genome.

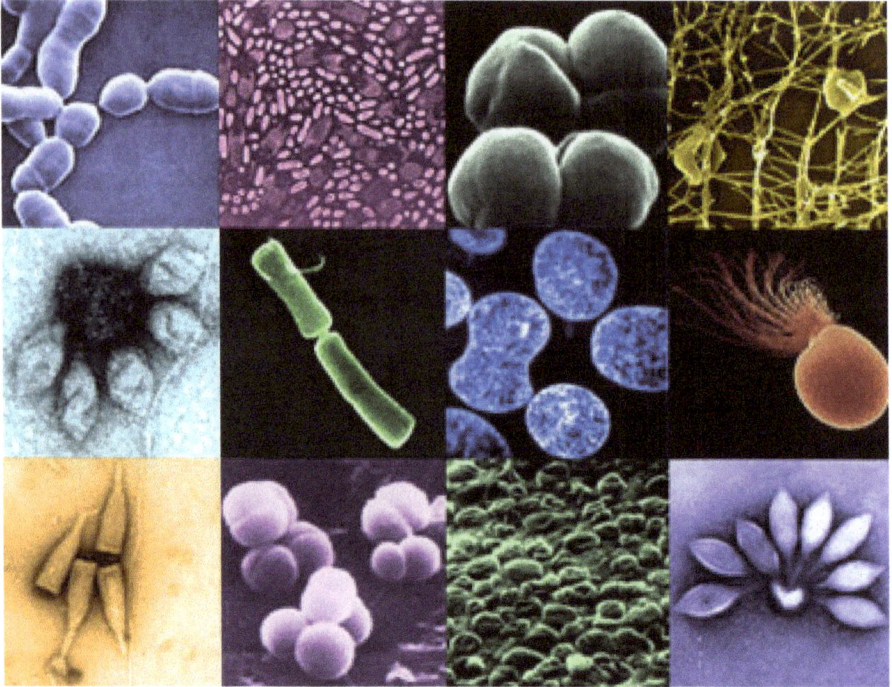

The human genome has twenty three thousand genomes and the human microbiome genome exceeds over one million and still counting. Any one or combination of these genomes, human and/or microbial, can play a very important role in health and disease. Alterations in an individual's flora may occur with changes in lifestyle, diet, illness, and age. The National Institutes of Health has embarked on the Human Microbiome Project to identify the organisms present in the human microbiome and their role in health and disease.

Anaerobic bacteria make up most of the flora in the colon and up to sixty percent of the dry mass of feces. These bacteria perform a variety of metabolic activities that benefit the host, so much so that some scientists refer to it as the "forgotten" organ. Their metabolic activity includes extracting energy from undigested carbohydrates by fermentation and absorption of short chain fatty acids. They also synthesize vitamin B and vitamin K as well as metabolizing bile acids and lipids. The gut flora also prevents pathogens from colonizing the intestines through competitive exclusion, also known as the "barrier effect". The bacteria stimulate the immune system lymphoid tissue to produce antibodies to pathogens, and to recognize and not develop an immune response to beneficial flora.

The human microbiome is normally established only after birth. Fetuses do accumulate a mass of sterile and odorless greenish feces called meconium, in their intestines. Fetuses usually pass meconium after birth but approximately twelve percent of pregnancies have yellow or green bile pigmented meconium stained amniotic fluid. The risk increases with the length of the pregnancy. In births occurring after forty-two weeks, described as post term, the rate of meconium staining approaches fifty percent. Fetuses have amniotic fluid in their lungs until they take their first breath of air after birth. In a minority of meconium stained amniotic fluid cases potentially fatal meconium aspiration syndrome occurs. If the newborn fails to pass meconium, a congenital abnormality of the colon needs to be excluded. Hirschsprung disease may involve failure of fetal development of the ganglions of the enteric nervous system. When it involves the colon, the bowel may not relax to allow the passage of meconium or feces and surgery may be required to remove the affected segment of bowel.

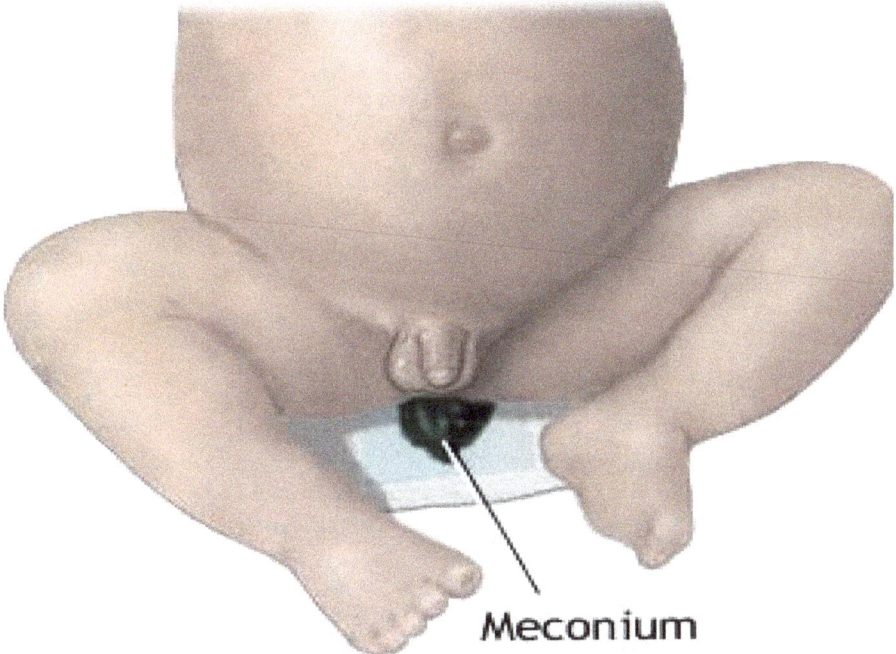

Meconium

www.healthcentral.com Creative Commons License

Since the digestive tract of the newborn is sterile, there are no microorganisms generating gas through cellular metabolism. All of the gas the newborn infant begins to pass is swallowed air. If an infant is bottle-fed rather than breast-fed they are much more likely to swallow even more air. Baby bottles are a common cause of aerophagia in infants as they suck in and swallow air if the formula does not always cover the nipple. Burping the baby after a feeding is the means of allowing the swallowed air to escape otherwise it will cause distension and discomfort. Some bottles are designed to use an internal plastic sleeve to prevent air from reaching the nipple when the formula is depleted the sleeve forms a vacuum so the infant is not sucking in air.

To 'Air' is Human

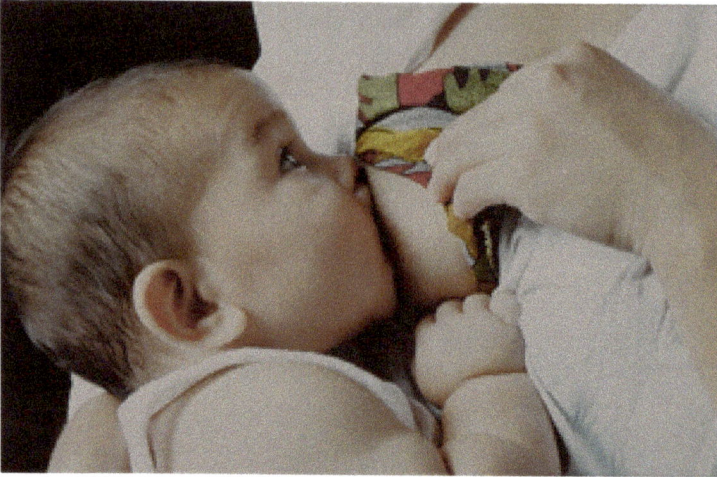

The first exposure to microorganism that will be swallowed and begin to colonize the infant digestive tract are from the birth mother if the delivery is vaginal and breast-feeding is initiated. The microorganisms that colonize the infant become its microbiome and play a major role in its ongoing health and wellness. The initial gut flora of the infant if born via a vaginal delivery and breast-feeding is identical to the vaginal and skin microbiome of the mother. This initial flora changes over the next few months especially if formula and other milks and foods are introduced. At about three months of age the gut flora is well established, and although changes will occur it is similar to the gut flora it will have as an adult.

The gut flora helps to set the infant's immune system, and it recognizes and tolerates microorganisms that are beneficial known as commensals. One of the theories why breast-feeding is preferable, as well as why a vaginal delivery is preferable to Caesarian section, is the natural microbiome exposure has advantages. The immunity of infants who did receive the natural microbiome from the mother is at a disadvantage. Some experts are advocating exposing the newborn to the mother's vaginal secretions and microbiome if the birth is via a Caesarian section.

The gut flora is one aspect of the microbiome, with skin, ears, mouth, genitourinary, and every surface of the body exposed to the external environment developing its own unique microbiome. Infants born by Caesarean section have exposure to different organisms, which establish a microbiome that is not believed to be as beneficial as via a natural vaginal delivery.

The microbiome is established rapidly upon exposure to the environment. Most people think that the digestive tract is an internal organ because it is located inside the body. They are often surprised to find out that that the digestive tract is actually considered an organ exposed to the external environment. It is a long hollow tube exposed to the external environment at both ends, and is transited by material that for the most part comes from outside of the body.

To 'Air' is Human

The results of cell division and multiplication are similar between cells of the body, and cells of the microbiome. Mathematically this growth pattern is described as exponential or logarithmic growth. For those more familiar with finance, it is more akin to compounding interest instead of simple arithmetic addition. If a single cell divides into two cells, those cells divide into four cells, those into eight cells, and the numbers increase rapidly. The colonization and establishment of the microbiome is extremely rapid. The limitation of cellular division and growth of human cells are controlled by genes, hormones, neurotransmitters, and a variety of other feedback control mechanisms. The microbiome is also under the influence of these mechanisms, as well as competition for habitat and nutrition.

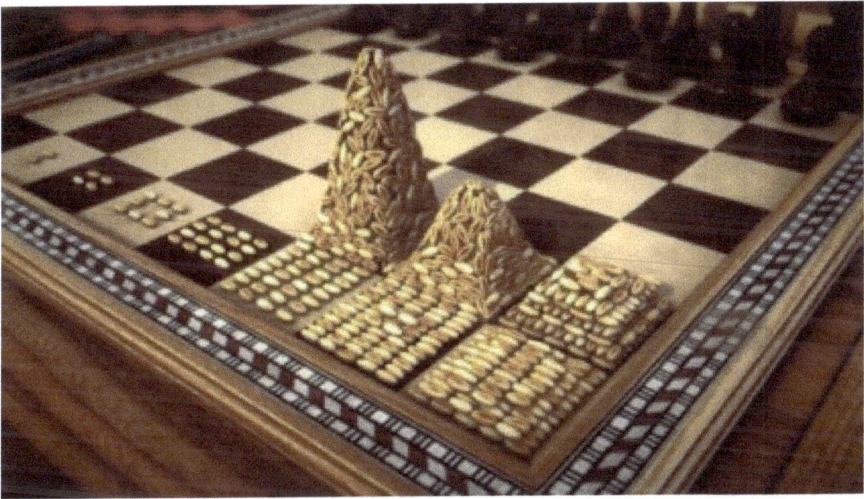

There is an apocryphal tale told of the invention of the game of chess. Long ago in an ancient land, there lived a very wise man that happened to be the Vizier at the court of a great Sultan. Months and years passed by and the great Sultan died, and his young prince replaced him. Being young, the prince lacked experience. He started spending more than what his father used to. The wise Vizier decided to teach the brash prince a lesson! The prince set a contest and as a reward, decided to give the winner whatever he wishes, boasting of his wealth, being under the illusion that his wealth is virtually endless. The Vizier won, and asked the prince for the prize: a single grain of wheat and a chessboard!

"What?! Just a grain of wheat! Are you insulting my wealth?" yelled the prince. "No! Your majesty!" The Vizier explained. "You have to promise to double that grain of wheat until the chessboard is full, so on the first day you give me one grain of wheat on the first square of the chessboard, on the second day you double it on the second square (giving me two grains), on the third, you double that on the third square (giving me four grains), and so on, until the sixty fourth square on the chessboard." "I would thought you being so smart", the young prince said. "You would ask for something more substantial. Anyway, if this is your wish I will grant you that."

And so, on the second day, the Vizier got 2 grains, on the third, he got 4 grains, and the young prince couldn't help himself making fun of the Vizier.
By the sixth day, the Vizier got 32 grains of wheat. By the eighth day and the end of the first row, he got a mere 128 grains. By the sixteenth day and the end of the second row, he got 32,768 grains. By the end of the game the prince could not provide enough grains to give the Vizier a chessboard's worth of grains because of the power of exponential growth. The last (sixty-fourth) square alone required 9,223,372,036,854,775,808 grains. The cumulative total of all of the squares was 18,446,744,073,709,551,615 grains. Indeed, that many grains would cover the entire earth several inches deep!

The gastrointestinal microbiome is also known as the gut microbiome and the gut flora. The gut microbiome is much more important than most people give it credit for. The microbes of the body far outnumber the number of human cells. The vast majorities are commensals or are engaged with us in a symbiotic relationship from which we both benefit. The normal flora is site specific so that the microbiome of the stomach is different from the small intestine, which is different again from the colon. The appendix serves as a reservoir of the normal large intestinal bacteria flora. It represents the healthy gut microbiome from which the gut flora can be replenished after a bout of intestinal dysentery.

The effect of the microbiome includes microbes, their genomes, and their environmental interactions. Gut flora consists of the microorganisms that live in the digestive tract and are the largest component of the human flora. The gut flora contains approximately one-hundred-trillion microorganisms in the intestinal tract, a number much greater than the ten trillion cells of the human body. The gut flora has approximately one hundred times as many genes as the human genome.

The human genome has twenty-three thousand genes and the human microbiome genome exceeds over one million genes and still counting. Any one or combination of these genes, human and/or microbial, can play a very important role in health and disease. Alterations in an individual's flora may occur with changes in lifestyle, diet, illness, and age. The National Institutes of Health has embarked on the Human Microbiome Project to identify the organisms present in the human microbiome and their role in health and disease.

Anaerobic bacteria make up most of the microbial flora of the colon and up to sixty percent of the dry mass of feces. These microorganisms perform a variety of metabolic activities that benefit the host, so much so that some scientists refer to it as the 'forgotten organ'. Their metabolic activity includes extracting energy from undigested carbohydrates by fermentation and absorption of short chain fatty acids. They also synthesize vitamin B and vitamin K, as well as metabolizing bile acids and lipids.

To 'Air' is Human

The gut flora also prevents pathogens from colonizing the intestines through competitive exclusion, also known as the 'barrier effect'. The bacteria stimulate the immune system lymphoid tissue to produce antibodies to pathogens, and to recognize and not develop an immune response to beneficial flora. One of the major advances in the understanding of microbial life has come about with the recent advances in genomics technology. This technology now allows the rapid and precise identification of organisms that could not be identified because they were too fastidious and difficult to culture from stool specimens.

These advances include the discovery of extremophiles, organisms that can live in extreme environments, and represent a previously undiscovered form of life called Archaea. This has prompted a reevaluation of the biological system of taxonomy, the categorizing of life forms. Most scientists now recognize six separate kingdoms: Animals (Animalia), Plants (Plantae), Fungi, Bacteria, Protozoan (Protista), and Archaea.

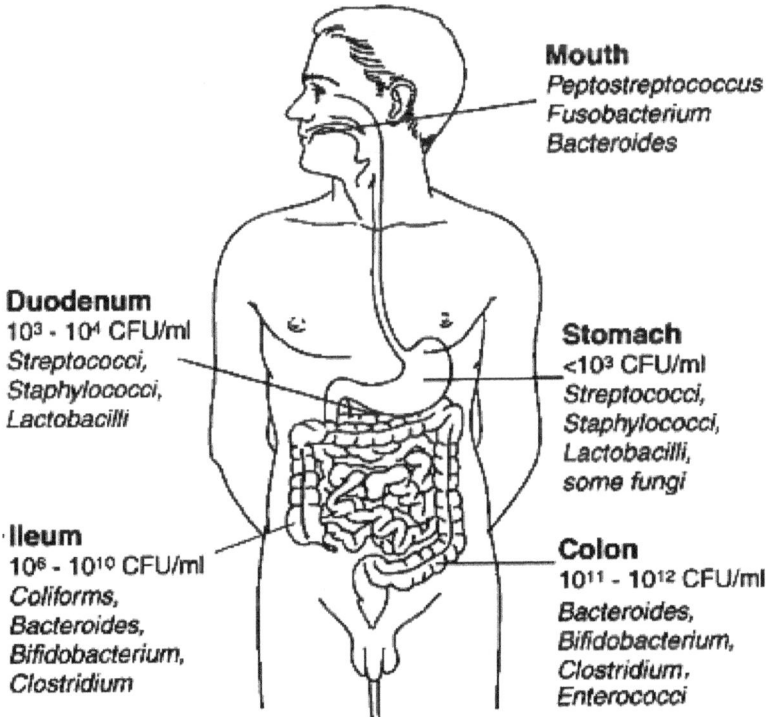

Mouth
Peptostreptococcus
Fusobacterium
Bacteroides

Duodenum
$10^3 - 10^4$ CFU/ml
Streptococci,
Staphylococci,
Lactobacilli

Stomach
$<10^3$ CFU/ml
Streptococci,
Staphylococci,
Lactobacilli,
some fungi

Ileum
$10^8 - 10^{10}$ CFU/ml
Coliforms,
Bacteroides,
Bifidobacterium,
Clostridium

Colon
$10^{11} - 10^{12}$ CFU/ml
Bacteroides,
Bifidobacterium,
Clostridium,
Enterococci

trialx.com/curetalk/wp Creative Commons License

Significant portions of the human microbiome are not bacteria at all and are actually Archaea. In fact, the methane produced in flatus comes from the methanogenic Archaea of the colon's microbiome. There will undoubtedly be major advances in the understanding of human health and diseases as the microbiome is explored and understood. The hygiene hypothesis proposes that a lack of early childhood exposure to infectious agents, parasites, and symbiotic microorganisms in the gut flora suppresses the development of the immune system. It is proposed that allergies, autoimmune disorders, and diseases seen at higher rates in the developed world may be due to excessive hygiene preventing the exposure necessary for optimal health. The hygiene hypothesis is supported by epidemiological data, yet the topic remains controversial with extensive research ongoing.

As a result of the hygiene hypothesis, helminthic infections emerged as a possible explanation of the low incidence of immunological disorders and autoimmune diseases in less developed countries. Helminthic therapy is the treatment of autoimmune diseases and immune disorders by means of deliberate infestation with a roundworm parasite. It is currently being studied as a promising treatment for several (non-viral) autoimmune diseases including Crohn disease, multiple sclerosis, asthma, and ulcerative colitis. The anti-inflammatory effects of helminth infection are also prompting research into diseases that are not currently considered to have an immune basis. For example, heart disease and arteriosclerosis both have similar epidemiological and inflammatory profiles to the autoimmune diseases. Presently the two versions of helminthic therapy being studied are *Trichuris suis* ova and *Necator americanus* larvae.

Dysbiosis (dysbacteriosis) refers to a condition with microbial imbalances on or inside the body. Dysbiosis is most prominent in the digestive tract or on the skin, but can also occur on any surface or mucous membrane exposed to the environment such as the vagina, lungs, mouth, nose, sinuses, ears, nails, or eyes. It has been associated with different illnesses, such as inflammatory bowel disease, as imbalances in the intestinal microbiome may be associated with bowel inflammation and chronic fatigue syndrome. Microbial colonies found on or in the body are normally benign or beneficial. These beneficial and appropriately sized microbial colonies carry out a series of helpful and necessary functions, such as aiding in digestion. They also protect the body from the penetration of and infection with pathogenic microbes. These beneficial microbial colonies compete with each other for space and resources.

When this balance is disturbed by any of a variety of causes, such as antibiotic exposure, the balance of the microbial populations becomes disturbed. This can lead to an overgrowth of one or more of the organisms, which then may have a negative effect on some of the beneficial organisms. The imbalance and negative impacts can initiate a vicious cycle with further disruption from the normal flora.

Small intestinal bacterial overgrowth (SIBO) is a disorder of excessive bacterial growth in the small bowel. Risk factors included decreased motility or anatomical changes that lead to stasis, immune deficiencies, and reflux of bacteria from the colon into the small bowel such as the surgical removal of the ileocecal valve. The symptoms of bacterial overgrowth may include nausea, vomiting, bloating, flatus, chronic diarrhea, constipation, abdominal discomfort, weight loss, malnutrition, and anemia from vitamin B12 deficiency. Irritable bowel syndrome (IBS) may have an association with small intestinal bacterial overgrowth with some studies showing improvement after treatment. Rosacea, a dermatological condition, also appears to have an association with improvement after treatment. Small bowel bacterial overgrowth syndrome is treated with antibiotics, and if retreatment is required, various antibiotics may be given in a cyclic fashion.

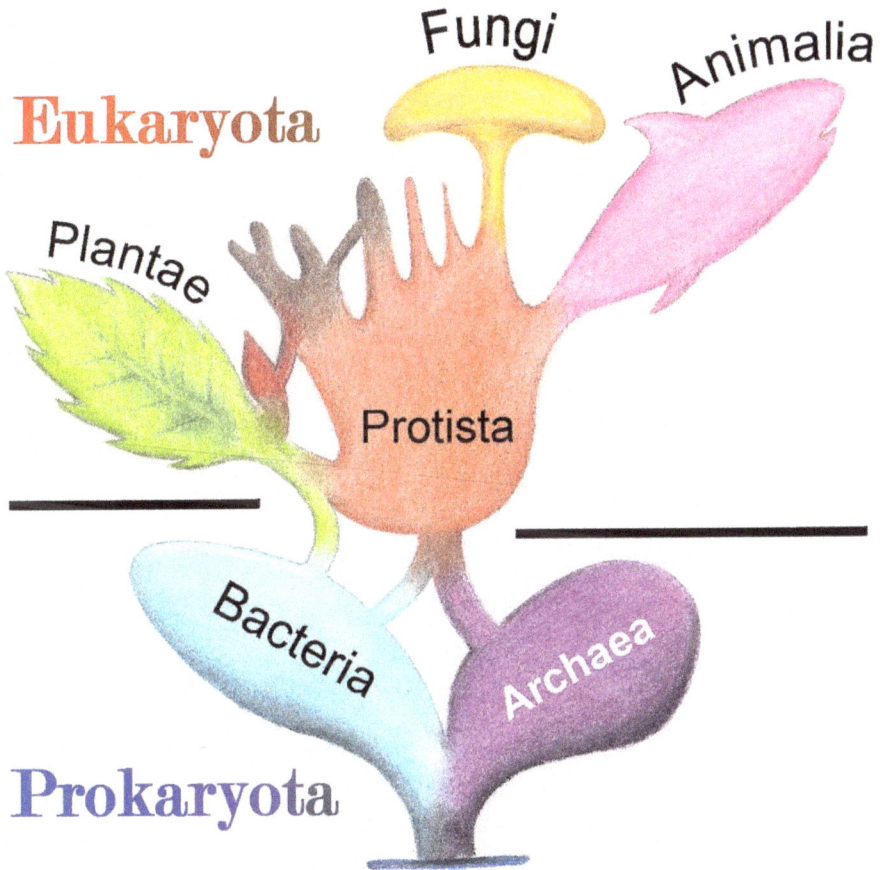

Maulucioni y Dorid Creative Commons License

Archaea

Phylogenetics was proposed in 1965 by Linus Pauling and Emile Zuckerlan using the sequences of the genes in organisms to determine how they are related to each other. Archaea were first classified as a separate group of prokaryotes in 1977 by Carl Woese and George E. Fox in phylogenetic trees based on the sequences of ribosomal ribonucleic acid (rRNA) genes. Archaea were first found in extreme environments, such as volcanic hot springs. The word *archaea* comes from the Ancient Greek ἀρχαῖα, meaning 'ancient things' as the first representatives of the domain Archaea were methanogens and it was assumed that their metabolism reflected Earth's primitive atmosphere and the

To 'Air' is Human

organism's antiquity. Archaea (singular *archaeon*) are prokaryote microorganisms, meaning that they have no cell nucleus or any other membrane-bound organelles in their cells. Archaeal cells have unique properties separating them from the other two domains of life: Bacteria and Eukaryota.

Archaea and bacteria are generally similar in size and shape, although a few Archaea have very strange shapes, such as flat and square-shaped cells. Despite a visual similarity to bacteria, Archaea possess genes and several metabolic pathways that are more closely related to those of eukaryotes. Archaea use more energy sources than eukaryotes. These range from organic compounds, such as sugars, ammonia, metal ions, hydrogen sulfide, elemental sulfur, and hydrogen gas. They can also utilize light without photosynthesis in a process known as photophosphorylation in salt-tolerant Archaea. Archaea reproduce asexually by binary fission, fragmentation, or budding.

Archaea were initially viewed as extremophiles living in extremely harsh environments, such as hot mineral springs, volcanic vents, salt lakes, and in glaciers. They have since been found in a broad range of habitats, including non-extreme environments such as soils, oceans, marshes, and the human colon and navel. Archaea are particularly plentiful in the oceans and in plankton. Archaea may play major roles in both the carbon and nitrogen cycles. There are no known examples of Archaea acting as pathogens or parasites. Archaea can also be commensals, benefiting from an association without helping or harming the other organism.

They are often found in the role of mutualism with a symbiotic benefit for both organisms. One example of mutualism are the methanogens found in the digestive tracts where they aid digestion. In anaerobic environments within ruminants and termites, cellulose is broken down by protozoans with the release of hydrogen gas. The Archaea methanogens reside within the protozoan and convert the hydrogen to methane within the protozoans organelle known as a hydrogenosome. Methanogens are also used in biogas production and sewage treatment. The heat stable enzymes from extremophile Archaea are used in biotechnology.

Archaea also associate with larger organisms such as corals, plant roots, and even in humans. For example, the methanogen *Methanobrevibacter smithii* comprises ten percent of the prokaryotes in the human gut flora. Archaea demonstrate a high level of horizontal gene transfer between species. The mitochondria which serve as the energy power source for human cells is thought to have originated as an independent organism that entered into a symbiotic relationship

Archaea are a relatively recent discovery that has revolutionized our understanding of the microbial world and in particular the human microbiome. One of the major advances in the understanding of microbial life has come about with the recent advances in genomics technology. This has been the discovery of extremophiles, organisms that can live in extreme environments and represented

To 'Air' is Human

a previously undiscovered form of life called Archaea. This has prompted a reevaluation of the biological system of taxonomy, the categorizing of life forms. Most scientists now recognize six separate kingdoms: Animals (Animalia), Plants (Plantae), Fungi, Bacteria, Protozoan (Protista), and Archaea.

Significant portions of the human micro biome are not bacteria at all and are actually Achaea. In fact the methane produced in flatus comes from the methanogenic Achaea of the colon's microbiome. Intense research activities are now being undertaken by the National Institute of health to identify and categorize the species and understand the activities of the flora in the Human Microbiome Project. There will undoubtedly be major advances in the understanding of human health and diseases as the micro biome is explored and understood.

Most people have not heard of the microorganisms called Archaea, which is a kingdom of single-celled microorganisms that have no cell nucleus or membrane-bound organelles within their cells. They were first discovered in extremely hot and acidic environments in which life was not thought possible to exist. It was like a science fiction story come to life that not only were organisms found to survive in this environment but also they were actually thriving in these extreme conditions. In the late 1970's, Dr. Carl Woese at the University of Illinois at Urbana Champaign used RNA sequences to determine how closely these newly discovered microbes were to other bacteria. He discovered that the prokaryotes were actually composed of two entirely different groups, the bacteria and a newly recognized group that he called Archaea. These three groups are now recognized as the three distinct domains of life.

Archaea and bacteria have a similar size and shape, which may have delayed their recognition as completely separate entities. Although a few Achaea have strange and unusual shapes, most look indistinguishable from bacteria by visual appearance. Their genetics and biochemistry are unique and there is no question but that they are an entirely different form of life. Archaea reproduce asexually by binary fission, fragmentation, or budding; unlike bacteria and eukaryotes, no known species form spores.

Initially, Achaea were thought to be limited to extremophiles having been found in geysers, deep ocean black smokers, and oil wells. Other extreme habitats included very cold art tic waters, and highly saline, acidic, or alkaline water. They have since been found in a wide variety of habitats including of soils, oceans, marshes, and the human colon and navel. Archaea are abundant in the oceans and may be active in both the carbon and the nitrogen cycle. They may represent up to twenty percent of the earths entire biomass.

Even acids with the extreme limit of a pH of zero were tolerable environments. Temperatures higher than that of boiling water which was thought to sterilize and kill al bacteria was comfortable for their reproduction. In fact they would survive in an environment as hostile as the planet Mars. Some scientists postulate that the first Achaea may have arrived on Earth on a meteorite and are actually extraterrestrial life that cane to earth from another planet or outside of our solar system. Science fiction could not be any more exciting than the actual science of studying Archaea.

There are no Archaea pathogens or parasites known, and they are often they are often commensals. One example of commensalism is the methanogens that inhabit the digestive tracts of humans and ruminants where they aid digestion. Methanogens are the primary source of the methane in the atmosphere and are major contributors to global warming. They are also used in biogas production and sewage treatment. The enzymes from extremophile Achaea can endure high temperatures and organic solvents and have contributed to major advances in biotechnology, environmental services, and the food service industry.

Extremophile Archaea are a source of enzymes that function under harsh conditions if temperature, salinity, acidity, or alkalinity. These enzymes have found many uses including research and industry. As an example amylases and galactosidases that function at over 100 °C (212 °F) may allow food processing at higher temperatures that usual. This may have commercial applications in the production of low lactose milk and whey. Archaea may also be hosts to new classes of antibiotics.

Extremophiles & Psychrophiles (Cryophiles)

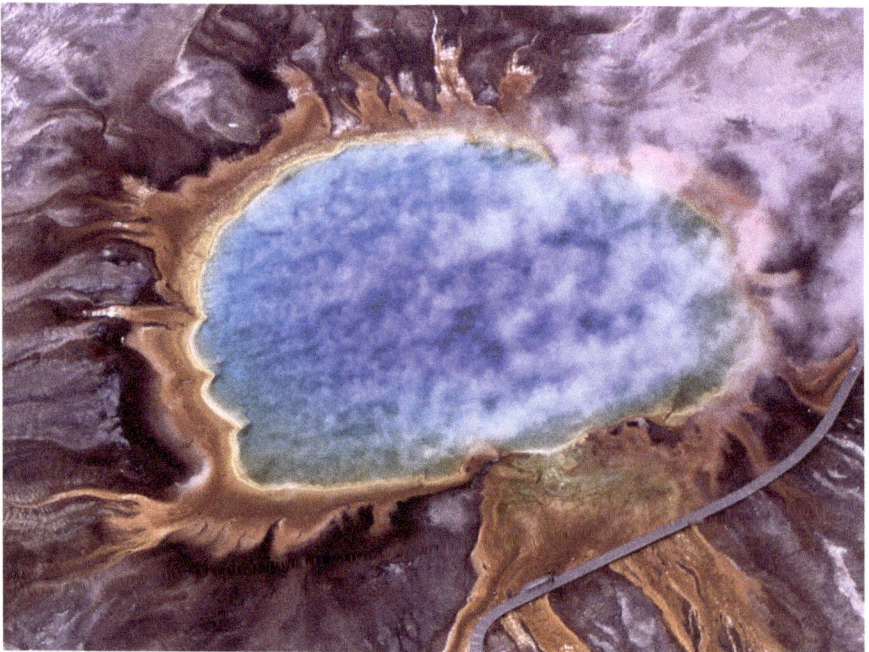

Grand Prismatic Mineral Hot Springs Yellowstone National Park. The striking coloration are from the extremophile Archaea that thrive in extreme environments that were previously thought to be incompatible with life. Creative Commons License

To 'Air' is Human

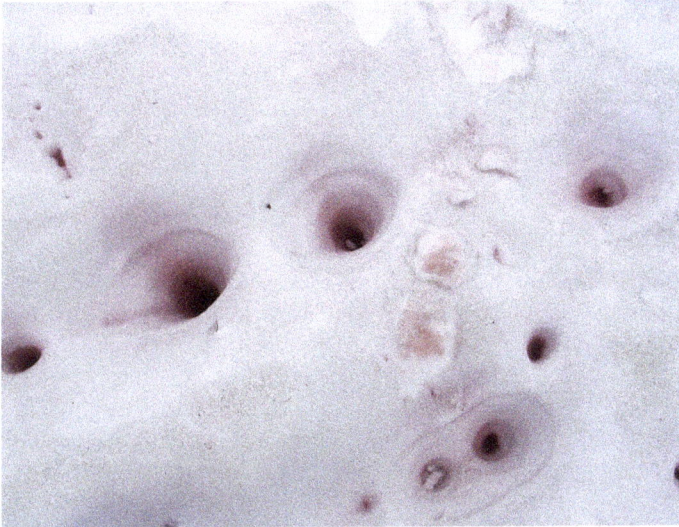

Unusual watermelon snow pits. 2206 Author Will Beback Creative Commons License

Psychrophiles also called cryophiles are extremophile organisms that are can successfully grow and reproduction in the cold temperature range from −15°C to +10°C. Temperatures as low as −15°C may be found in regions of high salinity water, known as brine, that is surrounded by sea ice. Thermophiles by contrast thrive at unusually hot temperatures. Psychrophiles are very adaptive and use a wide variety of metabolic pathways to survive. These include the processes of photosynthesis, chemoautotrophy (also known as lithotrophy), and heterotrophy. This adaptive strategy allows them to survive and thrive in diverse communities throughout the colder climate zones. They are found in diverse extreme environments including soil in alpine and arctic environments, deep ocean waters at very high latitudes, polar ice fields, glaciers, and snowfields.

They are of particular interest to astrobiology, the science of potential extraterrestrial life, and to geomicrobiology, the scientific study of microbes active in geochemical processes. In a research study at the University of Alaska Fairbanks a one thousand liter biogas digester using psychrophiles produces two hundred to three hundred liters of methane per day. Although it is only about twenty to thirty percent of the output from those in warmer climates, it is still a significant amount of biological activity in extreme cold climate zones. Most psychrophiles are either bacteria or Achaea present in widely diverse microbial lineages. Novel groups of psychrophilic fungi live in oxygen poor areas under alpine snowfields. Aristotle 384 BCE − 322 BCE wrote the first descriptive accounts of watermelon snow. It has puzzled mountain climbers, explorers, and naturalists for thousands of years.

The dramatic appearance of Watermelon snow, also called snow algae, red snow, or blood snow, is *Chlamydomonas nivalis* (Latin nivalis − snow), is the visible mark of the psychrophilic species of green algae. Compressing the snow by walking on it, or making snowballs, gives it a red color from a secondary red carotenoid pigment (astaxanthin), which it has in addition to chlorophyll. Psychrophiles have lipid cell membranes chemically resistant to the stiffening effect of extreme cold. They often create protein 'antifreezes' to maintain their intracellular space as liquid to protect their nuclear DNA in temperatures below the normal freezing point of water.

Methanogens

Methanogens are microorganisms of the Kingdom Archaea, not bacteria as previously thought. They produce methane as a metabolic byproduct in anaerobic conditions when oxygen is not present. Methanogens have been identified in a wide variety of extreme environments. Methanogens can thrive and reproduce in boiling water, as well as in ice cores taken miles down in arctic glaciers. They are common in wetlands, where they produce marsh gas, and in the digestive tracts of animals and humans where they generate the methane content of flatulence as well as the ruminant belch.

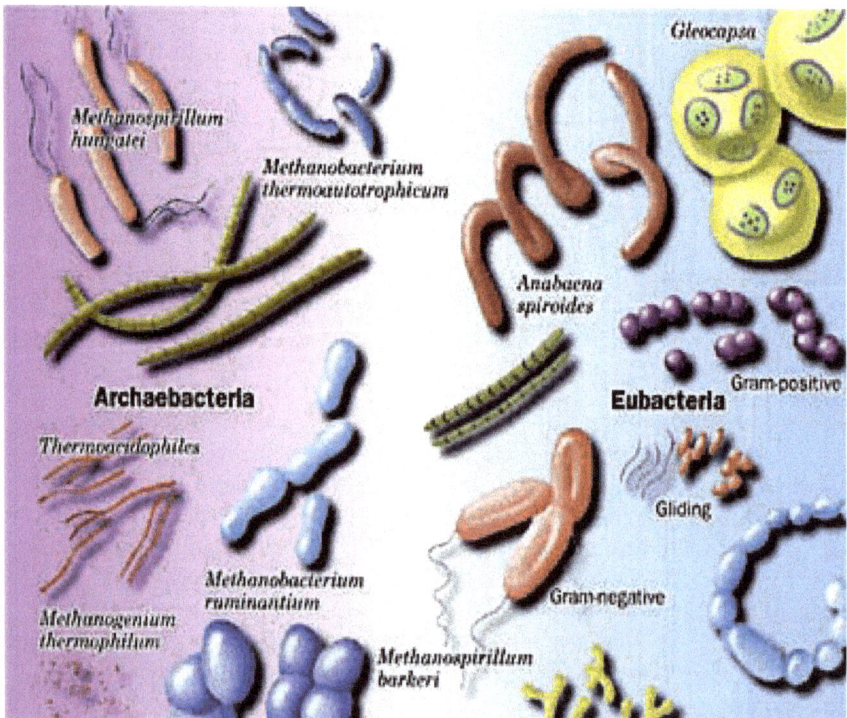

Most of the methanogenic bacteria are Archaea lawrencekok.blogspot.com Creative Commons License

Archaea are a relatively recent discovery that has revolutionized our understanding of the microbial world and in particular the human microbiome. One of the major advances in the understanding of microbial life has come about with the recent advances in genomics technology. This has been the discovery of extremophiles, organisms that can live in extreme environments and represented a previously undiscovered form of life called Archaea. This has prompted a reevaluation of the biological system of taxonomy, the categorizing of life forms. Most scientists now recognize six separate kingdoms: Animals (Animalia), Plants (Plantae), Fungi, Bacteria, Protozoan (Protista), and Archaea.

Significant portions of the human micro biome are not bacteria at all and are actually Achaea. In fact the methane produced in flatus comes from the methanogenic Achaea of the colon's micro biome. Intense research activities are now being undertaken by the National Institute of health to identify and categorize the species and understand the activities of the flora in the Human Microbiome Project. There will undoubtedly be major advances in the understanding of human health and diseases as the micro biome is explored and understood.

Most people have not heard of the microorganisms called Archaea, which is a kingdom of single-celled microorganisms that have no cell nucleus or membrane-bound organelles within their cells. They were first discovered in extremely hot and acidic environments in which life was not thought possible to exist. It was like a science fiction story come to life that not only were organisms found to survive in this environment but also they were actually thriving in these extreme conditions.

Bacteria

Bacteria (Greek bakterion rod) are categorized as a large kingdom of prokaryotic microorganisms. Typically just a few micrometers in length bacteria have a wide variety of shapes including, rods, spirals, and spheres. Bacteria were among the earliest forms of life to appear on Earth, and are ubiquitous. They inhabit soil, water, acidic hot springs, radioactive waste, and can reside deep within rocks miles underground in portions of Earth's crust. Bacteria also live inside of plants and animals and have survived in outer space during space flights. A gram of soil typically contains forty million bacterial cells and a single milliliter of fresh water may contain a million bacterial cells. There are approximately five nonillion, or to use a numerical version 5,000,000,000,000,000,000,000,000,000,000 (5×10 to the 30th power) bacteria on Earth. The enormous quantity of bacteria on Earth forms a total biomass that exceeds that of all plants and animals on the planet combined.

Bacteria are critical to life on Earth actively participating in many steps in the nutrient cycles that depend on these organisms, such as the fixation of nitrogen from the atmosphere. Most bacteria have yet to be identified and characterized. The science and study of bacteria is the field known as bacteriology, and is a branch of microbiology.

To 'Air' is Human

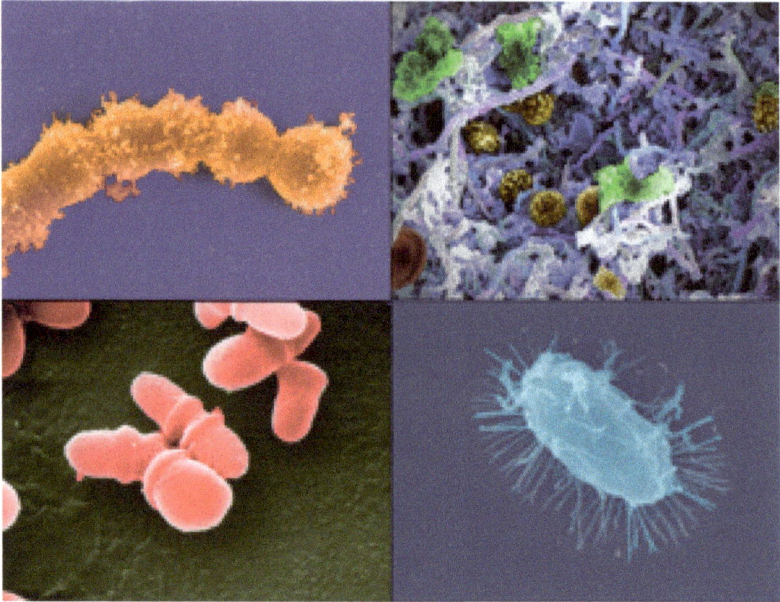

There are more than ten times as many bacterial cells in the human microbiome flora as there are human cells in the body. Very large numbers of bacteria are on the skin, and even more dramatic numbers are present as gut flora. The overwhelming majority of the bacteria in the body are commensals and do not cause disease. They are prevented from becoming pathogenic because of the protective effects of the immune system. Some bacteria are beneficial and engage in a symbiotic relationship with their human host.

Most people are not aware of the beneficial nature of the vast majority of bacteria. The recognition that several bacteria can be pathogenic and lead to disease and death has been well publicized. Several of the species of bacteria that are pathogenic and cause infectious diseases include cholera, syphilis, anthrax, leprosy, and bubonic plague. Many fatal bacterial diseases are respiratory infections, with tuberculosis alone killing about two million people a year. Antibiotics are utilized to treat bacterial infections, and are often also used in livestock farming. This has allowed antibiotic resistance to become increasingly common. In industry bacteria are important in sewage treatment, breakdown of oil spills, production of cheese and yogurt through fermentation. They have also been utilized in the mining industry in the recovery of gold, palladium, copper and other metals. Newer uses include biotechnology, the manufacture of antibiotics, and other proteins and chemicals.

Bacteria in the past were classified as plants in the class Schizomycetes. They are no longer considered members of the plant kingdom and at the present time bacteria are classified as prokaryotes. Prokaryotes are unlike the cells of animals and other eukaryotes. The cells of bacteria do not have a nucleus that contains the DNA based genetic information, and rarely have membrane bound organelles.

To 'Air' is Human

The term bacteria historically included all prokaryotes. About two decades ago a major scientific breakthrough occurred with the discovery that prokaryotes actually consist of two very different groups of organisms. They are presently classified as two distinct evolutionary kingdoms, Bacteria and Archaea. The prehistoric ancestors of both bacteria and Archaea were unicellular microorganisms that first appeared on Earth about four billion years ago. For about three billion years the dominant forms of life on Earth were microscopic bacteria and Archaea. Bacteria also played a major role in the evolutionary branching of eukaryotes from Archaea.

Eukaryotes developed from ancient bacteria physically entering the cells in an internally symbiotic association. This process, which began as the engulfment of symbiotic bacteria, progressed to the development of either mitochondria or hydrogenosomes. Some eukaryotes that already contained mitochondria that had previously developed from bacteria also engulfed cyanobacteria-like organisms. This symbiotic relationship developed into the formation of specialized chloroplasts in algae and plants.

Bacteria have a very wide diversity of shapes and sizes and are typically much smaller than eukaryotic cells. Most bacteria are between one half and five micrometers in length. The genus Mycoplasma has the smallest size of any bacteria, measuring only one third of a micrometer. They are so small that they are the same size as the largest viruses. Most bacterial species are either spherical cocci (Greek kókkos, grain) or rod shaped bacilli (Latin baculus stick). Elongation is commonly associated with motility. The bacteria called vibrio are rods with a slightly curved comma shape. Others bacteria called spirilla and spirochetes can be spiral shaped and tightly coiled. Several unusual species have a tetrahedral or cuboidal shape.

Recently discovered bacteria were identified deep under the Earth's crust. They grow as a branching filament with a star-shaped cross-section. These bacteria have a large surface area to volume ratio, which may be beneficial as these organisms exist in nutrient poor environments. A number of species of bacteria are found as single cells. Other species are often found in groups of multiple organisms that may associate in characteristic patterns. Neisseria organisms form pairs, Streptococcus organisms form chains, and Staphylococcus organisms group together in bunches and clusters that have the appearance of grapes. Less common species such as the genus Nocardia form complexes of branched filaments that have an appearance similar to that of fungal mycelia.

Bacteria frequently adhere to surfaces and may form a dense biofilm layer. These films may be as thin as just a few micrometers and may range up to thick bacterial mats up to half a meter in depth. These film layers and mats may contain a multitude of species of bacteria, protists, and Archaea. Many bacteria living in biofilms have a complex arrangement of both cells and extracellular components. These may form complex secondary structures comprising microcolonies with networks of channels to allow the diffusion of nutrients.

To 'Air' is Human

A lipid membrane known as a cell membrane or plasma membrane surrounds the bacterial cell. The cell membrane envelops and contains the contents of the cell. It acts as an environmental barrier and holds nutrients, proteins, and the other metabolically essential components of the cytoplasm within the cell. Bacteria, as prokaryotes, have few large intracellular structures and lack a true nucleus. They do not usually have membrane bound organelles in their cytoplasm such as mitochondria and chloroplasts that may be present in eukaryotic cells. Cyanobacteria may also produce gas within the cell, which forms into membrane bound vesicles. The gas vesicles may be used for locomotion by regulating their buoyancy. This allows the cell to move up or down in an aqueous environment, traveling to water layers with different light intensity and nutrient levels.

A special staining technique for the microscopic examination of bacteria was developed in 1884 by Hans Christian Gram. The Gram stain characterizes bacteria based on the structure of their cell walls. The thick layers of peptidoglycan and teichoic acids in the Gram-positive cell wall stain purple. The relatively thin Gram-negative cell wall consists of just a few layers of peptidoglycan. These layers are surrounded by a second lipid membrane containing lipoproteins and lipopolysaccharides appear pink. The endotoxin lipopolysaccharides are composed of lipid A and polysaccharides that contribute to the toxicity of Gram-negative bacteria.

A bacteria in which the cell wall has been entirely removed is called a protoplast. If the cell wall is partially removed it is called a spheroplast. ß-Lactam antibiotics, such as penicillin, interfere with the formation of peptidoglycan cross links disrupting the bacterial cell wall. The enzyme lysozyme, which is found in human tears, also disrupts and digests the cell wall of bacteria. This property of the tear lysozyme is the body's main defense against eye infections.

Swimming and motile bacteria frequently move between ten and one hundred body lengths per second. On a relative scale this makes them at least as fast as fish. Flagella are whip like rigid protein structures about twenty micrometers in length and twenty nanometers in diameter that are used for motility. Fimbriae are fine filaments of protein that are found all over the surface of the cell. They appear to be involved in the bacterial cell's ability to attach to solid surfaces or to other cells. The fimbriae are essential for the virulence of some pathogens. Pili are cellular appendages that are slightly larger than fimbriae and can transfer genetic material between bacterial cells in a process called conjugation in which they are called conjugation pili or sex pili.

Certain bacteria, such as Sporohalobacter, Clostridium, Heliobacterium, Anaerobacter, can form dormant structures that are highly resistant to destruction. These structures are called endospores and have a central cytoplasm core containing the DNA and ribosomes. They are surrounded by an impermeable and rigid protective coat. Endospores appear to be in a state of suspended animation and do not exhibit any signs of metabolic activity. They can survive extreme physical and chemical stresses that would kill metabolically active organisms. They have exhibited the ability to withstand high levels of UV light, gamma radiation, heat, freezing, detergents, disinfectants, pressure, desiccation, and outer space without any reduction in their pathogenicity. Endospores in this dormant state these organisms may remain viable for many millions of years. Viable spores that are over forty million years old have been identified that have maintained the ability to cause disease. Examples of disease caused by dormant spores include anthrax, which can be contracted by the inhalation of *Bacillus anthracis* endospores, and tetanus, which can be contracted by contamination of deep puncture wounds with *Clostridium tetani* endospores.

In unicellular organisms growth is manifested by increases in cell size until a fixed point where asexual reproduction by binary cell division takes place. Under ideal conditions bacteria can grow and undergo cell division very rapidly. Bacterial populations can double in size as quickly as every ten minutes. This exponential growth rate allows one cell to become 64 cells in one hour, 4,096 cells in two hours, 262,144 cells in three hours, 16,777,216 cells in four hours, over a billion cells in five hours, over four trillion cells in seven hours, etcetera. Certain infections can overwhelm and kill previously healthy humans and animals in a matter of just a few hours. The same power of exponential growth makes using microbes as miniature factories to produce biologic agents such as hormones, antibiotics, nutrients, etc. extremely attractive and efficient.

Bacteria are organisms that grow and multiply quickly. This feature, along with the relative ease to manipulate their DNA content, has made bacteria a model for many studies of genetics, molecular biology, and biochemistry. By creating a mutation in the DNA of bacteria a specific gene can be inactivated. By examining the effect of gene mutations, the function of genes, enzymes and metabolic pathways in bacteria can be identified. As many genes have identical functions in different organism the knowledge gained in experiments on bacteria can often be applied to more complex organisms such as humans. The scientific understanding of bacterial genes and metabolism has allowed the use of biotechnology to be commercialized. Bacteria can be bioengineered to produce a variety of therapeutic proteins, such as insulin, growth hormone, enzymes, antibodies, and other vital products.

Certain bacteria form close associations that are essential for their survival. One such mutualistic association occurs between anaerobic bacteria that metabolize a variety of organic acids. When organic acids such as butyric acid or propionic acid are metabolized hydrogen is produced as a byproduct. Increasing concentrations of hydrogen would be detrimental to the survival of these bacteria. In an association with mutual benefits methanogenic Archaea consume the hydrogen and allow the bacteria to thrive. The rhizosphere is the zone of soil that includes the root surface and soil that adheres to the root after gentle shaking. This zone contains a multitude of microorganisms that may carry out nitrogen fixation converting nitrogen gas to nitrogenous compounds. This provides an easily absorbable form of nitrogen for many plants, which cannot absorb and fix nitrogen from the atmosphere themselves.

There are many bacteria that have developed a symbiotic relationship with other organisms, including humans. In the human gastrointestinal tract, the gut flora also known as the microbiome, is predominantly beneficial organisms. There are over one thousand different species of bacteria in the normal human gut flora of the intestines. The organisms of the normal gut flora may contribute to gut immunity, synthesize vitamins such as vitamin K, folic acid, and biotin, convert sugars to lactic acid (Lactobacillus), as well as ferment complex indigestible carbohydrates. The presence of the normal gut flora inhibits potentially pathogenic bacteria from becoming established by the process of competitive exclusion. Supplements of beneficial bacteria may be provided as probiotic dietary supplements.

Pathogenic bacteria are the cause of a number of human diseases that may lead to illness and death and cause infections such as diphtheria, tetanus, syphilis, typhoid fever, leprosy, tuberculosis, cholera, and foodborne illness. A number of known medical diseases were discovered to be caused by pathogenic bacteria many decades or centuries after the disease was first described. A recent example was the discovery that peptic ulcer disease, long thought to be caused by excess gastric acidity, was actually caused by the pathogenic organism *Helicobacter pylori*. Bacterial diseases are also have a major impact on agriculture with bacteria causing fire blight, leaf spot, and wilts in plants, as well as mastitis, anthrax, Johne disease, and salmonella and in farm animals.

A number of species may exist in small numbers within the normal gut flora and microbiome. They become pathogenic and cause disease with a characteristic pattern of signs and symptoms when their numbers increase substantially. Some organisms can cause a variety of signs and symptoms dependent on the location of the infection. For example, Staphylococcus or Streptococcus can cause skin infections, pneumonia, meningitis and even overwhelming sepsis. Sepsis is a systemic inflammatory response that can lead to vascular collapse and death. At the same time, in smaller numbers, these organisms are part of the normal human microbiome that is present on the skin or in the nose without causing any illness.

Microorganisms have been utilized by humans for thousands of years in food production and preparation. Lactic acid is a metabolic byproduct of bacteria such as Lactobacillus and Lactococcus. These bacteria have been used for this property in combination with yeasts and molds in the preparation of fermented foods such as sauerkraut, cheese, soy sauce, pickles, wine, yogurt, and vinegar.

Antonie van Leeuwenhoek, a Dutch lens maker, was first to observe bacteria using a microscope he designed in 1683. His scientific observations were published in a series of reports to the Royal Society of London. Scientists were fascinated by his description of animalcules in human semen and pond water. Identification and study of bacteria did not begin until over a century had passed. Christian Gottfried Ehrenberg has been credited with being the scientist who introduced the word "bacterium" in 1828.

Louis Pasteur demonstrated in 1859 that the theory of spontaneous generation was incorrect. He also demonstrated that the fermentation process is caused by the growth of microorganisms, yeasts, and molds. Along with Robert Koch, Pasteur was an early advocate of the germ theory of disease. Koch was a scientific pioneer in the medical application of microbiology, and investigated the infectious causes of cholera, anthrax, tuberculosis and other life threatening conditions. Koch's research into the cause of tuberculosis proved that the germ theory was correct, for which he received Nobel Prize in 1905. Koch's postulates remain important scientific criteria to this day to prove that a specific organism is the cause of a disease.

By the nineteenth century, bacteria were known to be the cause of many diseases. Unfortunately, treatments for infections with antibiotics had yet to be developed, although there were some reports that moldy foods might be helpful. In 1910 Paul Ehrlich developed the first effective antibiotic by studying and modifying dyes that selectively stained the organism *Treponema pallidum*. This is the spirochete bacteria that causes syphilis, and a dye compound Ehrlich developed selectively killed the pathogen. Ehrlich received the 1908 Nobel Prize for his work on immunology and the use of various stains to identify bacteria.

Fungi

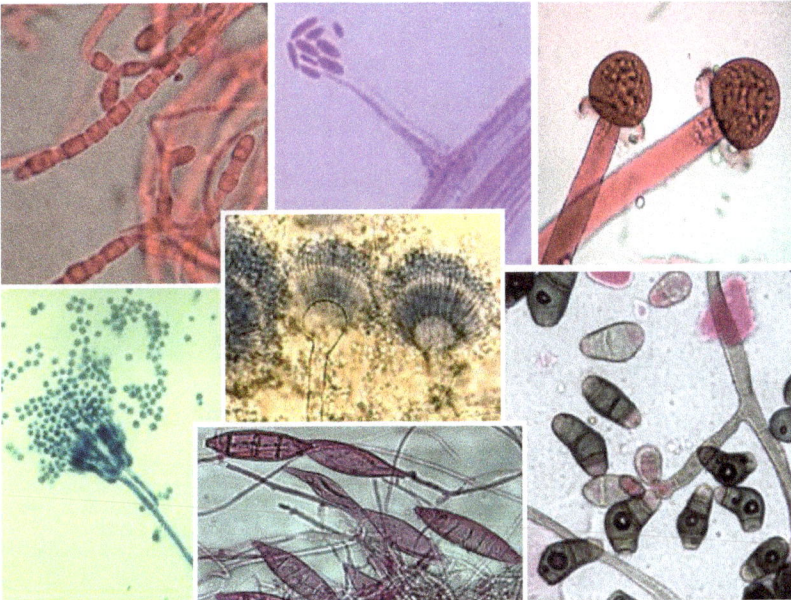

Collage of fungi. Public Health England

Fungi are eukaryotes and include yeasts, mold, mushrooms. Their cell walls contain chitin, not cellulose. The science of fungi is called mycology and was once considered a subsection of botany. Genetic studies have revealed that fungi are actually more closely related to animals than plants.

Parasite

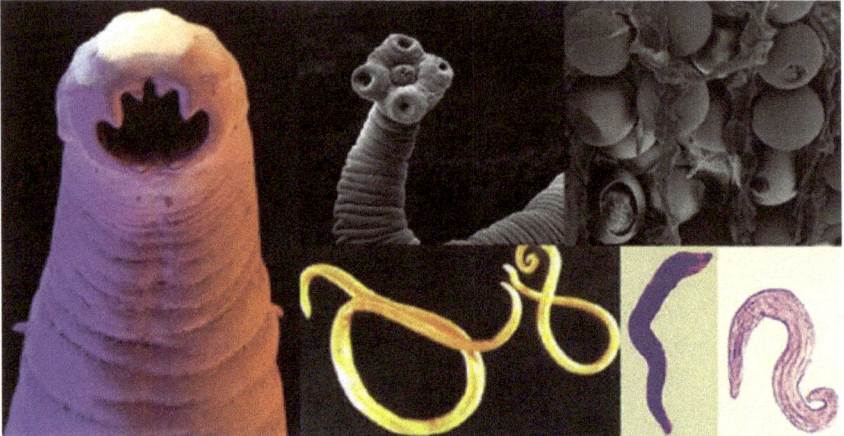

A variety of human parasites. Creative Commons License

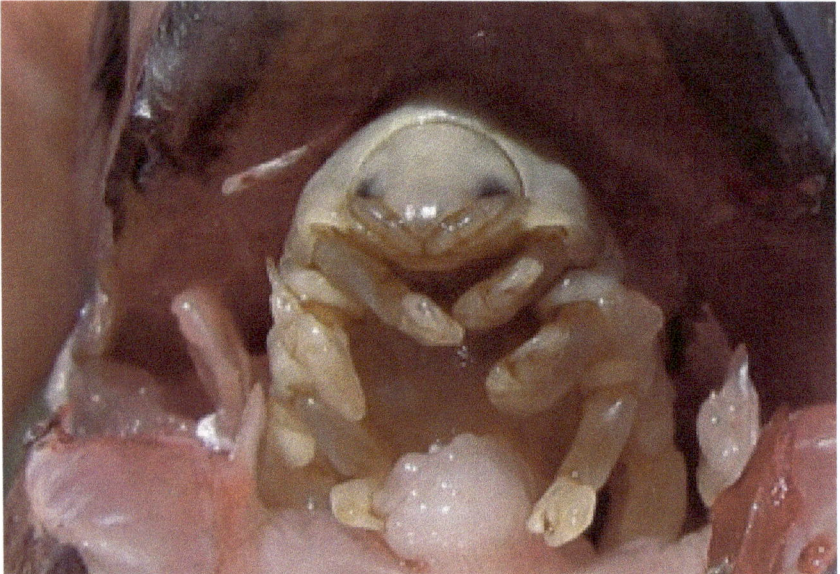

Fortunately for humans this nasty parasite is only found in fish. It eats the tongue of the fish and stays in its mouth ready to eat anything the fish consumes. Creative Commons License

Prion

Prions are fundamentally different than virus and contain and transmit infectious protein molecules that do not contain DNA or RNA. They can cause infections such as scrapie in sheep, bovine spongiform encephalopathy also known as mad cow disease in cattle, and chronic wasting disease in deer. In humans prion diseases include Kuru, which is acquired by cannibals eating the brain of a human infected with the virus. Other prion disease in humans includes Creutzfeldt–Jakob disease, and Gerstmann–Sträussler–Scheinker syndrome.

A prion is an infectious agent composed of protein in a misfolded form. The word prion was coined in 1982 by 1997 Nobel laureate Stanley B. Prusiner and is derived from the words protein and infection. Prions are responsible for the transmissible spongiform encephalopathies in a variety of mammals, including bovine spongiform encephalopathy also known as "mad cow disease". In humans, prions cause Creutzfeldt-Jakob Disease (CJD), Fatal Familial Insomnia, and kuru. All known prion diseases affect the structure of the brain or other neural tissue and all are currently untreatable and universally fatal.

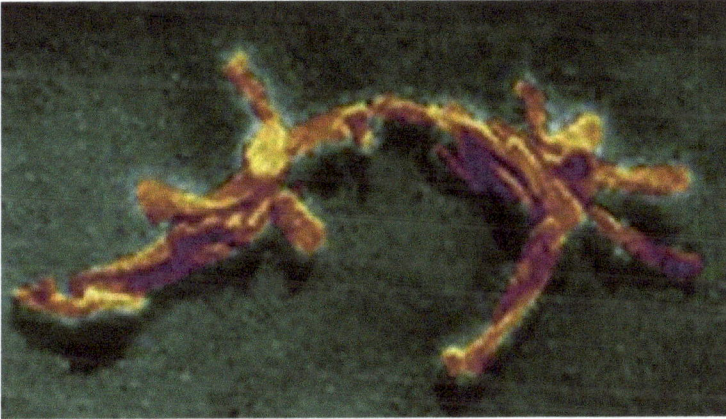

c0116801.cdn.cloudfiles.rackspacecloud.com Creative Commons License

Prions cause neurodegenerative disease by aggregating extracellularly within the central nervous system to form plaques known as amyloid, which disrupt the normal tissue structure. This disruption is characterized by "holes" in the tissue with resultant spongy architecture due to the vacuole formation in the neurons. Other histological changes include astrogliosis and the absence of an inflammatory reaction. While the incubation period for prion diseases is relatively long (5 to 20 years), once symptoms appear the disease progresses rapidly, leading to brain damage and death. Neurodegenerative symptoms can include convulsions, dementia, ataxia (balance and coordination dysfunction), and behavioral or personality changes. All known prion diseases, collectively called transmissible spongiform encephalopathies (TSEs), are untreatable and fatal.

Current research suggests that the primary method of infection in animals is through ingestion. It is thought that prions may be deposited in the environment through the remains of dead animals and via urine, saliva, and other body fluids. They may then linger in the soil by binding to clay and other minerals. A University of California research team led by Stanley Prusiner, has provided evidence for the theory that infection can occur from prions in manure. And since manure is present in many areas surrounding water reservoirs, as well as used on many crop fields, it raises the possibility of widespread transmission. Preliminary evidence supporting the notion that prions can be transmitted through use of urine-derived human menopausal gonadotropin, administered for the treatment of infertility, was published in 2011.

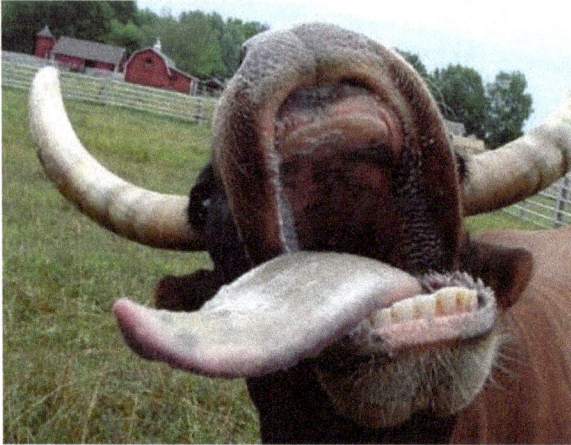

malialitman.files.wordpress.com Creative Commons License

Mad cow disease

Bovine spongiform encephalopathy, or mad cow disease, appears to cause a fatal human brain disease.

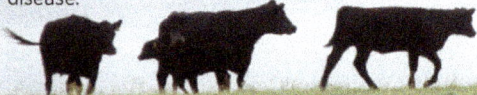

• **Severity** Cow begins "mad" seizures months or years after infection

• **Other livestock** Related disease called scrapie affects sheep

• **Prevention** Destroy infected farm animals; don't use animal products containing brain or central nervous system tissue as livestock feed

How it spreads

1 Person or animal eats food contaminated with brain or spinal cord tissue from infected animal

2 Disease attacks nervous system

Outer layer of brain develops tiny holes, looks spongy

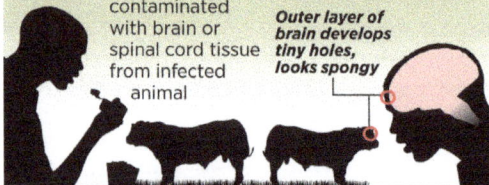

SOURCES: U.S. Centers for Disease Control and Prevention, U.S. Agriculture Department, MCT Photo Service

Creative Commons License

One of the recent illnesses identified as being caused by prions is mad cow disease also known as bovine spongiform encephalopathy. It is a fatal

To 'Air' is Human

neurodegenerative disease in cattle that causes an encephalopathy characterized by a spongy degeneration of the brain and spinal cord. Bovine spongiform encephalopathy has a long incubation period from about 30 months to 8 years. It usually affects adult cattle at a peak age of onset of four to five years with all breeds being equally susceptible. In the United Kingdom, the country worst affected, more than 180,000 cattle have been infected and 4.4 million slaughtered during the eradication program. The disease may be transmitted to human beings by eating food contaminated with the brain, spinal cord or digestive tract of infected cattle. In humans it is known as new variant Creutzfeldt–Jakob disease and by 2010 had killed more than 200 humans. Up to 500,000 bovine spongiform encephalopathy infected animals had entered the human food chain before controls on high-risk offal were introduced in 1989.

The epizootic condition was caused by feeding cattle the remains of other cattle in the form of meat and bone meal, which caused the infectious agent to spread. The infectious agent is remarkable for the high temperatures at which it remains viable, over 600 degrees Celsius (about 1100 degrees Fahrenheit). The infectious agent in bovine spongiform encephalopathy is a specific type of misfolded protein called a prion. Prions are not destroyed even if the beef or material containing them is cooked or heat-treated. Prion proteins carry the disease between individuals and cause deterioration of the brain.

Transmission can occur when healthy animals come in contact with contaminated tissues from others with the disease. In the brain, these proteins cause native cellular prion protein to deform into the infectious state, which then goes on to deform further prion protein in an exponential cascade. This results in protein aggregates, which then form dense plaque fibers, leading to the microscopic appearance of "holes" in the brain, degeneration of physical and mental abilities, and ultimately death. Cattle are naturally herbivores eating grass in pastures. Modern industrial and commercial cattle farming use various feeds are which may contain additional ingredients and supplements including antibiotics, hormones, pesticides, fertilizers, and protein additives. Meat and bone meal from the leftovers of the slaughtering process as well as from the carcasses of sick and injured cattle or sheep was often used as a protein supplement in cattle feed in Europe prior to about 1987.

In order to control potential transmission of bovine spongiform encephalopathy related variant Creutzfeldt–Jakob disease within the United States the American Red Cross has established strict restrictions on individuals' eligibility to donate blood. Because of the very long incubation period individuals who have spent a cumulative time of 3 months or more in the United Kingdom between 1980 and 1996, or a cumulative time of 5 years or more from 1980 to present in any combination of countries in Europe, are prohibited from donating blood.

Cows affected by bovine spongiform encephalopathy show progressively deteriorating behavioral and neurological signs. One notable sign is an increase in aggression with cattle reacting excessively to noise or touch. With time the cattle become ataxic and may also develop a drop in milk production, anorexia and lethargy. At the slaughterhouse in the United Kingdom the brain, spinal cord, trigeminal ganglia, intestines, eyes and tonsils from cattle are classified as specified risk materials and must be disposed of appropriately without entering the human food chain.

In the US regulations prohibited the feeding of mammalian byproducts to ruminants such as cattle and goats since 1997. However byproducts of ruminants can still be legally fed to pets or other livestock, including pigs and poultry, such as chickens. The US Department of Agriculture (USDA) has recalled of beef supplies that involved the introduction of sick and dying downer cows into the food supply. Because the US standards and testing requirements are less rigorous than believed necessary to combat bovine spongiform encephalopathy many countries are hesitant to import its meat products. Sixty-five nations implemented full or partial restrictions on importing U.S. beef products. Beef consumption in the US was also affected by public concerns about food safety.

Protist

The protist are a eukaryotic microorganism that may be unicellular or multicellular and includes protozoa and amoeba.. A number of these organisms may be pathogenic to humans such as chlamydia, trichomonas, and giardia. The majority are considered commensals in that they do not harm nor do they provide benefit.

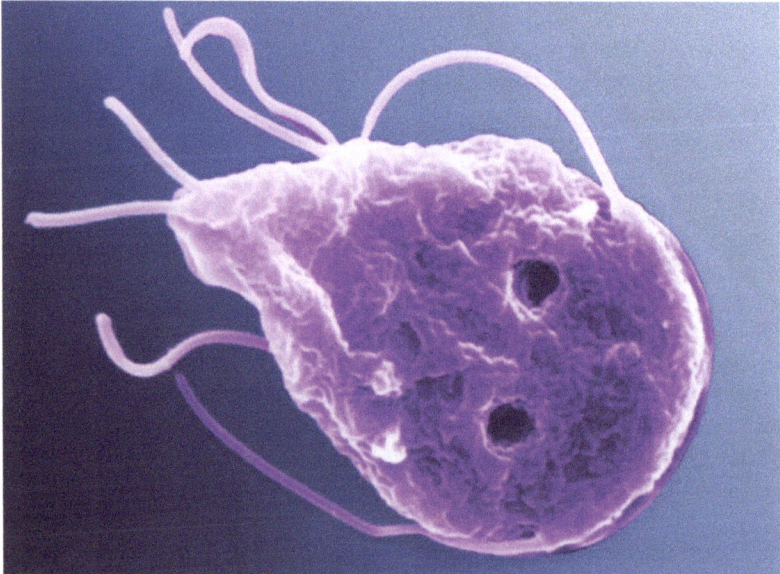

http://wellcomeimages.org/indexplus/obf_images/99/db/d408763f6cfcd8e0cc232c74db20.jpg
Giardia lamblia Creative Commons License

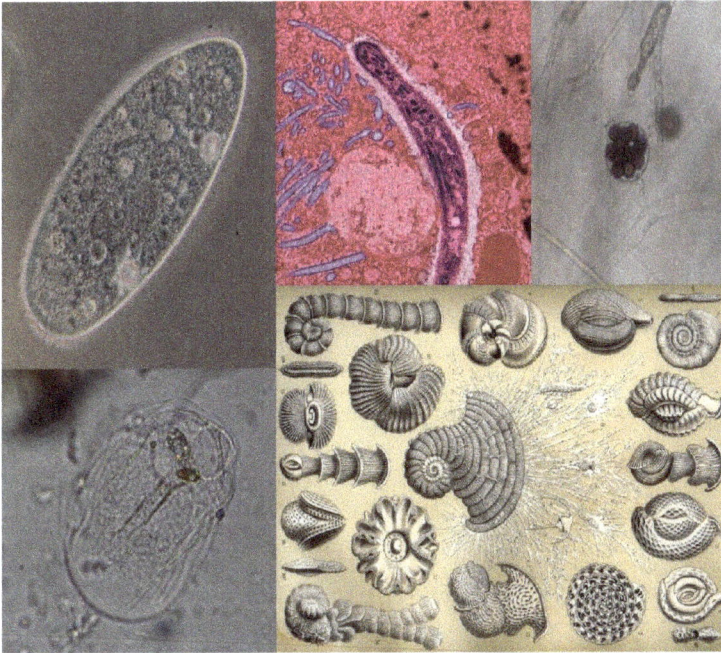

柑橘類 • Creative Commons License Protist collage

Virus

Virus (Latin virulentus poisonous) is a term that originally referred to poison and other noxious substances and was named by their discoverer Dmitri Ivanovsky in 1892. He mistakenly thought the illness transmitted from fluid filtered free of bacteria was a poisonous substance that the bacteria released. He did not realize that it was actually a living infectious agent much smaller than the bacteria that could not pass by the filter. Louis Pasteur was unsuccessful in his attempt to identify a bacterial cause for rabies. He speculated that the rabies pathogen may be too small to be seen using a microscope. In 1898 the Dutch microbiologist Martinus Beijerinck recognized that it was a new form of infectious agent but mistakenly thought that a virus was a liquid.

There is some controversy as to whether viruses should be considered a form of life, or nonliving organic structures that interact with living organisms. Some experts have described them as 'organisms at the edge of life' since they resemble organisms in that they possess genes, they evolve by the process of natural selection, and reproduce by creating multiple copies of their genetic code. Viruses have genes but they do not have the cellular structure that many define as the basic unit of life. Viruses do not have an independent metabolism and must invade a host cell to make new products and replicate. There are more viruses on Earth than stars in the universe. If you stacked every virus end to end they would stretch over one hundred thousand light years.

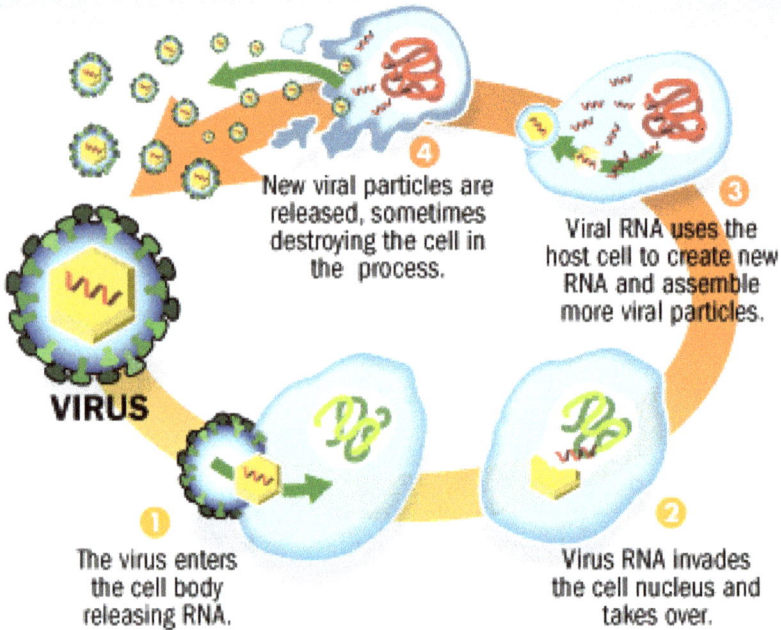

How a Virus Works ©2010 HowStuffWorks

4 New viral particles are released, sometimes destroying the cell in the process.

3 Viral RNA uses the host cell to create new RNA and assemble more viral particles.

VIRUS

1 The virus enters the cell body releasing RNA.

2 Virus RNA invades the cell nucleus and takes over.

Creative Commons License

A virion is a complete virus particle. It consists of the genetic material in the form of a nucleic acid that is enveloped by a protein protective coat called a capsid. The capsid is formed from the assembly of identical protein subunits, each of which is called a capsomere. Some viruses have a protective lipid envelope that was derived from the host cell membrane. The capsid is made from proteins, the nature of which are determined by the viral genome. The shape of the virion serves as the characteristic basis for the morphological distinction and classification of viruses. The shape can range from a simple helical structure to more complex structures such as an icosahedral forms. The average virus is only about one percent of the size of the average bacterium. Most viruses are so small that they cannot be seen directly with a standard optical microscope.

A very wide diversity of genomic structures can be seen among viral species. Viruses exhibit more genomic and structural diversity than bacteria, plants, Archaea, or animals. There are many millions of different types of viruses, yet to date only about five thousand have been described in detail. A virus may have either a DNA based or a RNA based genome, and is called a DNA virus or an RNA virus on this important distinction. The majority of viruses have RNA based genomes.

Viruses are the most numerous living organisms on Earth and they outnumber all of the other life forms combined. Viruses can infect all types of cellular life including plants, animals, fungi, and bacteria. Each specific type of viruses can infect only a limited range of hosts, and a number of viruses are species-specific. For example, the smallpox virus can infect only humans and it is therefore described as having a narrow host range. Other viruses that are described as having a broad range include the rabies virus, which can infect different species of mammals. The viruses that infect plants are nearly always harmless to animals. Most viruses that infect other animals are not pathogenic to humans.

Viruses may spread in a wide variety of ways including blood sucking insects and animals. When these animals or insects serve to transmit the disease bearing organisms they are known as vectors. Influenza viruses are spread through the aerosolization of the virions by coughing and sneezing. Norovirus and rotavirus are two of the most common causes of viral gastroenteritis and are transmitted by the fecal oral route. They are transmitted by direct contact or by entering the body through contaminated food or water.

A bacteriophage (Greek φαγεῖν*phagein* phage devour) is a virus that infects and replicates within bacteria. Bacteriophages consist of various proteins that envelope and encapsulate a DNA or RNA genome. The bacteriophage may have a relatively simple or an elaborate structure. The bacteriophage genome may be small and encode as few as four genes, or it may be very large and contain hundreds of genes. The bacteriophage genetic material is injected into the cytoplasm and replicates within the bacteria cell.

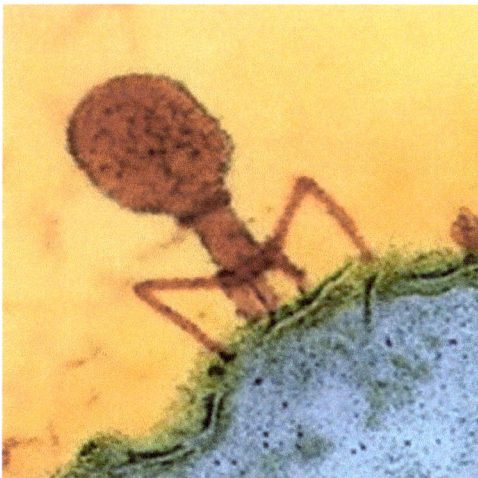

dennehylab.bio.qc.cuny.edu Creative Commons License

Bacteriophages are distributed widely and found in virtually all environments that harbor bacteria, such as soil or the gastrointestinal tracts of humans and animals. Seawater has one of the highest concentrations of bacteriophages in a natural nonliving environments. Bacteriophages and other viruses have a density in seawater of up to 9×10^8 virions per milliliter. These concentrations have been found in seawater microbial mats at the ocean surface. Up to seventy percent of marine bacteria may be infected by bacteriophages. Bacteriophages have also been used for over ninety years in the treatment of bacterial infections as an alternative to antibiotics in Russia, Central Europe, and France. Bacteriophages may have a role as a possible antimicrobial therapy against strains of bacteria that have developed resistance to many antibiotics.

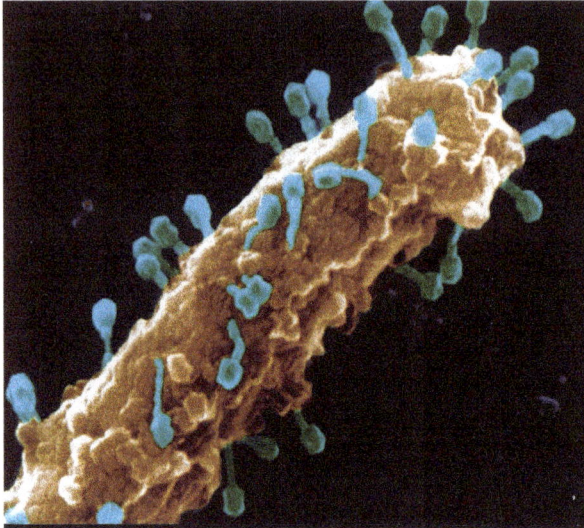

Swarm of bacteriophages attacking a bacterium rafefurst.files.wordpress.com Creative Commons License

Drinking the waters of various rivers as an effective treatment to cure infectious diseases has been documented since ancient times. In 1896, Ernest Hanbury Hankin reported that drinking the waters of the Ganges and Yamuna rivers in India could be effective in the treatment of cholera. The antibacterial action of the river water against cholera remained even if the water was passed through a very fine porcelain filter.

The antibacterial action was transmitted via the presence of microscopic viral bacteriophages in the river water. The discovery of the nature of viruses and their genetic structure and replication resulted in scientists Max Delbrück, Alfred Hershey and Salvador Luria being awarded the Nobel Prize in Physiology and Medicine in 1969. Bacteriophages are a very common and remarkably diverse group of viruses. In aquatic environments, they are the most abundant form of biological life comprising ninety percent of the biomass in the sea. In seawater they outnumber bacteria and Archaea by more than fifteen to one, reaching levels of two hundred and fifty million bacteriophages per milliliter of seawater. Most of the bacteriophages are harmless to plants and animals, yet are essential to the regulation of saltwater and freshwater ecosystems. It is estimated that viruses kill approximately twenty percent of the aquatic biomass each day.

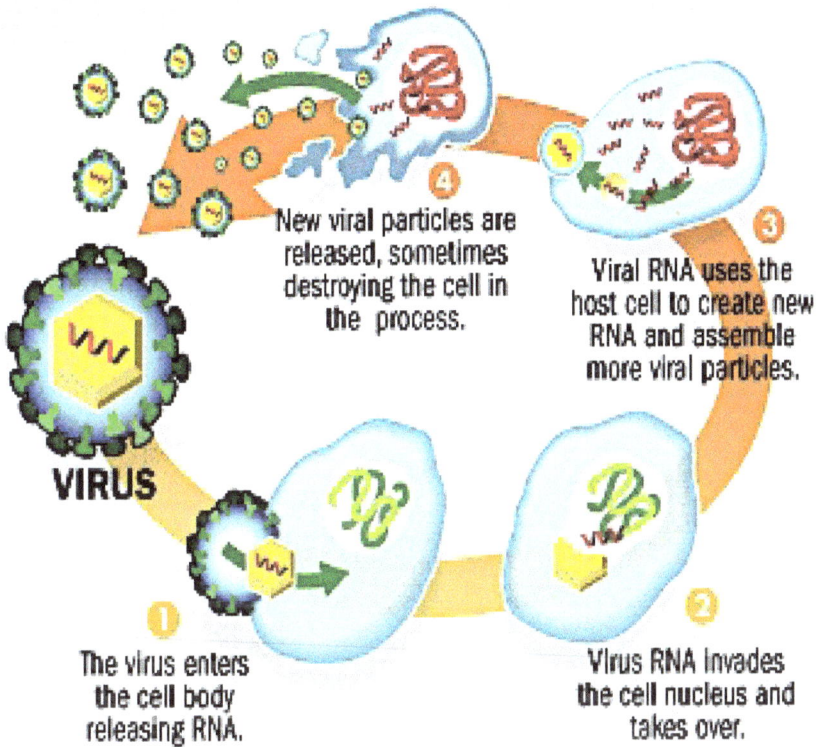

New viral particles are released, sometimes destroying the cell in the process.

Viral RNA uses the host cell to create new RNA and assemble more viral particles.

VIRUS

The virus enters the cell body releasing RNA.

Virus RNA invades the cell nucleus and takes over.

static.ddmcdn.com Creative Commons License

The bacteriophage viruses infect specific bacteria by binding to surface receptor molecules on the surface of the bacteria and then entering the cell. Within a short amount of time, often measured in minutes, bacterial polymerase starts translating viral mRNA into protein. These proteins may be new virions within the cell, helper proteins that assist in the production and assembly of new virions, or proteins involved in cell lysis. Viral enzymes may aid in the breakdown of the cell membrane. In the case of the T4 phage, overtaking the bacterial cell and producing and releasing over three hundred new virion phages could take place in less than twenty minutes from the time of infection.

Human immunodeficiency virus (HIV) is one of several viruses that may be transmitted via several bodily fluids, including through sexual contact and by exposure to infected blood. Antibiotics are not effective in the treatment of conditions caused by a virus viruses, but several antiviral drugs have been developed. Several examples of common human diseases caused by viruses include chickenpox, the common cold, and cold sores. And influenza. Viruses cause many serious diseases such as Ebola, AIDS, avian influenza, and SARS. The term virulence is used to describe the relative ability of viruses to cause disease. Some viruses can lead to chronic and even lifelong infections.

In chronic infections the virus is able to continue to survive and replicate in spite of the host defense mechanisms. This is seen commonly in untreated hepatitis B virus and hepatitis C virus infections. People chronically infected are known as carriers, and they can serve as an infectious reservoir for the virus to infect others. In populations where the proportion of the population that are carriers is high, the disease is said to be endemic.

Epidemiology is the area of science that deals with the study of health and disease in specific populations. Study of the transmission of viral infections in humans has demonstrated two different general categories. In the category of vertical transmission the virus is transferred from mother to child such as via the placenta or through breast milk. In horizontal transmission the virus is transmitted from person to person. An example of the vertical transmission of a virus occurs with the hepatitis B virus and HIV. With vertical transmission occurring in utero the baby has already been infected by the virus before it is born.

The most common form of the transmission of viruses in a given population is by means of horizontal transmission. Horizontal transmission can occur with the exchange of bodily fluids during sexual activity, blood transfusion, needle sharing, saliva from the mouth, etc. Horizontal transmission may also occur via contaminated food or water, aerosolized virions being inhaled, insect vectors such as mosquitoes, etc.

The incubation period, between the introduction of the virus to host and the first signs and symptoms of illness. Incubation periods are often of a characteristic duration for different viral diseases, and may range from a few days to weeks. The communicability period is the time when the infection can be passed from an infected individual or animal to another noninfected human or animal. It is during the communicability period that the illness is considered contagious. The knowledge of the length of time of both the incubation and communicability periods of specific viral infections is important in the control of outbreaks. An outbreak is described as an epidemic when there is an unusually high proportion of cases in a specific region, population, or community. A pandemic is the term used when the epidemic outbreaks occur on a worldwide basis.

Isolated populations that have not developed immunity to viruses can be decimated by epidemics. Among examples historically documented are the Native American populations that were devastated by contagious diseases. Smallpox was one of the infections brought to the Americas by European colonists that was particularly virulent in the native populations. The precise number of how many Native Americans were killed by infectious diseases after the arrival of Columbus in the Americas is not known, but numbered in the hundreds of thousands. It has been estimated that close to seventy percent of the indigenous population was destroyed. The decimation of the native population by diseases to which they had no natural immunity played a major role in the successful European colonization of native lands.

The catastrophic 1918 influenza pandemic lasted until 1919 and was caused by an extremely virulent and deadly influenza A virus. Unlike most influenza outbreaks that target the ill and elderly, most of the victims were healthy young adults. The influenza pandemic of 1918 may have killed as many as one hundred million people comprising five percent of the world's population at the time. The human immunodeficiency virus (HIV) is believed to have originated in primates in sub-Saharan Africa during the 20th century. HIV is a pandemic viral infection with approximately forty million people now living with the chronic disease worldwide. The United Nations and the World Health Organization (WHO) estimate that HIV has killed more than twenty five million people since it was first recognized in 1981. It has become one of the most devastating epidemics in recorded history, but has also led to research and therapeutic breakthroughs in the management of viral diseases.

Viruses are a known cause of cancer in humans and other species. Viral cancers can arise from both RNA and DNA viruses and occur in only a minority of infected persons (or animals). The risk of developing cancer is influenced by a number of factors including host immunity and genetic mutations. Viruses that are known to cause human cancers include several genotypes of the human papillomavirus, human T-lymphotropic virus, Epstein-Barr virus, hepatitis B virus, Kaposi's sarcoma-associated herpes virus, and the hepatitis C virus.

When the host immune system encounters a virus, it produces specific antibodies that bind to and inactivate the virus, making it non-infectious. This process is known as humoral immunity and is dependent two important classes of antibodies. The first class of antibodies are known as immunoglobulin M (IgM) and are effective at neutralizing viruses. Immunoglobulin M is produced by the cells of the immune system for only the first few weeks of an infection. The second class of antibody is called immunoglobulin G (IgG) and its production can be maintained as long as necessary. The presence of IgM antibody in the blood of the host indicates a recent acute infection, whereas IgG antibody indicates the infection occurred sometime in the past.

The host immune system second line of defense of is known as cell-mediated immunity and involves immune cells known as T cells. The host cells of the body display self-markers consisting of short fragments of their proteins on the cell surface that identify the cells as belonging to the host. A host cell infected with a virus may also display the foreign protein from the infecting virus, which may act as an antigen to stimulate the immune response and identify the cell as being infected. The immune system T cell mediated response recognizes the foreign viral fragment on the surface of the infected host cell. As the cell has been recognized as infected it is destroyed by killer T cells. The T-cells that identify the host cells as being infected by the specific virus proliferate and intensify the immune response to the virus. Macrophages are immune cells that are specialized at antigen recognition.

Interferon production is an important component of the host defense mechanism. Interferon stops viral reproduction by killing the infected cell and its close neighbors. Human immunodeficiency virus (HIV) is often able to successfully evade the immune system by frequently altering the sequence of the amino acid components of the proteins on the virion surface. With the antigenic markers on the cell surface changing regularly, the antibodies the body produced for earlier versions of the antigen are no longer effective.

Because viruses use the host cell metabolic pathways to replicate, drugs toxic to the pathway of viral replication are often toxic to all host cells as well. The most effective approach to controlling viral diseases are utilizing vaccinations to provide immunity, and the use of antiviral drugs that are able to selectively interfere with viral replication. Vaccination is an inexpensive and effective way of preventing infections by viruses. Their use has resulted in the significant decline in mortality and morbidity of serious viral infections such as mumps, smallpox, rubella, measles, and polio. Vaccines are commercially available for the prevention of over one dozen major viral infections of humans, and even more vaccines are available to prevent viral infections of animals such as livestock and pets.

Vaccines may consist of live but attenuated viruses, killed viruses, or antigens derived from viral proteins. Attenuated live vaccines contain forms of the virus that have been weakened to such a degree that they do not cause disease but can nonetheless confer immunity. Live vaccines have the potential of actually causing the disease they are meant to prevent, and can be particularly dangerous in causing active disease when given to people who are immuno-compromised. Antiviral drugs are often nonfunctional imitation analogues of the DNA nucleoside base building blocks. When a virus mistakenly incorporates a nonfunctioning analogue into its genome during replication, its life cycle is halted because the newly synthesized DNA is inactive.

Mountain Climbing (see Atmospheric Pressure, Ideal Gas Law)

Those who travel to higher altitudes, whether by climbing a mountain, driving up a mountain road, or traveling by air, experience an increase in flatulence. The underlying principle is the same, according to the gas laws of physics a reduction in atmospheric pressure results in an increase in the volume of intestinal gas. For those climbing hills and mountains with fellow travelers the incline usually means person behind has their nose at about the same level as the butt of the person in front. The practical take home message that is your advantage, if you understand the laws of physics, is to always be in the lead.

Another important consideration for those engaged in high altitude activities is the recognition that the oxygen content of air decreases with an increase in altitude. For those with underlying circulatory or lung conditions the additional stress of low oxygen content of the air can be potentially life threatening. Altitude sickness can also develop rapidly and is a life-threatening condition requiring an immediate descent in altitude.

Many air travelers are under the false impression that pressurization of the aircraft means the oxygen content of the air is the same as that on the ground at sea level. The aircraft is typically pressurized to maintain a cabin pressure equivalent to an altitude of approximately eight thousand feet. This leads to a reduction in the oxygen content of the air on the aircraft. Some normal individuals find this reduction in oxygen uncomfortable and develop headaches and other symptoms. Others are more sensitive, or recognize that their underlying medical condition requires that they have access to supplemental oxygen for their safe travel.

Nitrogen

Nitrogen is a chemical element with symbol N and atomic number seven is a colorless, odorless, tasteless, gas constituting seventy-eight percent by volume of Earth's atmosphere. The element nitrogen was discovered by Scottish physician Daniel Rutherford, in 1772. Nitrogen is the largest volume component of atmospheric air, and as would be expected, represents an identically high proportion of the gasses swallowed through aerophagia. Once in the body the carbon dioxide of the air is absorbed and eliminated as discussed above. The nitrogen however is a very poorly absorbed gas, and in essence will either come back up as a burp, or will sooner or later, comes out the other end as a fart.

The oxygen in the air, representing nearly twenty-one percent of the air gasses swallowed during aerophagia, is absorbed slowly, as the gut is not nearly as efficient as the lungs for respiration. As the carbon dioxide and oxygen are absorbed the percent of the gastrointestinal tract air that is nitrogen increases. As soon as the digestive process begins, hydrochloric acid of the stomach is neutralized by bicarbonate of the duodenum and pancreas. Large volumes of carbon dioxide gas are generated, as are smaller quantities of hydrogen, methane and other aromatic gasses discussed later.

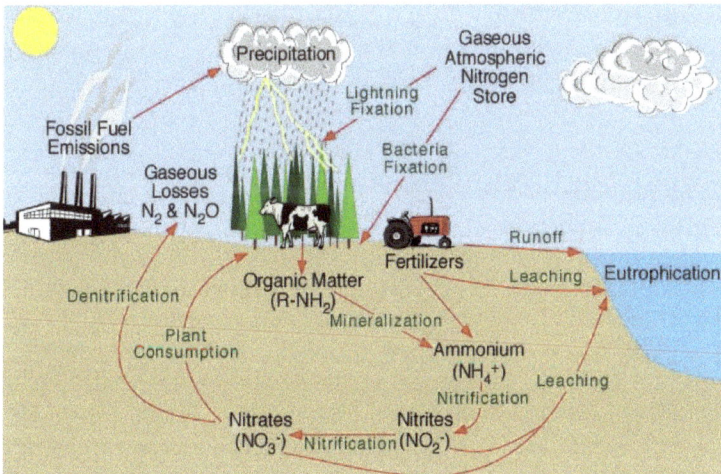

Pidwirny, M. "The Nitrogen Cycle" www.physicalgeography.net Creative Commons License

To 'Air' is Human

The nitrogen cycle is one of the most important nutrient cycles found in ecosystems. Living organisms use nitrogen in the production of complex organic molecules like amino acids, proteins, and nucleic acids. The nitrogen found in the atmosphere as a gas is about one million times larger than the nitrogen contained in living organisms. Nitrogen is often the most limiting nutrient for plant growth because most plants can only take up nitrogen in two solid forms: ammonium ion (NH_4^+) and the ion nitrate (NO_3^-). Animals receive the required nitrogen they need for metabolism, growth, and reproduction by the consumption of living or dead organic matter that contains material partially composed of nitrogen. The characteristic odor of animal flesh decay is caused by putrescence and cadaverine, which are breakdown products of the amino acids ornithine and lysine, respectively.

Nitrogen occurs in all organisms, primarily in amino acids, proteins, and in the nucleic acids DNA and RNA. The human body contains about three percent by weight of nitrogen, the fourth most abundant element in the body after oxygen, carbon, and hydrogen. It is a large component of animal waste (for example, guano) in the form of urea, uric acid, and ammonium compounds, which are valuable fertilizers. Nitrogen compounds were well known by the Middle Ages. Alchemists knew the mixture of nitric and hydrochloric acids, called aqua regia (royal water) could dissolve gold (the king of metals). Nitrogen compounds were used in saltpeter for gunpowder, and later as fertilizer. Nitrogen is used in beer due to the smaller bubbles it produces, which makes the beer smoother and headier.

When inhaled at pressures higher than four atmospheres nitrogen can act as an anesthetic agent causing nitrogen narcosis, a temporary semi-anesthetized state of mental impairment similar to that caused by nitrous oxide. Nitrogen also dissolves in the bloodstream and body fats. Rapid decompression (in the case of divers ascending too quickly, or astronauts decompressing too quickly can lead to life threatening decompression sickness (formerly known as caisson sickness or the bends), when nitrogen bubbles form in the bloodstream, nerves, joints.

Olestra

Olestra is a fat, cholesterol, and calorie free fat substitute that offers the mouth feel of fat without its nutritional consequences. It has been used in the preparation of otherwise high-fat content snack foods such as potato chips since it gained Food and Drug Administration (FDA) approval for use as a replacement for fats and oils in 1996. A popular olestra containing snack named Wow became the source of reports of gastrointestinal complaints including oily anal leakage and pungent intestinal gas. Subsequent studies suggested the gastrointestinal side effects might have been due to excessive intake of the product. Consumer concerns contributed to prohibition of the use or sale of olestra products in the European Union and Canada.

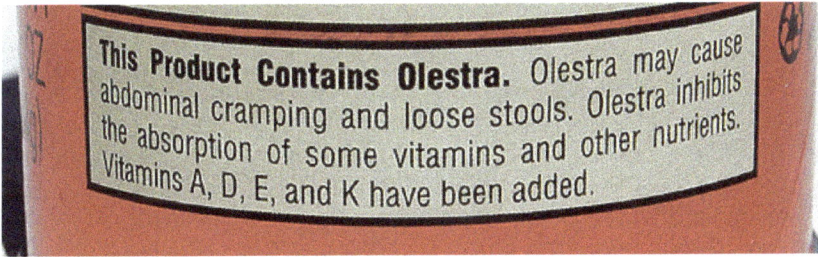

This Product Contains Olestra. Olestra may cause abdominal cramping and loose stools. Olestra inhibits the absorption of some vitamins and other nutrients. Vitamins A, D, E, and K have been added.

Triglycerides consist of three fatty acids bonded to glycerol, which acts as its backbone. Olestra uses the sugar sucrose as its backbone and bonds between six to eight fatty acids in a radial arrangement. This makes the molecule too irregular and too sizable to be absorbed by the intestinal lining, and it passes through the gut undigested. As it is not absorbed, it has no nutritive or caloric value. Because it contains fatty acids it can absorb and carry fat-soluble vitamins such as Vitamins A, D, E, and K with it as it transits the gut. Most products containing olestra are fortified with lipid soluble vitamins because of this effect, which could otherwise lead to malabsorption of these necessary nutrients.

Orlistat

Orlistat is a pharmaceutical designed to treat obesity. In the United States it is marketed as a prescription drug under the trade name Xenical, and is sold over-the-counter as Alli. Orlistat is a local inhibitor of gastric and pancreatic lipases and prevents the hydrolysis of triglycerides into absorbable free fatty acids. The triglycerides are excreted undigested in the feces along with the orlistat, which is not absorbed systemically. Taken three times daily before meals it prevents approximately 25% of dietary fat from being absorbed, resulting in modest weight loss in conjunction with a reduced calorie diet.

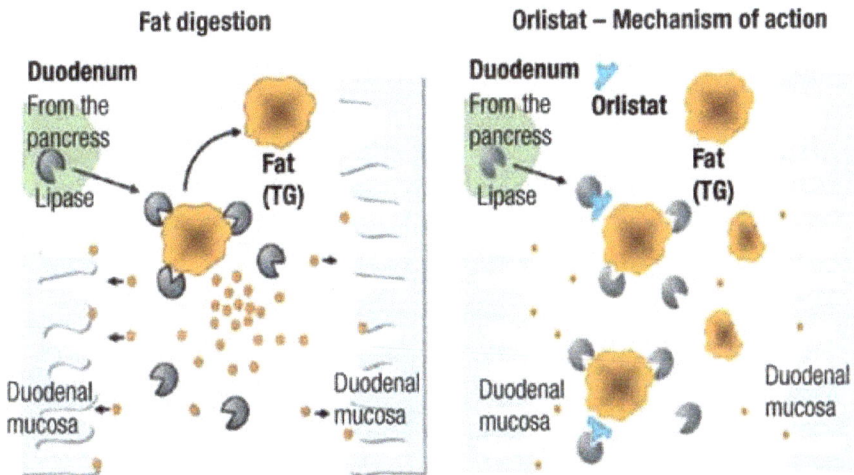

Orlistat – mechanism of action.
Creative Commons License

To 'Air' is Human

As expected with inhibition of fat absorption, Orlistat is notorious
for steatorrhea, oily, loose, and foul smelling stools. These decrease with time,
especially with the learned aversion of fatty foods, one of the behavioral
modifications that lead to the desired weight loss. Absorption of fat-
soluble vitamins and other fat-soluble nutrients are inhibited by the use of
orlistat. A multivitamin tablet containing vitamins A, D, E, K, and beta-
carotene should be taken once a day as a supplement when using orlistat.

Oxygen

Oxygen is a chemical element with symbol O and atomic number 8 that firms
dioxygen a colorless odorless, and tasteless gas. It was mistakenly named Oxygen
(the Greek ὀξύς (oxys) "acid", and γόνος (gonos) "producer"), by Antoine
Lavoisier who thought that all acids required oxygen (they require hydrogen). It
was discovered by Carl Scheele Sweden in 1773 but his publisher delayed
publication for two years. This inadvertently allowed British clergyman Joseph
Priestley, who independently discovered it a year later, to be given priority as its
discoverer because his work was published first.

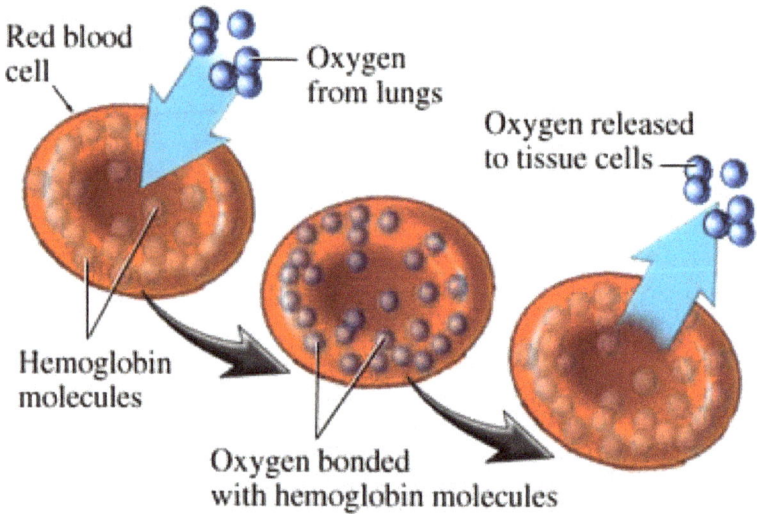

Red blood cell — Oxygen from lungs — Oxygen released to tissue cells — Hemoglobin molecules — Oxygen bonded with hemoglobin molecules

Oneminutecure.com Creative Commons License

Oxygen is a highly reactive element that forms compounds with most elements
except the noble gases. Oxygen is a strong oxidizing agent and only fluorine has
greater electronegativity. Oxygen is the third-most abundant element in the
universe, after hydrogen and helium. On Earth surface it is the most abundant
element making up half of the earth's crust, and makes up nearly twenty-one
percent of the air.

For free dioxygen to remain in Earth's atmosphere it needs to be replenished by the photosynthetic action of cyanobacteria, algae and plants. Free elemental O2 only began to accumulate in the atmosphere about 2.5 billion years ago with the Great oxygenation event. Towards the end of the Carboniferous period 300 million years ago O2 levels reached their highest levels of 35% and allowed insects to grow to a size with over a two-foot wingspan. I suspect that a mosquito that size would cause a human to pass out from blood loss if there were any humans to bite back then.

Cold water holds more dissolved O2 which is the reason the polar waters support a much higher density of life then tropical waters.
The marine Cyanobacteria and green algae generate up to 70% of the free oxygen produced on Earth. In humans and vertebrates the O2 changes the oxygen carrying hemoglobin to a bright red color. In mollusks and some arthropods like crabs hemocyanin gives a deep blue color when oxygenated. Hemocyanin uses copper, which has only one quarter of the oxygen carrying capacity as hemoglobin iron. If an iron nail is allowed to rust it will gain weight as it demonstrates its oxygen binding.

Parasite (see Microbiome)

Personalized Medicine

As with all issues of health and wellness each person needs to be assessed individually. With the advances in the human genome project it is now recognized that it is not just the genetic blueprint in the DNA that makes up the individuals uniqueness. Although humans have approximately 23,000 genes these genes are also controlled by external factors in a process described as epigenetics. It is also now recognized that the human body is in essence more than just human cells. The human system includes the microbiome, the microorganisms that live on and within us. The gut-brain-microbiome-food axis demonstrates the intimate interconnectivity of these four elements. If one were to analyze the human system by the number of cells a human is comprised of approximately 10% human cells and 90% microbial cells. If one were to analyze the system on the basis of the number of genes, humans are approximately 1% human genes and 99% microbial jeans.

The era of personalized medicine will advance the understanding of both health and disease. The previous approach of using population-based medicine will be abandoned as technology and bioinformatics allows treatments to be specifically tailored to the individual's genome, microbiome, and metabolome. The effectiveness of therapy should increase dramatically along with a significant reduction in adverse reactions to medications. This approach will also avoid the time and monetary expense of medications that did not provide a benefit, even if fortunately they did not cause an adverse reaction. In the interval as these advances are being brought into clinical practice it remains the best approach to tailor the treatment plan to the individual. What works for one may not work for another. Until the science and technology sufficiently evolve it often takes a trial and error approach to find the best treatment approach for the individual. And it is the individual who can be the only judge if the treatment is successful or the search for a solution must continue.

Physics

The laws and principles of physics apply to living as well as inanimate systems. An understanding of these principles explains many natural phenomena that are otherwise a source of mystery and confusion. When it comes to intestinal gas in particular, understanding the gas laws goes a long way in helping to manage this very common concern. Using Boyle's law, you can calculate how much the volume will compress as you go deeper underground or underwater. You can likewise calculate how much a gas will expand, as you go higher in altitude and the atmospheric pressure decreases. Using Charles Law you can calculate what happens to the gas in a cold drink when it is swallowed and is raised to body temperature

Boyle's Law

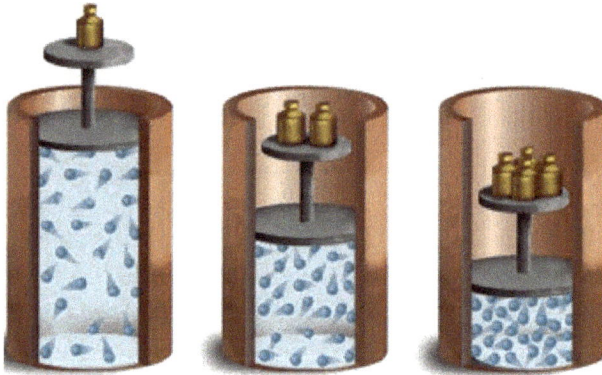

Charles's Law

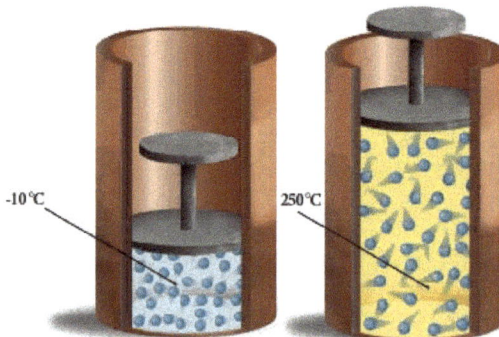

Prion (see Microbiome)

Protist (see Microbiome)

Rumination Syndrome

Rumination syndrome is an unusual condition and can lead to excessive air swallowing. Because the initiation of the rumination process itself requires the relaxation of the lower esophageal sphincter burps and belches are common findings. Rumination is typically seen in herbivorous livestock, which have compartmented stomachs to aid in the fermentation and digestion process. These animals regurgitate what is called the cud or partially digested food from the foregut stomach compartment to be chewed and swallowed again for further processes sings.

Humans can develop voluntary control of the esophageal musculature to retrieve stomach contents and swallow them again as if they were ruminant animals. The ability to train the esophageal muscles is most noted in yogi masters and circus performers but it is a learnable skill. Postprandial regurgitation is a symptom of rumination syndrome.

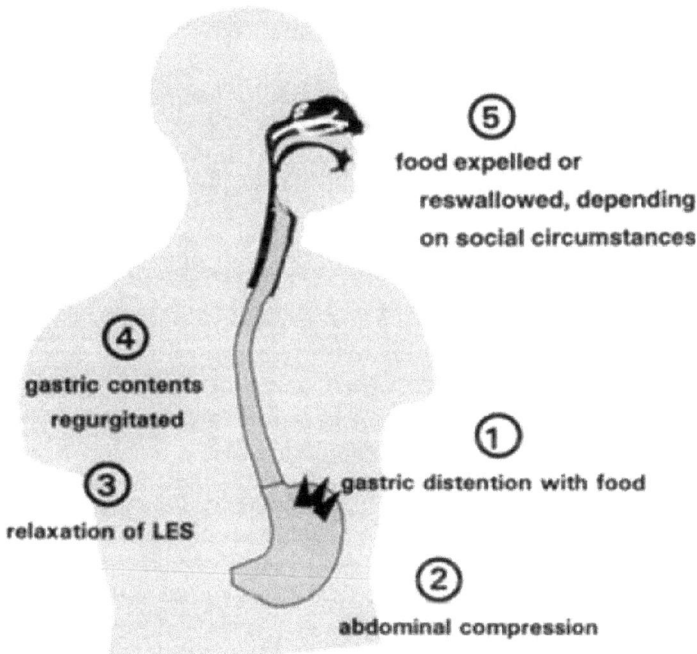

Rumination syndrome. Creative Commons License

For the others who subconsciously develop the rumination habit excessive air swallowing is simply the unavoidable result of the excessive swallowing that is part and parcel of the rumination syndrome. There are considerable psychological and psychiatric aspects of rumination disorders.

Scuba Diving (see Atmospheric Pressure, Ideal Gas Laws)

Scuba diving can be a very enjoyable activity, but it does require an understanding of the behavior of gasses and the laws of physics for safety. The atmospheric pressure changes associated with diving activity are pronounced and require close attention. Unfortunately, errors in judgment in scuba diving can be very unforgiving, and lead to fatal consequences if safety precautions are overlooked.

Boyle's Law was named after Robert Boyle, a chemist and physicist who published his discovery in 1662. The law describes that the pressure and volume of a gas are inversely proportional, if the temperature is kept constant. As the pressure on a gas increases its volume decreases, and vice versa, if you increase the volume of the gas, the pressure decreases.

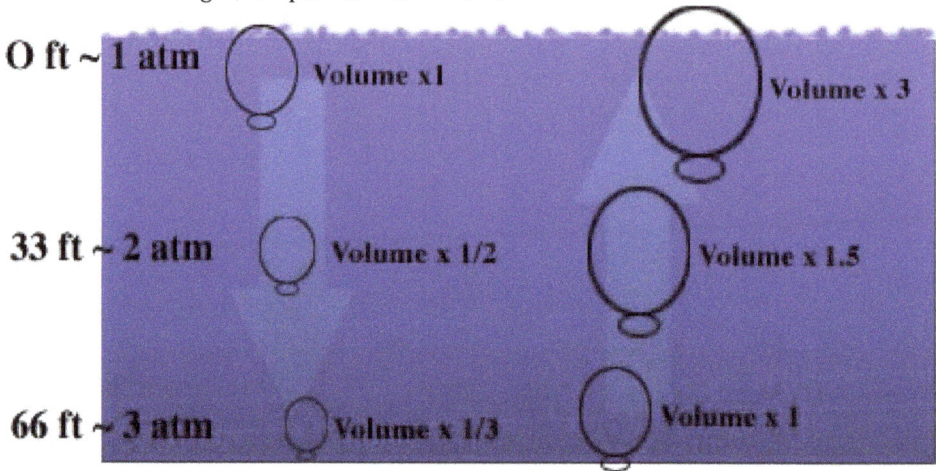

O ft ~ 1 atm — Volume x 1 — Volume x 3
33 ft ~ 2 atm — Volume x 1/2 — Volume x 1.5
66 ft ~ 3 atm — Volume x 1/3 — Volume x 1

At the surface (0 feet) the pressure is 1 ATM (atmosphere). At a depth of 33 feet underwater the pressure is 2 ATM, the sum total of 1 ATM of air pressure and 1 ATM of water pressure. If a balloon with gas at the surface is submerged it will be one-half of the original volume at 33 feet depth, and one-third the volume at 66 feet depth. On ascent the balloon volume will be one and one-half times greater on going from 66 feet depth to 33 feet depth. It will have a volume three times greater at the surface than it did at 66 feet depth.

The diver experiences the effect of these pressure changes firsthand. As one descends the air in the facemask is compressed giving rise to the phenomenon known as mask squeeze. The pressure changes in the air spaces of the ear canal can be very significant if they are not purposefully equalized during descent and ascent. Severe ear injury including perforated or ruptured eardrum can result from unequaled air pressure. Head cold, allergies, sinus congestion, and other conditions that reduce the patency of the Eustachian tubes can prevent equalization of air pressure and should preclude diving activity.

The air volume in buoyancy control devices requires adjustment to maintain neutrality. The gas laws also explains why divers are advised to exhale while ascending as the gasses in the lung can over expand if the breath is held and result in severe internal injury. Dive bubbles increase in size as the gasses expand because of the reduced atmospheric pressure as they ascend. The gasses in the bubble are following the gas laws that dictate their behavior with changes in pressure, temperature and volume.

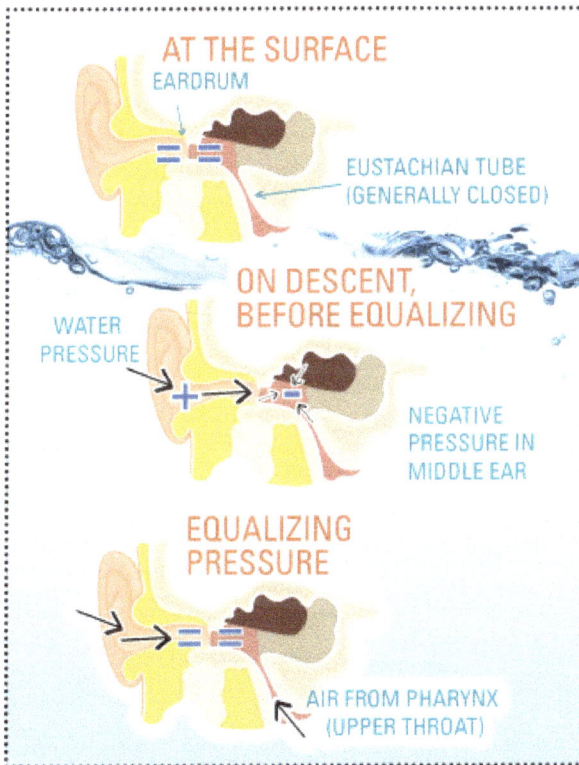

Creative Commons License

William Henry was an English physician and chemist who proposed what is now called Henry's law in 1803. The law states that at a constant temperature, the amount of a given gas dissolved in a liquid is directly proportional to the pressure of that gas. As the gas pressure increases, the solubility of the gas in the liquid increases. As the temperature increases, the solubility of gas in liquid decreases. The greater the pressure, the greater the quantity of a gas that can be absorbed by a liquid. The cooler the liquid, the greater the amount of gas that it can absorb. As the temperature of liquid increases, the solubility of the gas decreases forming bubbles that allow it to escape. Henry's Law explains why carbon dioxide in a pressurized container, such as in a can or bottle of a carbonated beverage remains

To 'Air' is Human

in solution until it is opened. As soon as the container is opened the pressure is reduced causing the carbon dioxide gas to lose its solubility and escape in the form of bubbles or fizz.

In a similar manner as a diver descends nitrogen inhaled is under increasing pressure and becomes soluble in the bloodstream, muscles and tissues. This is not a problem until the diver begins an ascent and the pressure is reduced allowing the nitrogen in the body to form bubbles. If the diver ascends too quickly this can lead to Decompression Sickness also known as the bends. This is the reason why divers are advised to ascend gradually, to allow the nitrogen to be exhaled out of the lungs rather than to form bubbles in the bloodstream or tissue. Henry's Law also explains why after a dive the diver should not be exposed to higher temperatures such as a sauna, hot bath or shower or engages in strenuous activities or exercise. The increase in body temperature may cause the nitrogen to become less soluble and increase the risk of Decompression Sickness. Likewise diving in colder water enhances the absorption of nitrogen into the body, which should be adjusted for by shorter dive times or shallower dives.

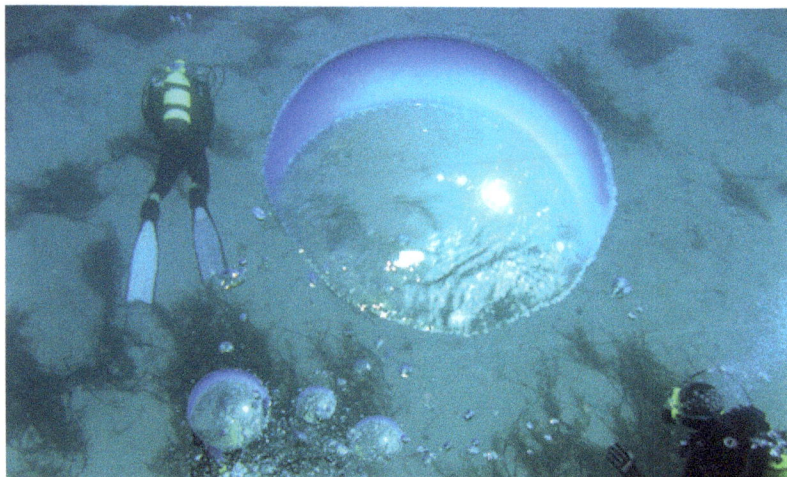

Charles' Law states that at a constant volume, the pressure of gas varies directly with the temperature. While a French philosopher named Joseph Louis Gay-Lussac published this law, Lussac attributed the law to an unpublished work by Jacques Charles. Jacques Alexander Charles was a French scientist, mathematician, inventor, and balloonist who studied the effects of temperature on the volumes of a gas. He formulated and published what became known as Charles' Law in 1787.

Charles wrote about the law after observing the effects of temperature on balloons. When a balloon is filled with gas and exposed to heat, the molecules of the gas cause the balloon to expand. When the balloon is exposed to colder temperatures, the molecules of the gas cause the balloon to deflate. The law states that at a constant pressure, the volume of a gas increases or decreases by the same factor as its temperature increases or decreases. Charles' law helps to explain the hazard of leaving scuba tanks out in the sun, or in the trunk of a car. The gas already under high pressure will have a further increase in pressure if subjected to heat, which can cause the tank to explode. The law also explains why scuba tanks increase in temperature when being filled with compressed air. Please see the entries on atmospheric pressure and ideal gas laws for more details.

Charles and Gay-Lussac's Law

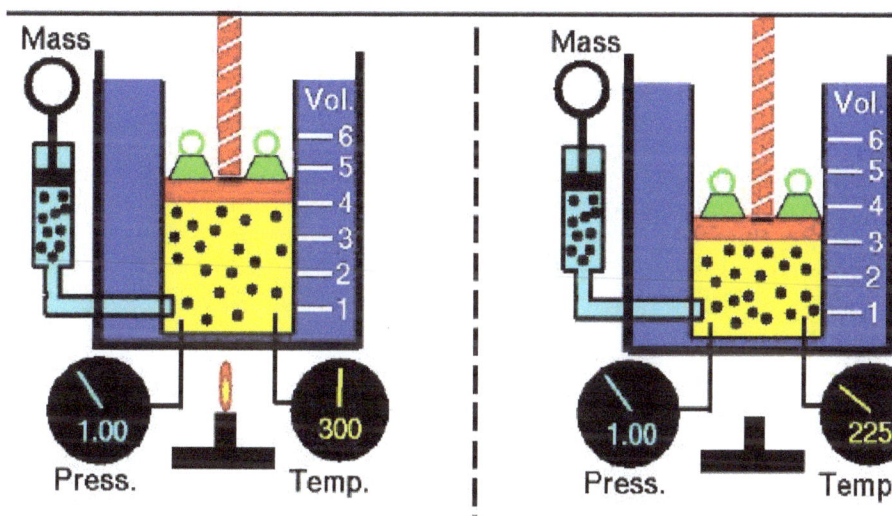

For a given mass, at constant pressure, the volume is directly proportional to the temperature

$$V = C\,T$$

Creative Commons License

Simethicone (see Bubbles, Surface Tension)

Simethicone is an oral over the counter product that is used as a treatment to reduce bloating, discomfort or pain caused by intestinal gas. Simethicone is a mixture of polydimethylsiloxane and hydrated silica gel, and is an anti-foaming agent that decreases the surface tension of gas bubbles. Surface tension is the property seen in water and other fluids that causes the formation of form semi-spherical droplets and bubbles. The reduction in surface tension does not eliminate the bubbles, nor does it cause them to become smaller.

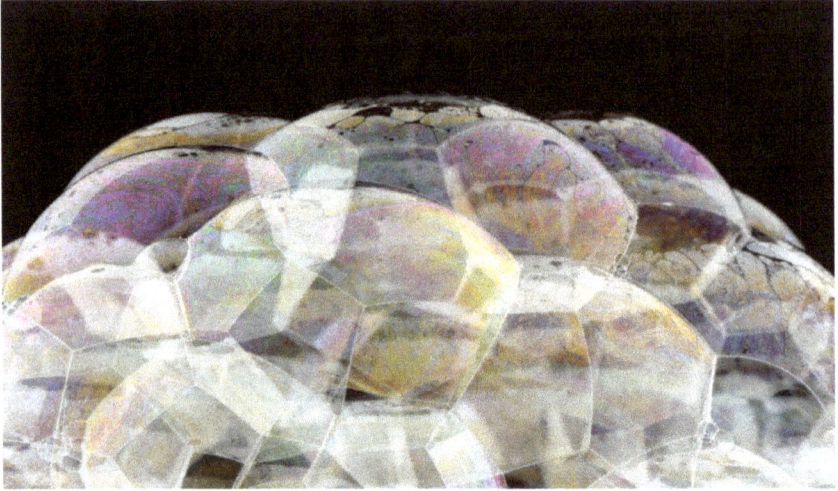

Creative Commons License

Counter intuitively, it actually causes them to combine into larger bubbles, and the presumptive relief is most often from being able to burp or belch up the larger bubble from the stomach more easily. There have been studies suggesting that simethicone increases the transit time so that intestinal gas may be more readily eliminated as flatus. Simethicone is not absorbed by the body and does not enter into the bloodstream.

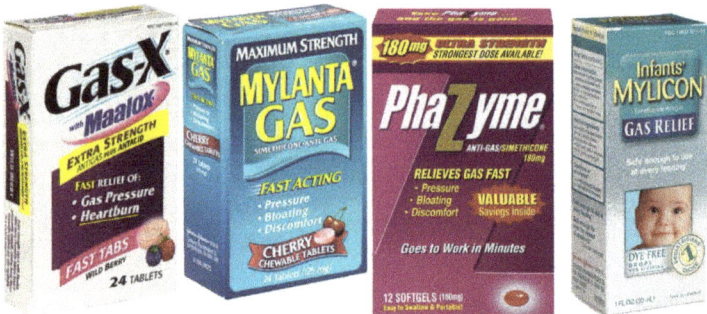

Creative Commons License

Simethicone has been promoted and marketed as a treatment for colic in babies, yet the actual cause of colic has yet to be clearly identified. Simethicone solutions of differing concentration also have industrial applications for reducing foaming in certain chemical processes, in detergents, as well as in medical imaging studies of the gastrointestinal tract.

Singultus (Hiccup)

Singultus, a hiccup, is an involuntary contraction of the diaphragm that may occur singly or in bouts. It is caused by a strong contraction, known as a myoclonic jerk, of the diaphragm. The diaphragm contraction increases the negative pressure in the chest cavity that cause the lungs to act as a vacuum inhaling a deep breath. Within milliseconds the epiglottis and vocal cords abruptly close creating a hic sound and cutting off the flow of air. A hiccup is an onomatopoeia, a word that was created to imitate the sound it is describing.

Hiccups are believed to be an evolutionary trait inherited from fish and tadpoles. The phrenic nerve which controls the diaphragm extends from the base of the skull and travels through the chest cavity. This design appears to have been derived from fish ancestors with gills closer to the neck. Interestingly enough as the human embryo develops the vestigial gills can be easily identified. The hiccup itself may have arisen from our evolution through the amphibian phase. The characteristic pattern of muscle and nerve activity of hiccups occurs in tadpoles that use both lungs and gills to breathe. When tadpoles use their gills they shut the glottis to close off the breathing tube while sharply inspiring. In essence tadpoles breathe with their gills using an extended form of a hiccup.

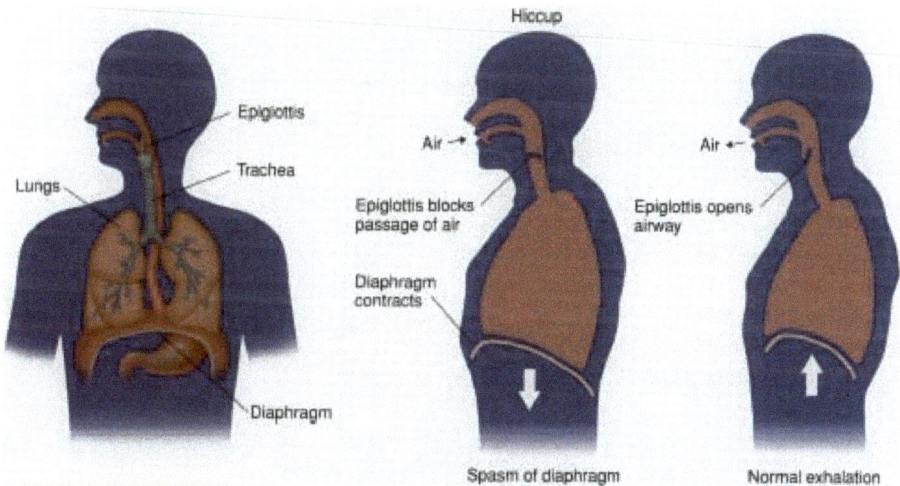

Creative Commons License

They resolve spontaneously in the vast majority of cases yet dozens of home and medical remedies exist that are not particularly effective. A recent theory proposes that hiccups developed as a reflex to allow the escape of swallowed air from the stomach during the suckling and feeding of infants. Pope Pius XII was seriously ill with a hiatal hernia and virtually uncontrollable hiccups in 1954.

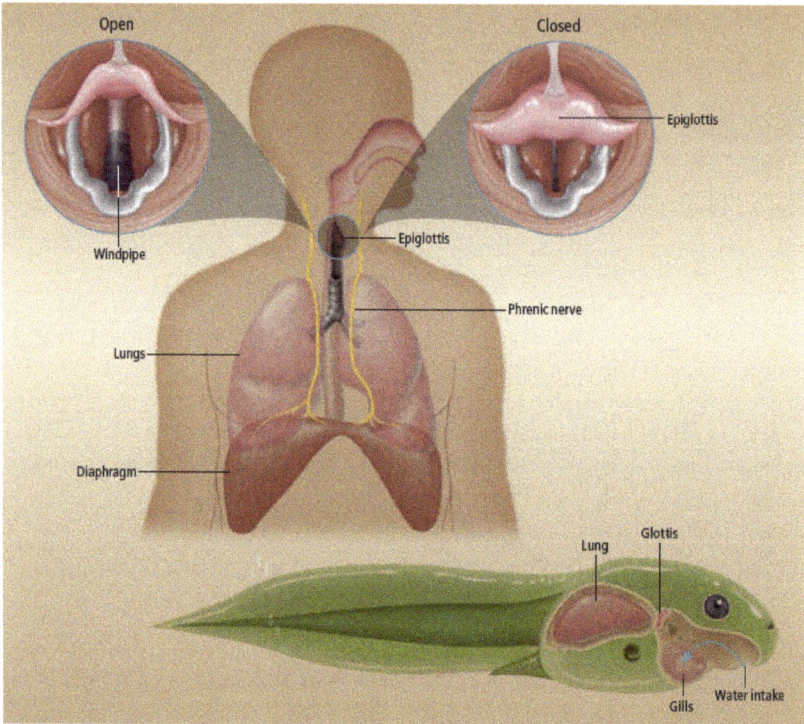

Creative Commons License

Common home remedies include: holding one's breath and exhaling slowly, holding the nose, breathing into a paper bag, sucking on ice cubes or hard candy, drinking water from the far side of a glass, gargling, pulling on the tongue, biting on a lemon, swallowing granulated sugar, swallowing hard bread crust, sneezing, peeling onions, bending over so that the head is lower than the chest, frightening the person with hiccups, slapping the person with hiccups on the back.

Spelunking

Spelunking, the exploration of caves, has become an increasingly popular activity and can take place above or below sea level altitudes. Some of the deepest explored caves have vertical drops in excess of one thousand feet. Although changes in atmospheric pressure are noticeable, this effect is one of the least dangerous aspects of the sport activity. The exploration of underwater caves known as cave diving, combines spelunking with scuba diving, and is a particularly demanding and challenging activity. In this activity understanding the potential effects of atmospheric pressure changes becomes critically important.

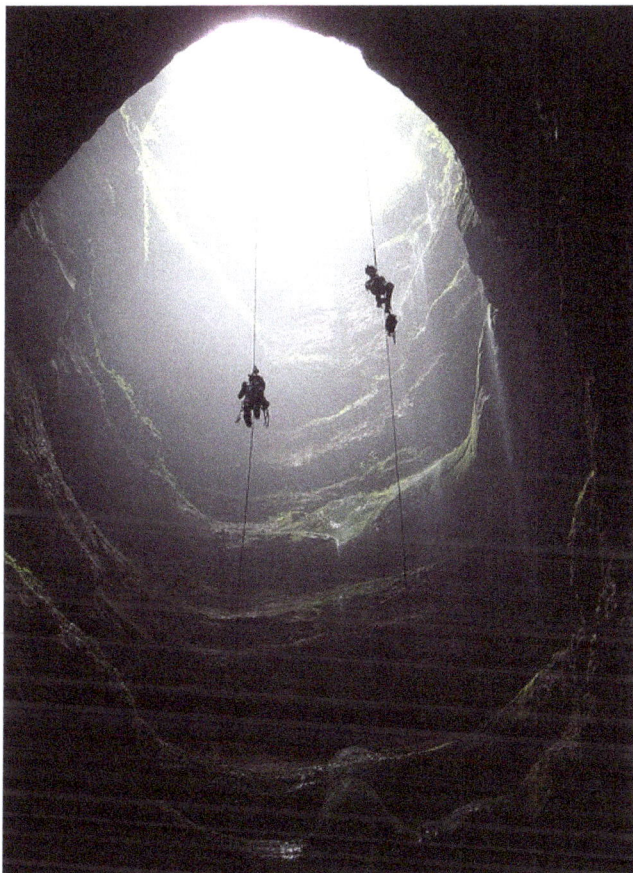

41.media.tumblr.com Creative Commons License

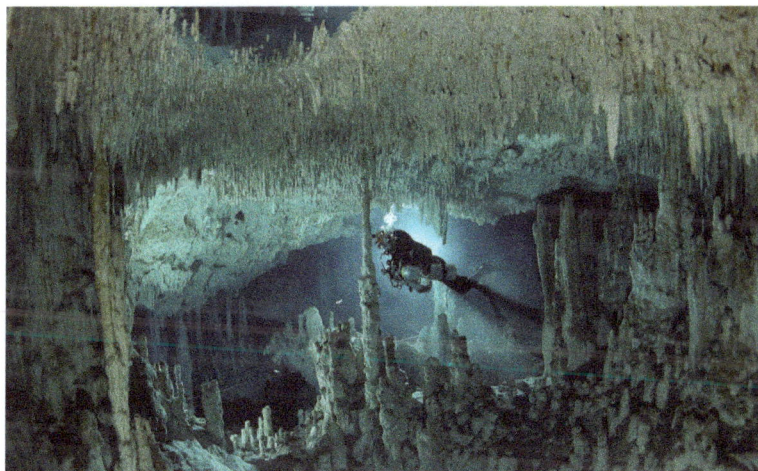

Creative Commons License

To 'Air' is Human

Surface Tension

Surface tension is a physical property exhibited when certain liquids are in contact with a gas. It is particularly pronounced when liquid water is in contact with the gasses of the air. Each water molecule contains two hydrogen atoms and one oxygen atom, giving rise to its familiar chemical shorthand of H_2O. Because of their atomic structure the negative charge of the electrons of the hydrogen atoms are attracted to the positive charge of the oxygen atom, creating was is known as a hydrogen bond. The electric charges also create an attractive force between water molecules, causing them to want to remain close together. These forces are balanced out when a water molecule is surrounded by other water molecules.

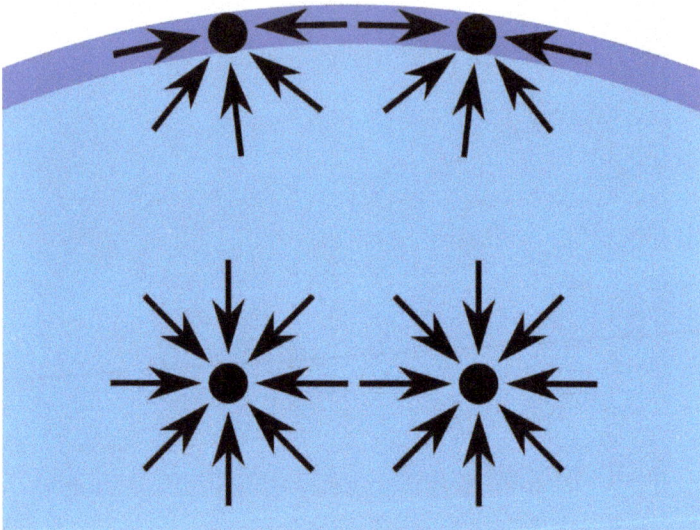

Booyabazooka Unbalanced charges on water molecules at the surface of a liquid gas interface.
Creative Commons License

When the water molecules on the surface are exposed to the gasses of the air above them they are no longer exposed to balanced charges. The water molecule on the surface exposed to the air is only subject to the electric charge pulling it down, keeping it in the liquid. This resistance to leaving its fellow water molecules behind gives it the property known as surface tension, a tension that prevents it from being separated from the remaining liquid. This surface tension is visible when you see water assume the shape of a droplet, or when you fill a glass to the brim and the fluid builds up above the lip of the glass before it begins to overflow. It is also the principle that allows insects heavier than water, such as the water glider, appear to walk on water because the surface tension acts as a walk able surface. Surface tension also is the force that allows the creation of bubbles. Surfactants are products that have the property of reducing surface tension and are used in detergents, as well as in anti-bubble and anti-gas products such as simethicone.

To 'Air' is Human

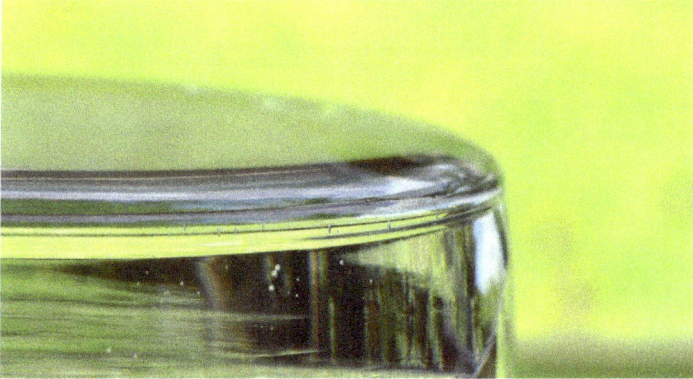

Surface tension allowing to go over brim of glass without spilling. Andre Roberto Doreto Santos www.flickr.com Creative Commons License

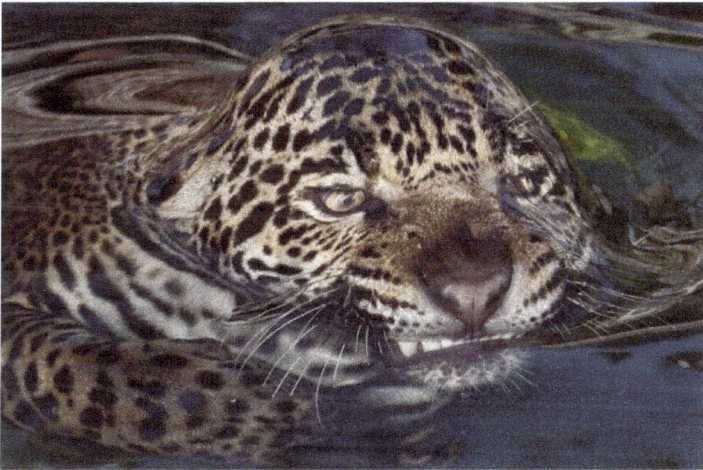

Photograph of surface tension effect. i.imgur.com Creative Commons License

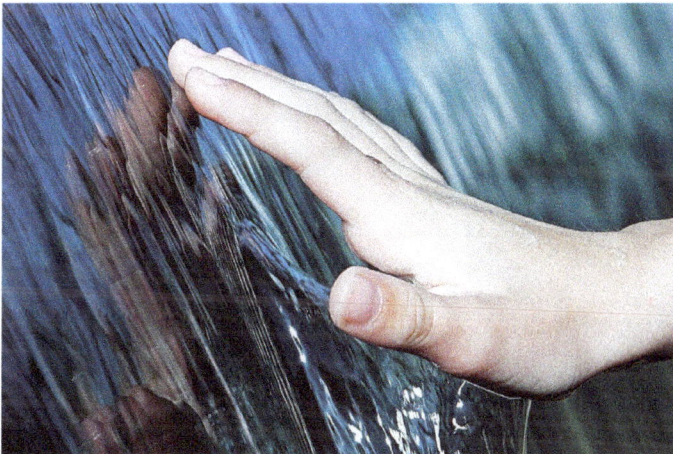

Photograph of surface tension effect. upload.wikimedia.org Creative Commons License

To 'Air' is Human

Underground Miners (see Atmospheric Pressure and Ideal Gas Laws)

Underground mining has significant occupational hazards. Some mines are subjected to pressurization to prevent the seepage of ground water into the mine. In other instances the mining activity may expose pockets of toxic gasses that can lead to injury or death. For those engaged in spelunking, the exploring of caves, descending to depths within the earth have hazards similar to mining related to atmospheric pressure changes. An understanding of the effects and dangers of changes in atmospheric pressure is critical to mine and cave exploration safety. Please see the entries on atmospheric pressure and ideal gas laws for further details.

Vagina (see Fart, Vagina)

Virus (see Microbiome)

Whoopee Cushion

A whoopee cushion is a device used as a practical joke which mimics the sound of flatulence when compressed. It is commonly placed on a chair or cushion so that the sound is generated when someone sits on it. It is typically constructed as a rubber bladder, which is inflated with air. A vibrating exit flap creates an audible fart like sound that is generated when sat upon. The modern commercially successful version was developed in the 1920's by the JEM Rubber Co. of Toronto, Canada. A more discrete alternate remote controlled version that can be hidden under a chair electronically generates prerecorded fart sounds

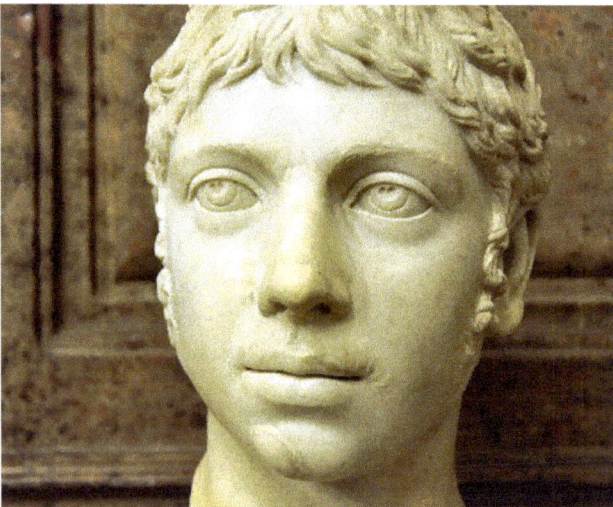

Elagabalus, Public Domain

Elagabalus, Marcus Aurelius Antoninus Augustus, (c. 203 AD – 222 AD) was Roman Emperor from 218 to 222. According to the findings of archeologist

To 'Air' is Human

Warwick Ball the Roman Emperor Elagabalus played practical jokes on his guests. At dinner parties he would place whoopee cushion like devices under their seats from which fart like sounds would emanate. He showed a disregard for Roman traditions and taboos, insulted the Roman Senate, the common people, and his own protectors the Praetorian Guard. It is therefore not terribly surprising that he was assassinated at age eighteen.

Yoga/Ayurveda

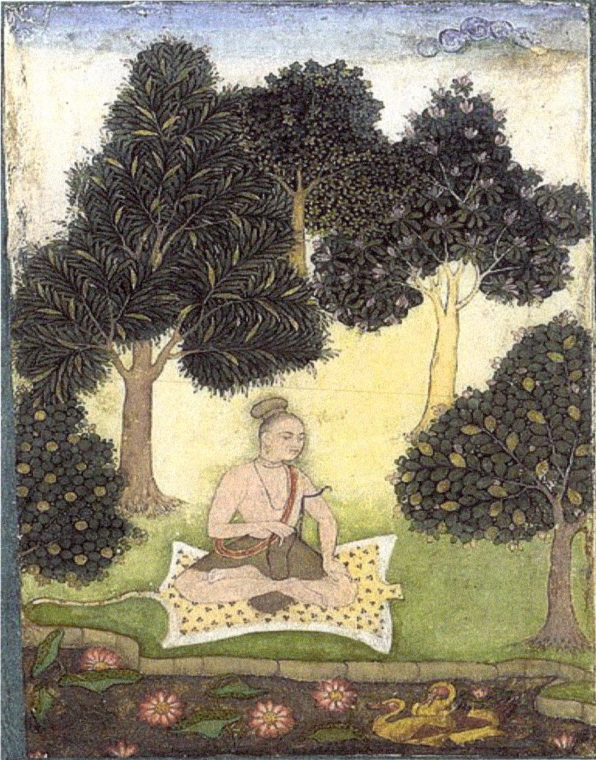

A yogi seated in a garden, North Indian or Deccani miniature painting, c. 1620-40
www.columbia.edu/itc Public Domain

Yoga is a physical, mental and spiritual practice that comprises many different schools and approaches. It has often been associated with the practice of Hinduism, Buddhism, Jainism and other belief systems that originated in the East. The origins of yoga are not clearly defined but were thought to arise in pre-Vedic Indian traditions. The first documents ascribed to yoga are found in the Buddhist Nikayas and the Yoga Sutras of Patanjali recorded around 400 AD. Recognizing its role in general health and wellness it is no longer an exclusive religious practice but has become increasingly adopted into the mainstream. Of course any general physical activity is beneficial as it increases bowel motility, yet there are a number of specific yoga postures that may provide additional benefit from compression and release of intra-abdominal pressure.

To 'Air' is Human

Yoga originally had been a religious practice and over thousands of years have become incorporated into secular wellness programs as well. Its effect on natural bodily functions, including intestinal gas were well recognized even in ancient times. Yogic masters and Brahmins in India practiced goze (flatus, eructation, belch) as a means of concentration in ridding the flesh of all evil. Yoga may provide benefit for some individuals with irritable bowel syndrome, especially poses that exercise the lower abdomen. It may also stimulate the passage of intestinal gas. In fact there is a specific yoga posture designed to aid in the release of intestinal gas. It is not unusual for participants in a yoga class to experience the auditory or olfactory consequences of someone else's, or their own, successful assumption of the yoga gas release pose.

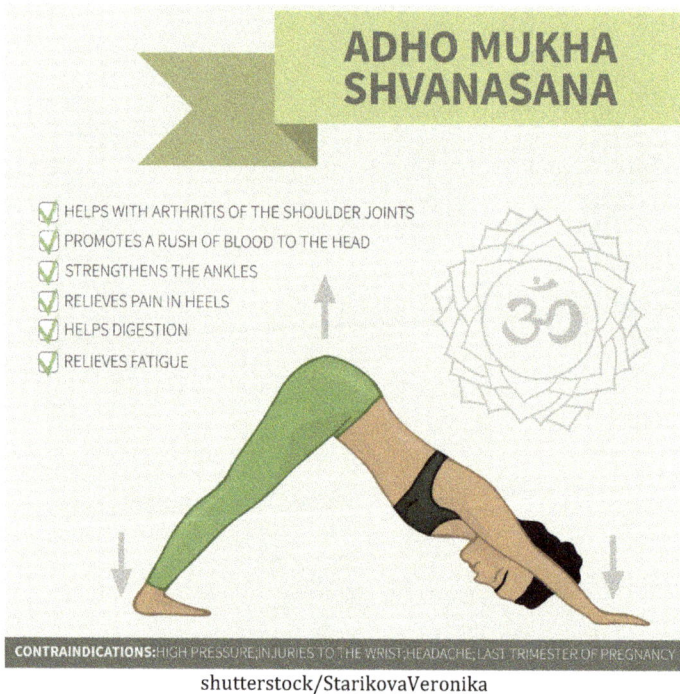

ADHO MUKHA SHVANASANA

- HELPS WITH ARTHRITIS OF THE SHOULDER JOINTS
- PROMOTES A RUSH OF BLOOD TO THE HEAD
- STRENGTHENS THE ANKLES
- RELIEVES PAIN IN HEELS
- HELPS DIGESTION
- RELIEVES FATIGUE

CONTRAINDICATIONS: HIGH PRESSURE; INJURIES TO THE WRIST; HEADACHE; LAST TRIMESTER OF PREGNANCY

shutterstock/StarikovaVeronika

It helped to achieving the suppression of consciousness and reaching towards enlightenment through union with the Supreme Being (Nirvana). Belching & forcing wind from the buttocks the yogi would chant: "Glory to those keen ebullitions which escape above & below!" (Allen Edwardes: The Jewel in the Lotus). Among certain Brahmins, a spiritual blessing was required after each bite of food: He takes a little rice soaked in melted butter and puts it into his mouth, saying: "Glory to the wind which dwells in the chest!' At the second mouthful, "Glory to the wind which dwells in the face!" At the third, "Glory to the wind which dwells in the throat!" At the fourth, "Glory to the wind which dwells in the whole body!" At the fifth, "Glory to those noisy ebullitions which escape above and below!" Any general physical activity is beneficial as it increases bowel motility, yet there are a number of yoga postures that may provide additional benefit from compression and release of intra-abdominal pressure.

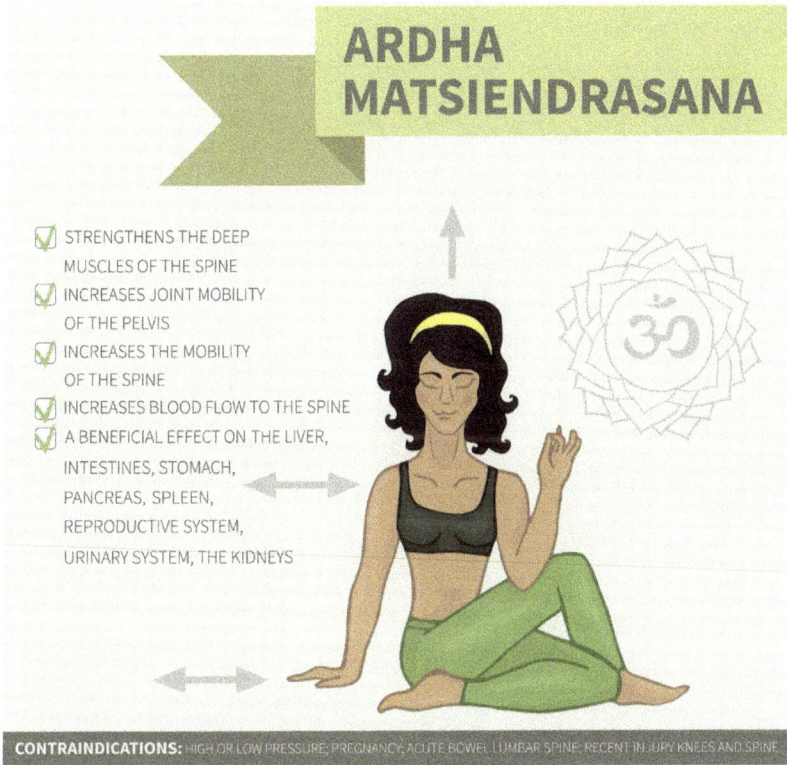

ARDHA MATSIENDRASANA

- STRENGTHENS THE DEEP MUSCLES OF THE SPINE
- INCREASES JOINT MOBILITY OF THE PELVIS
- INCREASES THE MOBILITY OF THE SPINE
- INCREASES BLOOD FLOW TO THE SPINE
- A BENEFICIAL EFFECT ON THE LIVER, INTESTINES, STOMACH, PANCREAS, SPLEEN, REPRODUCTIVE SYSTEM, URINARY SYSTEM, THE KIDNEYS

CONTRAINDICATIONS: HIGH OR LOW PRESSURE; PREGNANCY; ACUTE BOWEL LUMBAR SPINE; RECENT INJURY KNEES AND SPINE.

shutterstock/StarikovaVeronika

The Wind-Relieving Pose (Pavanamuktasana) is particularly effective . (Sanskrit: Pavana wind, mukta relieve , Asana Posture) Technique: Lie on your back, arms by your side and feet together. Inhale and as you exhale bend your right knee and flex your right leg bringing the right thigh up pressing on the abdomen. Inhale again and as you exhale lift your head and chest up off the floor and touch your chin to your right knee. Hold this position for several more cycles of inspiration and expiration. Then relax and after a rest repeat the sets with the opposite side. After a second period of rest and relaxation repeat the exercises using both legs at the same time. Avoid practicing the Wind-Relieving Pose (Pavanamuktasana) if you have high blood pressure, heart problems, excess acidity reflux or GERD, hernia, slip disc, neck or back problems, or are pregnant or if you feel any ill effects from the exercise. Other yoga positions and moves that may be helpful include Balasana (Child's Pose) supported, Paschimottanasana (Seated Forward Bend), Supta Baddha Konasana (Reclining Bound Angle Pose) supported, Janu Sirsasana (Head of the Knee Pose) supported, and Jathara Parivartanasana (Revolved Abdomen Pose).

Sthala Basti, also called Vata Basti, Air Basti, Air Enema, is an advanced Hatha yoga technique that is best learned from an expert teacher. There are a number of different approaches and techniques but mastery of anal sphincter is a challenging practice. Once you master this technique you may not become as famous as the Petomane of the Moulin Rouge but you will certainly be able to entertain your soon to be former friends.

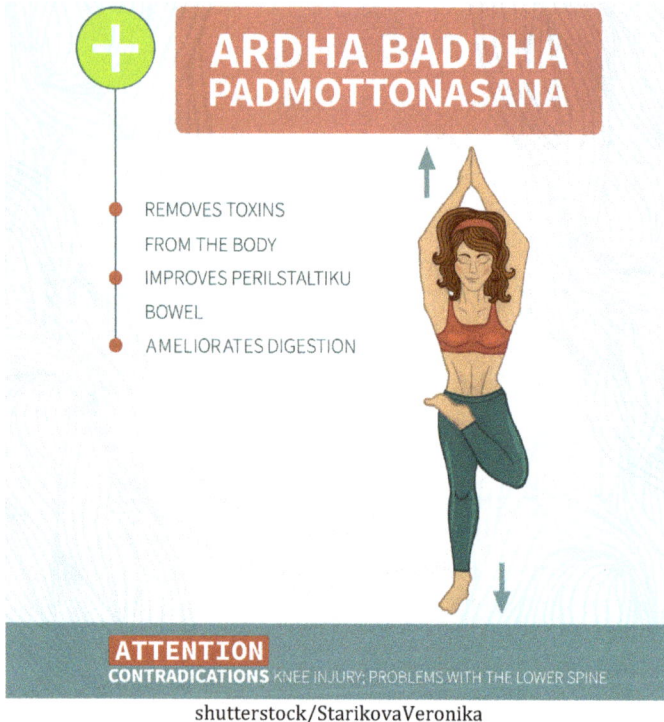

ARDHA BADDHA PADMOTTONASANA

- REMOVES TOXINS FROM THE BODY
- IMPROVES PERILSTALTIKU BOWEL
- AMELIORATES DIGESTION

ATTENTION
CONTRADICATIONS KNEE INJURY; PROBLEMS WITH THE LOWER SPINE

shutterstock/StarikovaVeronika

Sthala Basti starting from Paschimottanasana technique. Sit with your legs stretched out in front of you and then bend forward halfway. You do not however fully place your upper body on your legs but only bend forward halfway. Perform Uddiyana Bandha by exhaling completely then taking a false inhalation while holding the breath. This flattens and pulls in the abdomen under the rib cage as if the chest was suctioning it. The process is repeated many times followed by relaxation of the anal sphincter muscles to allow air to be drawn in with the uddiyanna Bandha maneuver. The air suctioned in is released as flatus.

Sthala Basti in lying Position technique. Lying on the back bend the knees up towards the chest and raise the buttocks. Practice developing control of the anal sphincter muscles by contraction and relaxation of the sphincter. When the sphincter is relaxed air suctioned into the colon is released as flatulence.

Sthala Basti in Utkatasana technique. Sit in Utkatasana, also called the chair or lightning bolt pose, by squatting while standing with the knees bent 90 degrees backwards to thighs. The back and upright arms form a forward facing 90-degree angle from the thighs. If necessary until sphincter control is mastered a hollow tube like bamboo or a catheter is placed in the anus and Uddiyama Bandha is performed. Air is sucked into the colon and released as flatus.

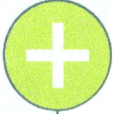

+

UTTANASANA

- STIMULATES THE KIDNEYS AND LIVER
- LOOSENS THE PELVIS AND THE CALF MUSCLES
- STRETCHES THE BACK OF THE THIGHS
- PULLS THE SPINE
- IMPROVES DIGESTION

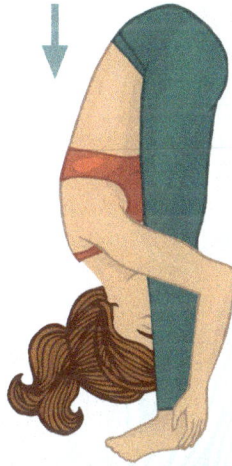

ATTENTION CONTRADICTIONS HIGH AND LOW BLOOD PRESSURE; CIRCULATORY DISORDERS OF THE HEAD

shutterstock/StarikovaVeronika

Yoga is often associated with the Indian medical system of Ayurveda. The word agni is Sanskrit term for 'fire'. Sanskrit is in the Indo-European family of languages as is Latin, English, Greek and others. The Sanskrit word 'agni' is the equivalent of the Latin 'ignis', which is the root of the English word ignite often used as descriptive action to start a fire. Agni is a central concept in Ayurveda, as it represents the fire energy equivalent produced by the metabolic process of digestion. It allows the breakdown, absorption, and assimilation of food nutrients while eliminating waste and toxins, known as the Ayurveda term 'ama', from the body. The accumulation of ama results in the slow but progressive deterioration of the body which ultimately leads to ill health and disease.

Agni also refers more broadly to our ability to process and digest all aspects of life, including food, experiences, memories, and sensory impressions. It transforms the physical matter of food into the useable forms of energy the cells of the body require. *Jathar-agni* determines the production of hydrochloric acid in the stomach, while *Bhuta-agni* determines the production of bile in the liver. *Kloma-agni* determines the production of the pancreatic enzymes, while *Jatru-agni* regulates the thyroid gland. *Dhatu-agni* is the agni at the level of tissue and cellular metabolism. The Ayurvedic concept of agni beliefs continues to an even subtler level of *Indrya-agni,* described as the door of perception, which transforms external information into internal knowledge. In Ayurveda a stronger agni allows for a stronger and clearer body and mind. The nature and quality of the various *agnis* depend on the individual's blend of the three doshas: vata, pitta, and kapha. In individuals with a predominance of the vata and kapha doshas the agni tends to be weak resulting in a digestive system that is cold, irregular, and sluggish. This is believed to contribute to signs and symptoms of constipation, malabsorption, and excess intestinal gas. In pittas the fires of agni is excessive and can result in heartburn, acid reflux, colitis, and other burning symptoms.

Culinary herbs and spices are used in Ayurveda to enhance the level of agni between and during meals. The meals should be balanced and provide a sampling of each of the tastes, sweet, sour, astringent, bitter, salty, and pungent. One popular Ayurvedic practice is to consume a small piece of fresh ginger with a few drops of lemon juice prior to eating a meal. This allows a slow and progressive awakening of the fire of digestive Agni. Other aromatic spices that aid in digestion include black pepper, cayenne pepper, cardamon, and liquorice. They are believed to aid in the cooking and predigestion of foods. The spices also stimulate the secretions of saliva and digestive enzymes which reduces the work load of the Agni and results in less fatigue after eating. By assisting digestion the Herb's and spices reduce gas and ama. When digestion is incomplete, fermentation takes place and it is this process which produces gas and ama which can contribute to gastrointestinal signs and symptoms. Fennel is a common herb offered in Indian restaurants as a carminative. The seeds are chewed, the juice swallowed, and the pulp spit out. It relaxes the lower esophageal sphincter to allow swallowed air to be released and may reduce gas, discomfort, and fatigue. Hing is also used in Ayurveda cooking to assist weak agni and digestion. It is a resinous sap from the asafetida plant and, when combined with other aromatic and carminative herbs in the Ayurveduc remedy hingavashtak, it is believed to promote the deeper assimilation of nutrients.

Ojas is the Ayurveduc term for the vital nectar of life. To achieve optimal health it is important to eliminate ama and focus on the production of Ojas, the Sanskrit term meaning 'vigor'. Ojas is the pure and subtle essence that has been extracted from food that has been completely and properly digested. It circulates throughout the body tissues and heart, sustaining the physical body, providing clarity to the mind, and nurturing emotional balance. A diet of pure easily digested foods, described in Ayurveda as 'Sattvic', promotes the creation and flow of Ojas. Sattvic foods include organic milk, almonds, honey, sesame, rice, and fruits.

Some foods are difficult if not impossible for the body to convert into ojas, including meat, poultry, fish, oily foods, cheese, processed food, and items with an excess of sour or salty tastes. Freshly prepared meals produce more Ojas than foods that has been canned, frozen, or reheated. Alcohol and tobacco use reduce and eliminate ojas. Signs of Ojas includ: You feel rested upon awakening, Your skin has a healthy glow, Your tongue is clear and pink, Your body feels light, regardless of the number on the scale, You feel centered throughout the day, Your digestion is strong without bloating, You feel energized & enthusiastic, Your mind is clear, Your body has a pleasant smell, You rarely get sick. Signs of Ama include: Bad breath, Coated tongue, Dull appetite, Delicate digestion, Sluggish or irritable elimination, Generalized pain, Fatigue, Depression, Susceptibility to infections, Difficulty manifesting intentions.

Oma's is the essence of the processing of all signals our body receives, not just the foods we eat. Much as important as the quality and character of the foods, is the quality of our experience and environment. If we are in a stressful or uncomfortable environment creating ojas cannot take place because we are experiencing what are basically indigestible emotions that are distributing distressed chemical messages throughout our cells and organs. To create a nurturing atmosphere for meals it is important to pay attention to all of the senses — taste, sound, sight, touch, and smell. Here are a few suggestions to enhance the production if ojas

- Eat in a comfortable environment and atmosphere
- Do not eat when you are upset.
- Sit down comfortably to enjoy your meal.
- Do not multitask while you are eating, do not eat while reading, watching television, or while on a computer or mobile device.
- Only eat when you are hungry.
- Dine at a moderate pace. Chew your food well and with enjoyment of the taste, texture, and aroma. Don't gulp down your food or eat too slowly.
- Moderate the quantity of raw foods, which are harder to digest than cooked ones.
- Include all six tastes (sweet, sour, astringent, bitter, salty, and pungent) with each meal.
- Drink water to maintain adequate hydration
- Use spices and herbs that assist the digestive process
- Enjoy pure Sattvic foods they are easily digestible, including organic milk, almonds, honey, sesame, rice, and fruits.

Afterword

To 'Air' is Human, Everything You Ever Wanted to Know About Intestinal Gas covers everything you ever wanted to know about the burp, belch, bloat, fart and everything digestive, but were either too afraid or too embarrassed to ask. It has a companion volume: ***Artsy Fartsy, Cultural History of the Fart*** is a fascinating and factually correct review of the common fart through human culture and history. The cough, sneeze, hiccup, stomach rumble, burp, belch, and other bodily sounds simply cannot compete with the notoriety of the fart. Whether encountered live and in person or through the medium of literature, television, film, art, or music it may leave a powerful and lingering memory. The intent of the book is to demonstrate that the ubiquitous fart has a more illustrious story to share than just lowbrow humor. The societal standards and cultural acceptance of this normal physiologic event have evolved over the years, and it is currently popular as a point of humor even in sophisticated circles. The history of the fart in culture and society is a seldom told but fascinating tale.

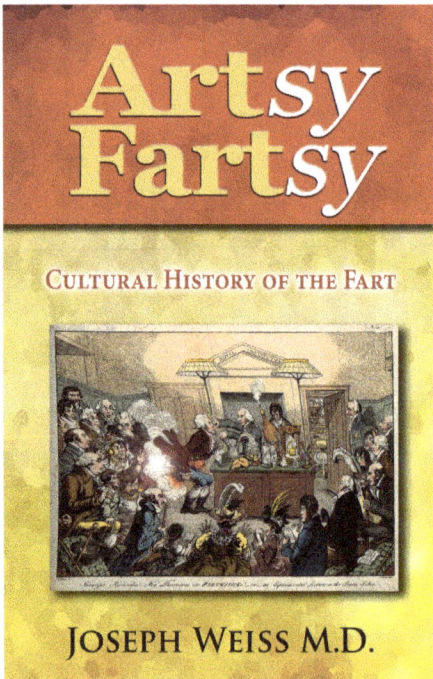

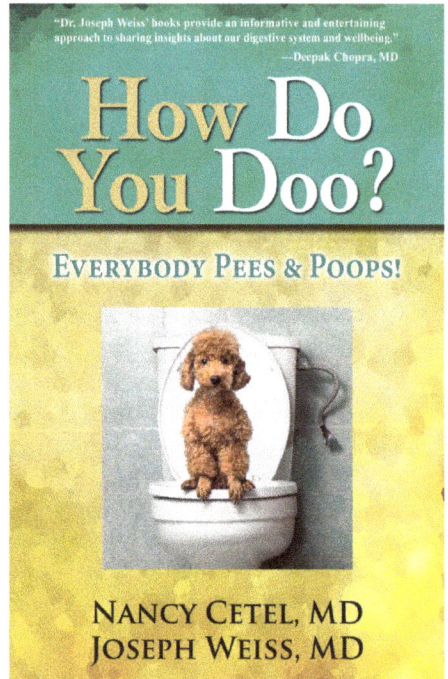

How Do You Doo? Everybody Pees & Poops! A delightfully informative, entertaining, and colorfully illustrated volume with valuable practical insights on toilet training. Tasteful color photographs of animals answering the call of nature allows the child to understand that everybody does it! Additional informative relevant content to entertain the adult while the child is 'on the potty' is included.

To 'Air' is Human

The Scoop on Poop! Flush with Knowledge is a uniquely informative tastefully entertaining, and well-illustrated volume that is full of it! The 'it' being a comprehensive and knowledgeable overview of all topics related to the remains of the digestive process. Whether you call it poop, feces, excrement, manure, dung, or the hundred plus other euphemisms, shit happens, and it happens a lot! Tens of billions of pounds and kilograms of it or deposited every day by while diversity of animal and microbial life. Humans alone contribute over three billion pounds a day, and only a small percentage of that is treated by a sewage system

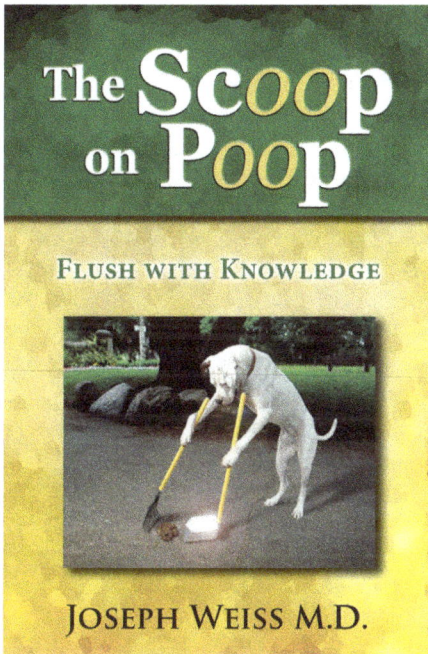

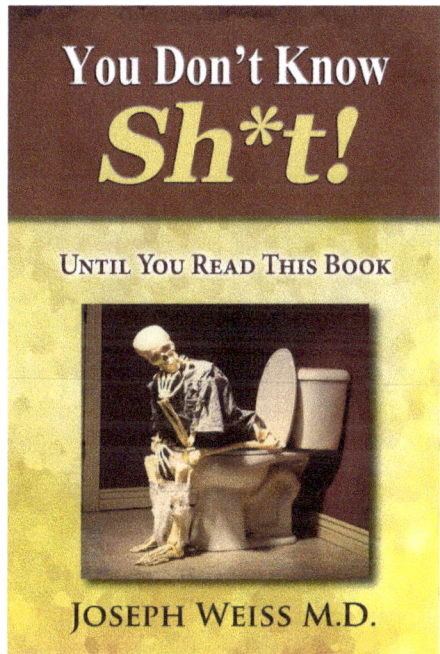

The identical content of The Scoop on Poop has been provocatively and cheekily retitled as ***You Don't Know Sh*t! Until You Read This Book***. This volume is an informative, entertaining and colorfully illustrated fountain of knowledge that is full of valuable information, including eccentricities and peculiarities, about the remains of the digestive process. Although this end result is politely described as feces or excrement, it is more commonly known by one of oldest words in the English language, shit. The book covers everything you ever wanted to know about this subject. Whether you disdain it, or appreciate it, it is part of the human (and animal) experience. The purpose of this volume is to share rarely discussed but very important knowledge about poop. The information ranges from the potentially life-saving to the sidesplitting descriptions of the eccentricities and peculiarities of human behavior on the subject matter. The wealth of information and trivia can sustain a long social conversation, or cut it short abruptly!

To 'Air' is Human

AirVeda: Ancient & New Medical Wisdom, Digestion & Gas covers the remarkable advances in the understanding of digestive health and wellness. New information about the critical role of genomics, epigenetics, the gut microbiome, and the gut-brain-microbiome-diet axis are opening new avenues to optimal whole body health and wellness. An appreciation of the ancient wisdom of Ayurveda and other disciplines shows that they had advanced insights into the nature of the human body and the holistic approach. Although intestinal gas, basic bodily functions, and feces have been topics culturally suppressed, knowledge and understanding are needed to achieve and maintain optimal health. This volume, and others in the series, provide an informative and entertaining in depth look at the amazing world of human health and digestion.

"Ayurveda is a 5,000 year old system of natural healing that reminds us that health is the balanced and dynamic integration between our environment, body, mind and spirit. In Dr. Joseph Weiss' book, AirVeda, he provides an informative and entertaining approach to sharing insights about our digestive system and wellbeing by applying the ancient wisdom of Ayurveda to everyday life." **Deepak Chopra, MD**

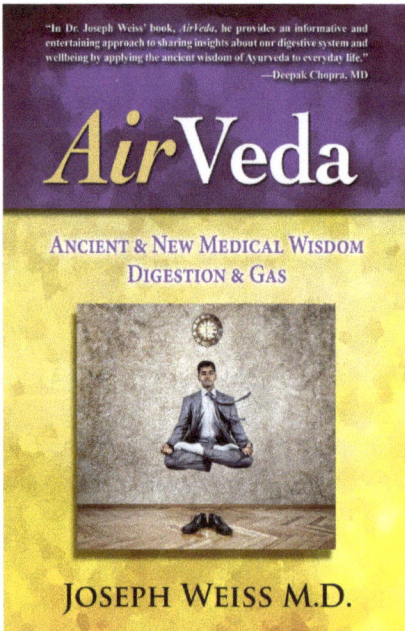

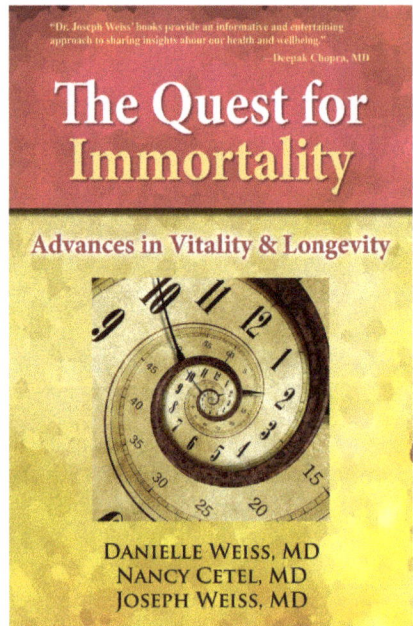

The Quest for Immortality, Advances in Vitality & Longevity provides an informative and enlightening overview of the remarkable advances in science and medicine that are dramatically enhancing human health and lifespan. The volume is written in clear, understandable, and engaging language with striking colorful illustrations. From groundbreaking nanotechnology to genomics and stem cells, the secrets of vitality and longevity are being uncovered along with more traditional advances and practical insights into disease prevention and health enhancement.

An even more comprehensive yet entertaining series are the extensive volumes of ***Digestive Health & Disease, An Illustrated Encyclopedia of Everything You Ever Wanted To Know About Digestion & Nutrition***. These volumes are a uniquely informative, entertaining, and lavishly illustrated compendium of alimentary knowledge and eccentricities. It covers everything you ever wanted to know about digestion and nutrition in health and disease. Volumes One through Five are available on Amazon.com.

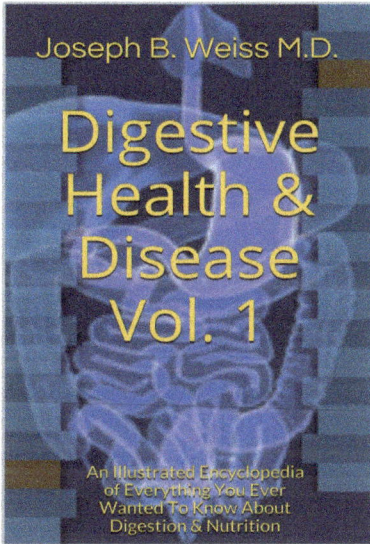

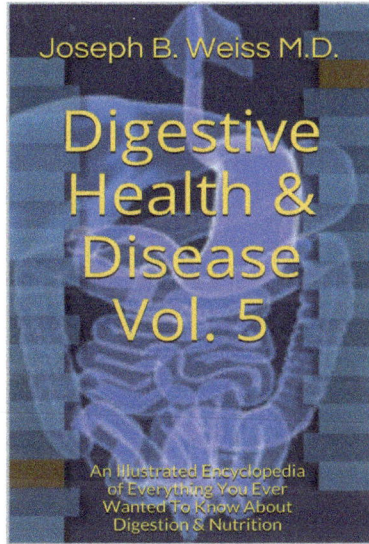

Organized as a reader friendly encyclopedia, the volumes cover over two thousand five hundred subject topics. Each volume may be utilized as an independent fully contained resource for the subjects it covers. The extensive size and scope of the series allows topics to be included that are rarely discussed in other books in the field and may be of great interest to the curious mind.

Written for the intelligent lay public, the medical and scientific terminology is translated into plain English. Practical and useful information and guidance are the primary goals, but entertaining and interesting information is included wherever possible. Designed for the visual learner as well, the clearly written text is supplemented by excellent photographs, illustrations, and charts. The reader will be informed, entertained, and the beneficiary of their newfound understanding of the universal process of digestion and metabolism that is the basis of all healthy living.

The website www.smartaskbooks.com has a complete list of books and programs by Joseph Weiss, MD, FACP, FACG, AGAF, Clinical Professor of Medicine (Gastroenterology), University of California, San Diego.

Appendix A: Colloquialism, Idiom, & Synonym of Fart

The word fart is one of the oldest words in the English language. One of the most important dictionaries in the long history of the language is Samuel Johnson's *A Dictionary of the English Language* published in 1755. An important innovation in his dictionary was the use of quotations from literature to illustrate the usage of the word defined.

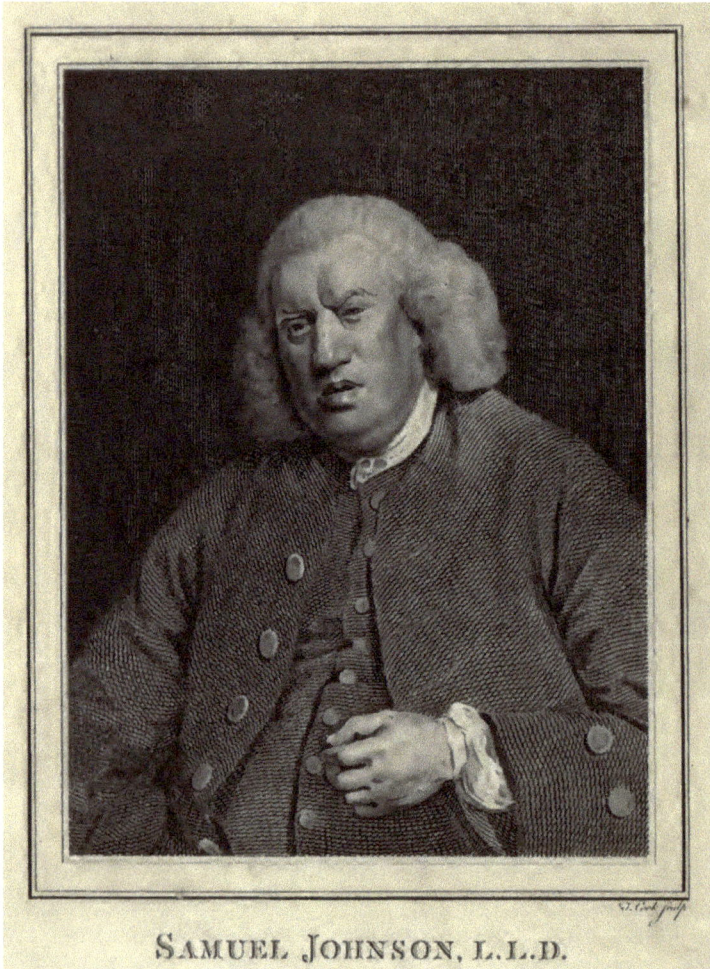

SAMUEL JOHNSON, L.L.D.

Public Domain

The word fart is proper English, and was in use for hundreds of years, before relatively recent polite and civil society considered it taboo. Without an alternative word, euphemisms were created and used. The number of terms that were synonymous with fart numbers in the many hundreds. The partial list that follows gives a good approximation of the wide variety of colorful alternatives.

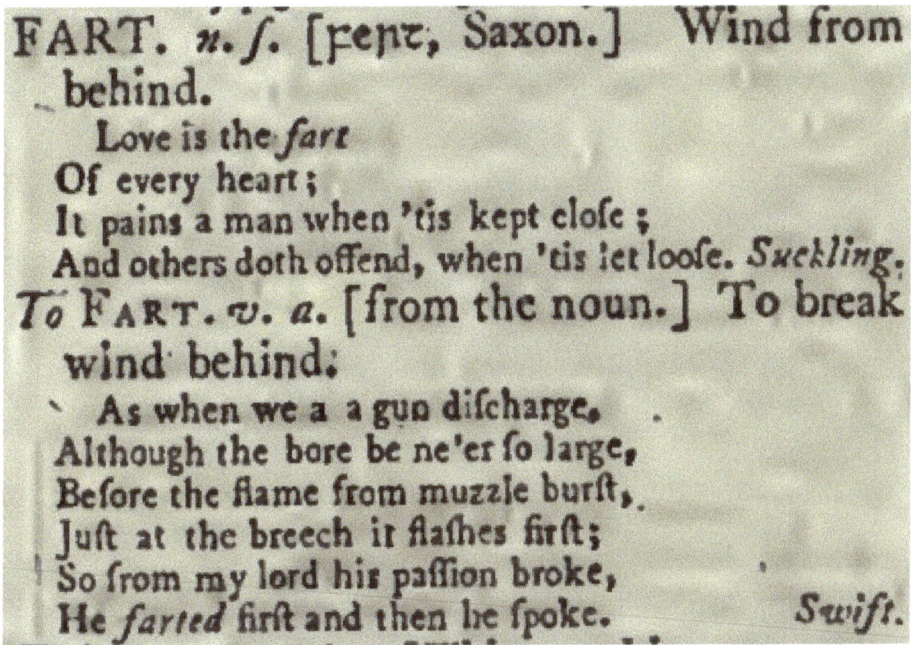

FART. *n. f.* [ᚠᛖᚾᛏ, Saxon.] Wind from behind.

> Love is the *fart*
> Of every heart;
> It pains a man when 'tis kept clofe ;
> And others doth offend, when 'tis let loofe. *Suckling.*

To FART. *v. a.* [from the noun.] To break wind behind.

> As when we a a gun difcharge,
> Although the bore be ne'er fo large,
> Before the flame from muzzle burft,
> Juft at the breech it flafhes firft;
> So from my lord his paffion broke,
> He *farted* firft and then he fpoke.   *Swift.*

Public Domain

The origins of these phrases, and their acceptance into the cultural lexicon, are often obscured. Sometimes new words are added simply by an author creatively using a newly invented word in a literary work. I am fond of a new word coined by David Gilmour, an entrepreneur and philanthropist. He described a word that combines the sense of anticipation and subsequent disappointment, when the experience is not as satisfying as expected. The word he crated 'anticipointment' is a portmanteau that should stand the test of time.

I am tempted to add to new words to the lexicon as well. I am using the author's prerogative to place the words in print below, and although I have not heard them elsewhere before someone may well have created them before me. The first word is fartigenic, or its alternative, fartogenic. Fartigenic is a portmanteau combining the word fart with the Latin root suffix -genic of genesis and creation fame. The word describes a substance, which induces the creation of a fart. Refried beans and chili con carne would be good examples of fartigenic foods. My second word creation choice would be related to the common phrase stomach flu when used to describe a viral gastroenteritis with diarrhea and farting. We often use the term flu when describing a viral illness even though in is not a true influenza virus. I am taking poetic liberty to borrow the influenza root word to describe a stomach flu as 'inflatuenza'. My third and final word would be an alternative word for bloating or distention. As one could consider this condition to be caused by the retention and delay of the necessary intestinal gas passage, I suggest the word 'gastipated'.

To 'Air' is Human

Okay, so maybe that word will not stand the test of time, and I should cease my word mining activities while I still have you as a reader.

What follows are the colloquialisms, idioms, and synonyms, that for better or for worse, are part of the lexicon.

A bit more choke and you would have started – an Australian phrase often addressed to the person responsible for an audible fart

Afflatus – Although it contains the word flatus this word has nothing to do with a fart. Flatus is Latin for a blowing, breathing, or a wind. Afflatus is a word first used by Cicero in his volume *De Natura Deorum* (*The Nature of the Gods*). In his book it is used as a phrase for a sudden rush of unexpected breath, a fresh inspiration. The word inspiration is derived from inspire, to breath as well as to have a creative thought or new idea. Afflatus thus can mean a divine inspiration. The only way to associate it with a fart is to consider it to be the exact opposite of a brain fart.

After thunder comes the rain – Phrase used when fart is passed just before urinating.

Air bagel – Fart

Air biscuit – Fart

Anal acoustics - Fart

Anal ahem - Fart

Anal audio - Fart

Anal salute - Fart

Anal volcano - Fart

Aqua fart - An underwater fart bubble, usually seen in the bathtub or swimming pool. The only way to clearly see an otherwise invisible fart.

Arse blast - Fart

Artsy Fartsy – Presented as art and culture but just as likely to be seen as pretentious, eccentric, eclectic, and unworthy of sophisticated cultural approval.

As much chance as a fart in a thunderstorm, windstorm, blizzard, hurricane, tornado, gale, etcetera - Means having no chance at all.

Ass blaster - Fart

Ass biscuit - Fart

Ass thunder - Fart

Ass whistle - Fart

Brain fart – Mental lapse, which usually results in an error while doing a repetitive activity.

Backdoor breeze - Fart

Backfire - Fart

Barking spiders - Fart

Bean blower - Fart

Blast off - Fart

To 'Air' is Human

Blowing a Raspberry (or Strawberry) – Imitating the sound of a fart by exhaling through pursed lips, usually as a sign of derision. Also known as a Bronx cheer.

Blowing the butt bugle - Fart

Blowing you a kiss - Fart

Bomber - Fart

Bottom blast - Fart

Bottom burp - Fart

Break wind - Fart

Breath of fresh air - Fart

Bronx cheer - Imitating the sound of a fart by exhaling through pursed lips, usually as a sign of derision. Also known as a Blowing a Raspberry or Strawberry.

Brown horn brass choir - Fart

Brown thunder - Fart

Bun shaker - Fart

Burnin' rubber - Fart

Buster - Fart

Busting ass - Fart

Butt bleat - Fart

Butt burp - Fart

Butt percussion - Fart

Butt trumpet - Fart

Butt tuba - Fart

Buttock bassoon - Fart

Cheek flapper - Fart

Cheesin' - Fart

Colonic calliope - Fart

Crack a rat - Fart

Crack one off - Fart

Crack splitters - Fart

Crop dusting - Farting while passing seated bystanders

Crowd splitter - Fart

Cut a stinker - Fart

Cut loose - Fart

Cut the cheese - Fart

Cut the wind - Fart

Death breath - Fart

Deflate - Fart

Drop a barking spider - Fart

Drop u bomb Fart

Drop ass - Fart

Dutch oven – Farting under the blankets while in bed, then covering up your bedmate to share the aroma.

Empty my tank - Fart

Eproctophilia – A fart fetish, the receiving of sexual pleasure and arousal from the fart of another. The author James Joyce (see separate entry) describes this fetish in letters published after his death.

Exploding bottom - Fart

Exterminate - Fart

Farst – Descriptive of a fast fart

Fart – (Foreign languages) – Unrelated to the English usage of the word, in the German and Scandinavian languages the word means speed, often used in speeding or speed control zones signs. in Danish a *fartcertifikate* means a trade certificate. In Norwegian a *fart plan* means a schedule. The Norwegian phrase *stå på fartin* pronounced as stop-a –fartin means ready to leave. Likewise, the phrase *farts måler* pronounced as fart smeller refers to a speedometer. In Swedish a speed bump is called a *farthinder*. *Fartlek* is speed training by running at alternate intervals of fast and slow paces. Likewise, if you travel on a Scandinavian marine vessel you may see the control of engine speed labeled as *half fart* and *full fart* for half speed and full speed respectively. Fart kontrol zones are speed zones. In Germany a similar word *fahrt* means a journey, trip, tour, or passage. It is often seen in signs that say *einfahrt* (sounds like in-fart) and *ausfahrt* (sounds like out-fart) denoting entrance and exit respectively. In Spanish and Portuguese *fart* means an excess of anything, especially a food. One of the richest deserts they offer is called a *farte*, which means a fruit tarte in Spain and usually a sugar almond or cream cake in Portugal. In Italy the word *farto* means mattress. In Hungarian *fartaj* means buttocks. In Poland if you want to buy a popular candy bar with a name that that means lucky you will be looking for a *Fart* bar.

Fartalito - Word for a small fart combining English and Spanish (Spanglish)

Fartable farter – An individual who can fart on command

Fart about – Waste time on silly or unnecessary activities

Fart absorption ratio – Humorous descriptive of the quantity of farts that a material can absorb and retain before the trapped gas escapes. Usually used to describe furniture such as a chair, sofa, ottoman, cushions, mattress, but can also be applied to rugs, carpets, clothing, etcetera.

Fart ache – Descriptive of a fart so potent that exposure to the fumes gives a headache. May also be used to describe pain after farting with anorectal disease such as fissures, abscess, fistula, hemorrhoids, and after delivery or surgery.

Fartachoo – A fart and sneeze occurring simultaneously

Fartacious – Ability to produce copious farts, either by volume or frequency.

Fartacrite – An individual who is hypocritical about farts, considering the farts of others as objectionable while their own farts are perfectly acceptable.

Fart addict – One who is obsessed with farting, usually used to describe an individual who produces farts in prodigious frequency and quantity.

Fartage - (French) Waxing of cross-country skis, unrelated to fart.

Fart against thunder – The fart equivalent of urinating (pissing) into the wind.

Fartagious – Contagious farting, often noted in preadolescent males.

Fartaholic – An individual who is described as being addicted to farting, often used to describe a husband.

Fart alarm – When the need to fart is misinterpreted as the need to defecate. Also when a baby's diaper is changed assuming a bowel movement occurred, only to find the diaper is empty as it was just a fart.

Fartalicious – A particularly attractive fart, either by acoustics, aroma, or quantity. Also may be used as a sarcastic compliment denoting that the taste of a food or drink was offensive.

Fart amnesty – A zone where unhindered farting is allowed without criticism or limitation. The zone is usually defined by the significant other, and may be in a remote location and different time zone.

Fart and dart – An individual who release a fart and quickly departs to let others experience their fart. Also known as fart and run.

Fart and flee – A practical joke, often executed spontaneously on releasing a fart in a crowded public place. The person immediately behind you is left standing in the aromatic wake of your fart, is assumed to be the culprit, and is the recipient of abhorrent glares from others.

Fart angels – Actively moving arms and legs in the same fashion as one makes snow angels by lying down in the snow. The activity is done in the standing mode to help circulate the air in the hope of dissipating the smell.

Fartanoid – A frantic sense of insecurity that an impending fart may allow the release of bowel contents.

Fartapalooza – A spasm of frequent, voluminous, and typically audacious farts over a short period of time. More often occurs following ingestion of a fart inducing meal, such as refried beans.

Fart app – An application for mobile phones and other electronic devices that reproduces sounds that imitate the various acoustic forms of the art of the fart.

Fart around – Waste time on silly or unnecessary activities

Fart arpeggio – A fart that changes tone at least twice so that three or more notes are produced during its course. A master of this technique was Joseph Pujol, known as Le Pétomane, during his performance career on the Moulin Rouge in Paris.

Fartarrhea – Similar to shart as a combination of shit and fart, but with diarrhea and fart. The fart often releases a mist of liquid feces, which soil the underwear or clothing if not released while on a toilet.

Fart arse – (British) To be stupid, farting or mucking around.

Fart art – Euphemism for abstract art appearance of soiling of underwear upon passing a particularly powerful fart that carried some organic fecal matter, mucus, or moisture. More common with a bout of dysentery or diarrhea.

Fart ass – Similar to smart-ass

Fart attack – Condition of pain related to intestinal gas, including intestinal gas in the pre-fart stage of bloating and distension. Play on words with similarity to heart attack, Unfortunately symptoms that suggest intestinal gas discomfort (fart attack) may actually be due to a heart condition (heart attack) and delay urgently needed medical care. In this situation a misdiagnosed fart/heart attack can be a true life threatening condition. A popular dark humor cartoon illustration shows a family member misinterpreting a cardiologist as saying that her spouse had a massive 'fart attack'

Fart baby – Descriptive term for abdominal bloating from intestinal gas, more noticeable in young thin women who develop visible distension that gives the impression of an early pregnancy.

Fart bag – A plastic or paper bag used to capture and seal in a fart, to be subsequently opened in the face of an unsuspecting victim.

Fart bellows – Farting under a blanket while in bed, and then trying to clear the fart by using the blanket as a bellow. The opposite of a Dutch oven, where the goal is to trap the fart under the blanket.

Fart blanche – To be given carte blanche to fart at will under the blanket or other locations.

Fart box – A euphemism for anus, rectum, and rectal cavity.

Fart brain – Used similarly to airhead, suggesting that farts rather than brains reside in the skull

Fart breath – Foul smelling breath

Fart bride – A woman who was very discrete about bodily functions, especially farts, before marriage, but loses all inhibitions after marriage.

Fart bubble – An underwater fart bubble, usually seen in the bathtub or swimming pool. The only way to clearly see an otherwise invisible fart.

Fart catcher – Nickname given to horsemen seated immediately behind the horses pulling a carriage. Also used to describe assistants and servants who walk a few paces behind them superior.

Fart buddy – A friend who is close enough that farting in their presence does not lead to any offense, and may contribute to an open farting atmosphere.

Fart burn – The burning rectal or anal sensation after extensive diarrhea and farting. Also may be experienced after eating hotly spiced foods.

Fart camouflage – Also known as fart camo. Making noise by an activity to hide the sound of a fart. The goal is to create a distraction to allow the noisy passage of a fart to go undetected. Using an air freshener, perfume, or other strong aroma may be used in an attempt to mask the smell. Opening windows and doors with the excuse that it is too warm is often used as a fart camouflage maneuver.

Fart candy – Candy that induces farting by having a high content of non-absorbable sugars. Dietetic candies often have this property.

Fart door - Colloquial term for anus.

Farter – A person who procrastinates by farting around. (British) Slang term for anus, also a sleeping bag which is warmed by farts.

Farterbox – (Irish) Slang for anus

Fartface – Facial expression that gives the impression that the wearer is smelling a noxious fart. Also slang for an idiot or stupid person.

Fart factory – Slang for anus, also to describe a frequent or voluminous farter.

Fart fetish – Formally known as eproctophilia, the receiving of sexual pleasure and arousal from the fart of another. The author James Joyce (see separate entry) describes this fetish in letters published after his death.

Farther, Farthest, Farthermost – These words denote greater distance from an object, an are unrelated to the word fart that is contained within their spelling. The only way they may be tied to the word fart is in vocabulary games like Scrabble, Boggle, and others where additional points may be gained by adding letters to a core word.

Fart higher than your ass – Arrogant and pretentious, translation of original phrase from the French *péter plus haut que son cul.*

Farthing – British coin currency with a nominal value. Benjamin Franklin uses the nominal currency as a double entendre at the end of his proposal to the Royal Academy of Brussels to create an award for an additive that word give farts a pleasant smell (see entry on Benjamin Franklin)

Farthingale – A hoop like structure worn under the skirt by women in the late 16th and early 17th centuries to give it the shape of a bell or cone. Originally introduced at the Spanish court it subsequently became popular fashion in Tudor England. Although the shape and structure may have been helpful to muffle the sound and contain the aroma of a fart, there is no evidence that the name was related to the word fart. One theory behind the development of the farthingale was to hide a pregnancy that may have resulted from illicit relationships.

Fart in a bottle – Description of restless movement suggestive of agitation or being flustered.

Fart in a thunderstorm or windstorm –Figure of speech suggesting the event is unnoticed or unidentifiable because of background activity. When in the phrase as much chance as a fart in a thunderstorm, windstorm, blizzard, hurricane, tornado, gale, etc. it means having no chance at all.

Farting clapper - Anus, or more pejorative asshole.

Farting fanny – Nickname given to heavy German artillery guns used during World War I

Farting shot – An action designed to show contempt.

Farting through silk –financially affluent, able to afford luxuries

Fart lighting – Ignition of flammable gas (methane and/or hydrogen) released in some farts. Serious injury and burns have resulted from this activity, most often seen in adolescent males.

Fartman – A fictional superhero popularized by television and radio personality Howard Stern (see separate entry).

Fart monkey – Term of endearment, usually for a pet such as a dog or cat that farts whenever it needs to. The fart monkey can also serve as fart camouflage and be designated as the source of an errant fart.

Fart sucker – A parasite or toady willing to do whatever it takes to curry favor. Analogous to ass kisser, brown-nose equivalent. Interesting tie in to French slang for criminal suspect. The French pronounce suspect as soos-pay, the same way they would pronounce the words *sucé pet*, which translates literally as fart sucker. The French authorities can use the double entendre to express their dislike of a suspect without being chastised.

Fart time – Describes employed hours per week that fall between full-time and part-time employment. Usually defined as between twenty-one and thirty-five hours of work time per week.

Fire a stink torpedo - Fart

Fire the retro-rocket - Fart

Firing scud missiles - Fart

Fizzler - Fart

Flamethrower - Fart

Flamer - Fart

Flapper - Fart

Flatulate - Fart

Flatulence - Fart

Flatus - Fart

Flipper - Fart

Float an air biscuit - Fart

Floof - Fart

Fluffy - Fart
Fog slicer - Fart
Fowl howl - Fart
Fragrant fuzzy - Fart
Free-floating anal vapors - Fart
Free Jacuzzi - Fart
Freep - Fart
Frequency Actuated Rectal Tremor - Fart
Fumigate - Fart
Funky rollers - Fart
Gas attack - Fart
Gas blaster - Fart
Gas from the ass - Fart
Gas master - Fart
Gaseous intestinal by-products – Fart
Ghost turd - Fart
Grandpa - Fart
Gravy pants - Fart
Great brown cloud - Fart
Heinus anus - Fart
Hole flappage - Fart
Hole flapper - Fart
Honk - Fart
HUMrrhoids - Fart
Hydrogen bomb - Fart
Ignition - Fart
Insane in the methane - Fart
Invert a burp - Fart
Jet propulsion - Fart
Joan of Fart – Artful nickname for a female who has farted audibly
    or aromatically.
Jockey burner - Fart
Jumping guts - Fart
Just calling your name - Fart
Just keeping warm - Fart
Just the noise - Fart
Kaboom - Fart
K-Fart - Fart
Kill the canary - Fart
Lay a wind loaf - Fart
Lay an air biscuit - Fart
Leave a gas trap - Fart
Let a beefer - Fart
Let a brewer's fart – To have diarrhea.
Let each little bean be heard - Fart
Let one fly - Fart

To 'Air' is Human

Let one go - Fart
Let the beans out - Fart
Lethal cloud - Fart
Letting one rip - Fart
Lingerer - Fart
Made a gas blast – Fart
Make a stink - Fart
Make a trumpet of one's ass – Fart
Mating call of the barking spider - Fart
Meteor – Fart
Methane bomb - Fart
Methane production experiment - Fart
Moon gas - Fart
Mud duck - Fart
Must be a sewer around - Fart
Nose death - Fart
Odor bubble - Fart
Odorama - Fart
Old fart – An old man, a person in authority very set in their ways,
    inflexible.
One-man jazz band - Fart
One-gun salute - Fart
Painting the elevator - Fart
Pant stainer - Fart
Panty burp - Fart
Parp - Fart
Party in your pants - Fart
Pass gas - Fart
Pass wind - Fart
Pet – Fart (French) The diminutive for fart in the French language. It
    makes the written English use of pet shop, pet food, love of pets,
    etc. an interesting translation. The pronunciation is different
    however, as pet is pronounced as pay in French
Pissed as a fart – Very drunk (British & Australian)
Play the tuba - Fart
Playing the trouser tuba - Fart
Plotcher (aka a wet one) – Fart
Poof - Fart
Poop gas - Fart
Poot - Fart
Pootie – Fart
Pop - Fart
Pop a fluffy - Fart
Preventing spontaneous human combustion – Fart
Puff, the magic dragon - Fart
Quack - Fart

To 'Air' is Human

Raspberry (Razz) - Slang for *'blowing a raspberry or strawberry'*,
  imitating the sound of a fart by exhaling through pursed lips,
  usually as a sign of derision. Also known as a Bronx cheer.
Rebuild the ozone layer one poof at a time - Fart
Rectal honk - Fart
Rectal shout - Fart
Rectal tremor - Fart
Release a squeaker - Fart
Release an ass biscuit - Fart
Release gas - Fart
Rep - Fart
Rimshot - Fart
Rip ass - Fart
Rip one - Fart
Ripple fart - Fart
Roast the Jockeys - Fart
Rotting vegetation - Fart
Royal fart – A fart of unusual distinction.
Safety - Fart
Salute your shorts - Fart
SAS (silent and scentless) – Fart
SBD (silent but deadly) – Fart
Set off an SBD - Fart
Shart – Fart passage that allows the escape of fecal material. The
  word shart is a portmanteau of shit and fart.
Shit fumes - Fart
Shit honker - Fart
Shit vapor - Fart
Shoot the cannon - Fart
Shoppin' at Wal-Fart - Fart
Silent and scentless (SAS) – Fart
Silent but deadly (SBD) – Fart
Singe the carpet - Fart
Singing the anal anthem - Fart
Sounding the sphincter scale - Fart
Sound of a barking spider - Fart
Sound of a wompus cat - Fart
Sparrow-fart - Denotes the earliest of daylight, early dawn, sunrise,
  sunup, first light of day. Although it uses the same word 'fart' it is
  not a reference to the passage of intestinal gas
Sphincter song - Fart
Spit a brick - Fart
Squeak one out - Fart
Squeaker - Fart
Steamer - Fart
Step on a duck - Fart

To 'Air' is Human

Step on a frog - Fart
Stink bomb - Fart
Stink burger - Fart
Strangling the stank monkey - Fart
Strawberry - Slang for imitating the sound of a fart by exhaling
    through pursed lips, usually as a sign of derision. Also known as a
    Bronx cheer or a raspberry
Stress release - Fart
Tail wind - Fart
The colonic calliope - Fart
The dog did it - Fart
The F bomb - Fart
The gluteal tuba - Fart
The Sound and the Fury - Fart
The stink's gone into the fabric - Fart
The third state of matter - Fart
The toothless one speaks - Fart
Thunder pants - Fart
Thunderspray - Fart
Toilet tune - Fart
Toot - Fart
Toot your own horn - Fart
Trelblow - Fart
Triple flutter blast - Fart
Trouser cough - Fart
Trouser trumpet - Fart
Turd honking - Fart
Turd hooties - Fart
Turn on the air conditioning in the colon - Fart
Uncorked symphony - Fart
Under burp - Fart
Venting one - Fart
Wet one - Fart
What the dog did - Fart
Who Cut the Cheese - Fart
Wrong way burping - Fart
Zinger – Fart

Appendix B: Fart in Foreign Languages

American Sign Language:

The non-dominant hand is an "A" or an "S" handshape. The dominant hand is a bent hand and is held so that the fingers are underneath the pinkie side of the non-dominant "fist." The dominant hand "unbends" and bends one time as if showing gas escaping. Here is a "one handed" version of fart, both versions are widely used. You start by opening up the pinkie, and then the ring and middle finger. The index finger stays curled up. Then you reverse and close the middle, then ring, then pinkie fingers. For comic effect or emphasis you can puff one cheek and force a bit of air through your lips at the corner of your mouth.

Afrikaans: fart
Albanian: pordhÃ«, pjerdh; pordhë, hajvan, pjerdh
Arabic: ضرطة, ضرط ضرطة نفخة , ضرطة , ha ridge
Armenian: fart, basz toe
Avestan: pərəδaiti
Azerbaijani: osurmaq
Basque: fart
Belarusian: Ð¿ÐµÑ€Ð´ÐµÑ‚Œ
Bulgaria: fart Флатуленция, пръдня
Catalan: pet, *colloq* pet, *colloq* torracollons, *colloq* tirar-se un pet, fer-se un pet
Chinese (Simplified): 屁, 放屁 屁 fom pee/ pie Chee
Chinese (Traditional): 屁, 放屁 屁 fom pee/ pie Chee
Croatian: prdnuti, vjetar, prdac, ispuštati vjetrove, prditi
Czech: prd
Danish: prut
Dutch: wind laten, winderigheid, een wind laten, een scheet laten, (slang) scheet (slang)
Esperanto: furzi, furzo
Estonian: pieru
Farsi: gooz bede, گوز ، گوزیدن
Filipino: umut-ot, kabag-gas oh mo toot ka
Finnish: pieru
French: péter, pet, dis gas, péter (argot); làcher une vesse; vesser pet (argot), vesse, merdeux
Galician: peidar
Georgian: fart
German: furz, flatulenz, fuhren sie gas, furzen, sich mit jedem dreck abgeben (Umgangssprache), scheißer (slang)
Greek: πέρδομαι (perdomai), Î°Î»Î±½Î¹Î¬, κλάνω, πέρδομαι κλανιά, πορδή
Haitian Creole: fart

To 'Air' is Human

Hebrew: "נאד" (סלנג), נפיחה (סלנג) "נאד לתקוע" ,"להפליץ"

Hindi: पादना

Hmong: tso paus, tawb paus

Hungarian: fing, fingik, szellentés

Icelandic: rÃ¦fill

Ilokano: uttot

Indonesian: kentut

Irish: fart

Italian: fart, flatulenza, pass il gas, scoreggiare scoreggio, peto

Japanese: おなら, 屁, おならをする, 屁をこく（俗語）おなら, 屁（俗語）

Korean: 방귀 뀌다, bung koo

Latin: pēdĕre

Latvian: fart

Lithuanian: bezdalius

Macedonia: Đ¿Ñ€Đ´ĐµĐ¶

Malay: kentut

Maltese: fart

Norwegian: fart

Persian: گوز ,گوز ،گوزیدن gooz bede

Philippine: kabag-gas, oh mo toot ka, umut-ot,

Polish: bpierd, pierdzieÄ‡, gazy jelitowe, parvee etra, vi pierdzieć, pierdnięcie, pierdnąć

Portuguese: peidar, pedo, flatulência, soltar um pum (gíria) peido,

Romanian: bÄfÅŸi, flatulenţă, gaze (vulgar), vint, a da vinturi,

Russian: пердеть (perdet'), издавать громкий треск, пукнуть громкий треск при выходе газов из организма, непристойный звук; пукание; старик зря терять время Đ¿ĐµÑ€Đ´ĐµÑ‚Œ, метеоризм, puk nee
The Russian words for fart include *perdyozh* (first act of breaking wind), *perdun* (perpetrator and outcome), *perdil'nik* (place from where it comes), *Perun* (ancient God of wind), *bzdun* (silent fart), *bzdyukha* (silent fart as well as a stupid jerk). Some of the Russian verbs for the action of farting are particularly colorful. *Perdet'* (to fart with or without sound), *bzdet'* (to fart silently), *pereperdet* (to fart repeatedly), and my favorite word *nabzdet'sya* (ton fart silently to one's complete and utter satisfaction!).

Sanskrit: pardate

Serbian: Đ¿Ñ€Đ´Ñ‹ÑfÑ‚Đ‚

Slovak: prd

Slovenian: prdec

Somali: doughso

Spanish: pedo, tirarse un pedo (familismo), peo, pasar gasses, peer, ventosear, ventoseo, cuesco

Swahili: fart, kyfoosi

To 'Air' is Human

Swedish: fart, fjärt , flatulens, prutta, fjärta (slang) prutt, fjärt (slang)

Tagalog (Philippine): kabag-gas, oh mo toot ka, umut-ot,

Taiwanese: 放屁 屁 funkee-pass gas

Thai: ตด, ฟาท, ลมตด (ผายลม),ตด,การผายลม,บตก,ผายลม

Turkish: osuruk, ul cer, osurmak, gaz yapmak osuruk, yellenme

Urdu: گوز, پاد- پھسکي باؤ- گوز, پادنا یا پاد پھسکي مارنا- باؤ سڑنا

Vietnamese: đánh rắm, trung tiện, dit, danh từ, đùi 0 rắm,
   nội động từ, chùi gháu

Visayan: otot

Welsh: basio gwynt

Yiddish: פֿאַרצן

Index

To 'Air' is Human

To 'Air' is Human

To 'Air' is Human

www.ingramcontent.com/pod-product-compliance
Lightning Source LLC
Chambersburg PA
CBHW051243020426
42333CB00025B/3025